Human Diseases
A Systemic Approach ----------------------------

fifth edition

Mary Lou Mulvihill, PhD
Professor Emeritus
William Rainey Harper College
Palatine, Illinois

Mark Zelman, PhD
Associate Professor
William Rainey Harper College
Palatine, Illinois

Paul Holdaway, MA
Professor
William Rainey Harper College
Palatine, Illinois

Elaine Tompary, PharmD
Instructor
William Rainey Harper College
Palatine, Illinois

Jill Turchany, PhD
Assistant Professor
Rock Valley College
Rockford, Illinois

Prentice
Hall

Upper Saddle River, New Jersey 07458

Library of Congress Cataloging-in-Publication Data

Human diseases: a systemic approach / Mary Lou Mulvihill ... [et al.].—5th ed.
    p. cm.
   Previous editions entered under author.
   Includes index.
   ISBN 0-8385-3930-0
   1. Pathology.   I. Mulvihill, Mary L.   II. Mulvihill, Mary L. Human diseases.
RB111.M83 2000
616—dc21

00-051491

Notice: The author and the publisher of this volume have taken care to make certain that the doses of drugs and schedules of treatment are correct and compatible with the standards generally accepted at the time of publication. Nevertheless, as new information becomes available, changes in treatment and in the use of drugs become necessary. The reader is advised to carefully consult the instruction and information material included in the package insert of each drug or therapeutic agent before administration. This advice is especially important when using new or infrequently used drugs. The publisher disclaims any liability, loss, injury, or damage incurred as a consequence, directly or indirectly, of the use and application of any of the contents of this volume.

Publisher: *Julie Alexander*
Executive Editor: *Greg Vis*
Acquisitions Editor: *Mark Cohen*
Editorial Managing Editor: *Marilyn Meserve*
Director of Production and Manufacturing: *Bruce Johnson*
Managing Production Editor: *Patrick Walsh*
Production Editor: *Gretchen Miller*
Project Liaison: *Janet Bolton*
Manufacturing Manager: *Ilene Sanford*
Creative Director: *Marianne Frasco*
Cover Design Coordinator: *Maria Guglielmo*
Cover Design: *Alamini Design*
Cover Photographer: *Nancy Kedersha/Photo Researchers, Inc.*
Marketing Manager: *David Hough*
Editorial Assistant: *Melissa Kerian*
Interior Design: *Janice Bielawa*
Composition: *York Graphic Services*
Printing and Binding: *R.R. Donnelley & Sons*

Prentice-Hall International (UK) Limited, *London*
Prentice-Hall of Australia Pty, Limited, *Sydney*
Prentice-Hall Canada Inc., *Toronto*
Prentice-Hall Hispanoamericana, S.A., *Mexico*
Prentice-Hall of India Private Limited, *New Delhi*
Prentice-Hall of Japan, Inc., *Tokyo*
Prentice-Hall Singapore Pte. Ltd
Editora Prentice-Hall do Brasil. Ltda, *Rio de Janeiro*

10 9 8 7 6 5 4 3 2 1
ISBN 0-8385-3930-0

To Mary Lou Mulvihill, friend, colleague, and educator,
whose vision began this work

and

To our students who inspired us to continue it

Brief Contents

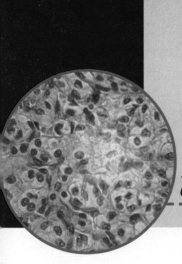

Detailed Contents

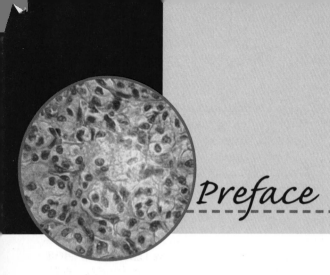

Preface

➤ WELCOME TO THE FIFTH EDITION

This thoroughly revised and updated fifth edition of *Human Diseases: A Systemic Approach* continues to meet the needs of instructors and students who have used its previous four editions, but has been revised to meet the changing needs of students and instructors by including new pedagogical features to enhance student learning. This edition includes a robust teaching/learning package that features a full range of multimedia tools for both students and instructors. Like the previous editions, this text is written for students entering allied health careers and for students interested in learning the fundamentals of human disease. It embraces the ideas of the original author, the late Dr. Mary Lou Mulvihill, whose vision guided and inspired us as we revised this text. Although the changes in some places are numerous and extensive, instructors will recognize Mary Lou's original purpose and organization. We believe the revisions will serve to greatly enhance understanding of human disease basics.

➤ TEXT ORGANIZATION

The text is divided into three parts. Part I, *Mechanisms of Disease*, introduces important terminology, the study of disease, inflammation and allergy, neoplasia, heredity and disease, dietary factors and disease, and includes a new chapter, Infectious Diseases. Part II, *Diseases of the Systems*, introduces students to the major diseases associated with each body system. Part III, *Stress, Aging, and Wellness*, discusses the role stress and aging play in health and disease. Students are also introduced to the concept of wellness.

➤ CHAPTER REVISIONS

In contemplating our plans for the revision we studied every word, figure, photograph, and chart. Changes in some areas are minor, in others extensive, and in some cases, passages were completely rewritten to better facilitate student understanding.

Chapter 3, *Infectious Diseases,* is new to this edition. This chapter discusses the nature of infectious disease and provides a framework for learning about the specific infectious diseases discussed throughout the text. It includes discussions of antibiotic resistance and emerging infectious diseases, which are of considerable medical importance. Some passages, such as those on tuberculosis and pneumonia (Chapter 13), benefited from complete rewriting. Other passages, such as those on cirrhosis and jaundice (Chapter 12), were improved through careful editing and updating. The text was scrutinized for currency and was carefully updated throughout (see AIDS/HIV discussion in Chapter 2).

Figures and photographs were added, deleted, or improved to comprise over 100 photographs. Over 150 full color line drawings illustrate and explain many difficult concepts. Revised and new charts throughout the text organize complicated information for students.

➤ ENHANCEMENTS TO THE FIFTH EDITION

Each chapter opens with an expanded Outline and with Student Objectives. Key terms are highlighted and appear in boldface when first introduced and a pronunciation guide appears in the margin for key terms where they are introduced. The end of each chapter contains a revised set of study questions as well as study aids. Each chapter also includes the following pedagogical aids to facilitate student learning:

- **Side by Side photographs and art** depicting normal and diseased organs and tissues are included in each systems chapter.

- *Fact or Fiction?* at the opening of each systems chapter questions popular wisdom and helps students debunk myths.
- *On the Practical Side* offers useful health tips throughout the text.
- *Epidemiology: Diseases by the Number* provides data that gives perspective on the incidence and importance of certain diseases.
- *Prevention Plus!* offers sound advice on disease prevention throughout.
- *Diseases at a Glance* charts summarize each chapter's diseases and their signs, symptoms, diagnosis, and treatments.

➤ TEACHING/LEARNING PACKAGE

For the Student

- **Companion Website**
  (www.prenhall.com/mulvihill)
  Tied chapter-by-chapter to the text, the Companion Website provides interactive student quizzes, complete with instant scoring and immediate user feedback, links to resources on the web, and case studies.

- **CD-ROM**
  Provides interactive activities organized by chapter, anatomy exercises, links to useful websites and an audio glossary of all key terms in the book.

For the Instructor

- **Instructor's Manual** (0-8385-3691-3)
  Contains lecture outlines, discussion questions, multimedia resources and a printed version of the testbank.
- **Test Manager** (Win, 0-13-032388-8; MAC, 0-13-032389-6)
  Computerized test manager contains approximately 500 questions in a customizable format.
- **Instructor's PowerPoint CD-ROM** (0-13-032738-7)
  Over 200 color illustrations from the text are available for projection in the classroom utilizing PowerPoint.

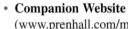

- **Companion Website**
  (www.prenhall.com/mulvihill)
  In addition to the student resources, the site links to appropriate online resources and provides a Syllabus Manager for instructors.

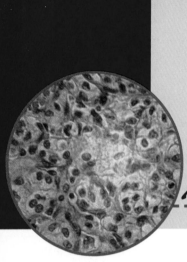

Acknowledgments

Prentice Hall Health is grateful to the knowledgeable and enthusiastic author team of *Human Diseases, A Systemic Approach,* Fifth Edition—Mark, Paul, Elaine, and Jill, we thank you. To Dr. Mark Zelman, we thank you for the extraordinary efforts and time you have invested, as lead author, to create and develop a text to help students succeed in their study of human diseases.

The making of this text represents a group effort. The authors thank all those who have contributed to this endeavor, many are known by name; many have worked quietly behind the scene. Thanks and appreciation is extended to the editorial staff, production staff, and support staff at Prentice Hall Health. In addition, thanks goes to York Graphic Services and their staff for the development and production services they have provided.

Major changes have been made in the art program for this edition; the authors thank Precision Graphics and Visible Productions for many of these new pieces of art.

► REVIEWERS

We wish to thank the following professionals who have reviewed manuscript for this Fifth Edition of *Human Diseases: A Systemic Approach.* Their fresh viewpoints, attention to detail, careful reading, and valuable feedback contributed greatly to the overall quality of this teaching tool.

William C. Bell
Professor of Health Sciences (Emeritus)
Grand Valley State University
Allendale, Michigan

Barbara L. Belyea, RN, BSN
Professor of Nursing
Saddleback College
Mission Viejo, California

Kirsten Berdahl, PT, A.T.C.
Physical Therapist Assistant Program
GateWay Community College
Phoenix, Arizona

Sue Biedermann
Chair and Associate Professor
Health Information Management Program
Southwest Texas State University
San Marcos, Texas

Rachelle Dorne, M.Ed, OTR
Assistant Professor
Occupational Therapy Program
Tennessee State University
Nashville, Tennessee

Mary Jo Gay, MN, RN
Assistant Professor of Nursing
Missouri Western State College
St. Joseph, Missouri

Louise C. Grim, MSEd, PT
Professor Emerita
Physical Therapist Assistant Program
Alvernia College
Reading, Pennsylvania

Chris Hollander, CMA, BSM
Medical Assisting Program Director
Westwood College of Technology
Denver, Colorado

Jennifer Horung, MBA, RHIA, CPHQ, CCS
Director, Health Information Program
Gwynedd-Mercy College
Gwynedd Valley, Pennsylvania

Diane Mack, MA
Associate Professor
Biology Department
William Rainey Harper College
Palatine, Illinois

Barbara McNeely, MSN, BSN, CMA
Medical Assisting Program Chair
Knoxville Business College
Knoxville, Tennessee

Mary T. Moretti, PT
Clinical Coordinator/Instructor
Physical Therapist Assistant Program Director
Stanly Community College
Albemarle, North Carolina

F. Lee St. John, Ph.D.
Associate Professor of Zoology
The Ohio State University at Newark
Newark, Ohio

Mary Ellen St. John, Ph.D
Professor
Division of Allied Health and Public Service
Central Ohio Technical College
Newark, Ohio

John R. Steele
Associate Professor
Ivy Tech State College
Gary, Indiana

Vincent G. Stilger, HSD, ATC
Assistant Professor
Undergraduate Athletic Training Program Director
West Virginia University
Morgantown, West Virginia

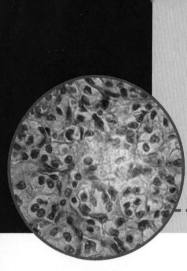

About the Authors

Mary Lou Mulvihill, PhD, was a dedicated author, writer, teacher, wife, and friend. Dr. Mulvihill authored Editions One, Two, Three, and Four of this text *Human Diseases, A Systemic Approach*. This book is dedicated to her memory; Dr. Mulvihill died during the final preparation of the Fourth Edition. It was an honor to have her as an author. She is remembered for her generosity of spirit and enthusiasm for life. May this text be a lasting tribute to a life lived fully, and in service to others.

Mark Zelman, PhD, is Chair of the Biology Department at William Rainey Harper College in Palatine, Illinois. He enjoys teaching a variety of biology courses, including Human Anatomy, Microbiology, and Introduction to Human Disease. At home, he teaches backyard bird- and bat-watching to his sons, Joseph and Thomas, who are his favorite students. In addition, Dr. Zelman is learning all about native gardening from his wife, Lisa, who is his favorite teacher.

Paul A. Holdaway, MA, a native of Indiana, a "Hoosier," attended and graduated from Indiana State University with a Master of Arts degree. Paul became an instructor at Indiana State University and later served as Head of Science at a community college. He is now a senior member of the Biology Department at William Rainey Harper College in Palatine, Illinois. He takes pleasure in a wide range of biological and clinical interests. At William Rainey Harper College, Professor Holdaway teaches Human Diseases, Human Anatomy, and Human Physiology.

Elaine Tompary, PharmD, is an accomplished pharmacist who has assisted various medical and pharmaceutical institutions. She has sought additional challenges and, in the process, has gained solace and satisfaction through teaching and encouraging others to reach higher plateaus. Dr. Tompary coordinates a pharmacy technology program and teaches classes in Pharmacy, Nursing, Biology, and Allied Health. She is currently on staff at William Rainey Harper College in Palatine, Illinois. She is a devoted wife to Drew, and a loving mother to Christopher and Andriana. Her hope and inspiration is her faith which aids in her desire to serve others.

Jill Turchany, PhD, received her PhD in Microbiology from the University of California at Davis. She received and completed a postdoctoral fellowship in infectious diseases at the University of California at San Diego, where she studied the parasite Giardia lamblia. Dr. Turchany has published several scientific papers, as well as a non-majors and a majors laboratory manual. She has been teaching for six years, the last five have been at Rock Valley College, Rockford, Illinois. Dr. Turchany teaches Biology for majors, Biology for non-majors, Anatomy and Physiology, Human Diseases, and Microbiology.

Mechanisms of Disease

Disease can be the result of many factors: infection, injury, or allergy, to name a few. Heredity and malnutrition cause many diseases as do abnormal cell growth or tumor formation. Part I treats these mechanisms of disease.

chapters

Microscopic Image of a Kidney Carcinoma

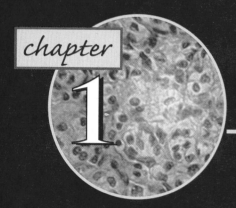

Introduction to Disease

The human body is a masterpiece of art. The more one understands the functioning of the body, the greater appreciation one has for it. Even in disease, the body is quite remarkable in attempting to right what is wrong and compensate for it.

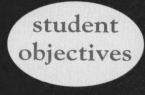

student objectives

After studying this chapter, students should be able to

➤ Define disease
➤ Discuss etiology of disease
➤ Discuss factors involved in the pathogenesis of disease
➤ Discuss abnormal growth patterns
➤ Explain diagnosis of disease

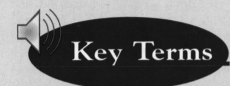

Key Terms

Acute

Aplasia

Atrophy

Bacteria

Chronic

Complications

Computed tomography (CT)

Congenital birth defects

Diagnosis

Disease

Dysplasia

Etiology

Exacerbation

Functional

Homeostasis

Hyperplasia

Hypertrophy

Hypoplasia

Idiopathic

Lesion

Magnetic resonance imaging (MRI)

Metaplasia

Mutated

Pallor

Pathogenesis

Pathology

Prognosis

Relapse

Remission

Sequela

Signs

Symptoms

Syndrome

Terminal

➤ CHAPTER OUTLINE

- Introduction
- Etiology of Disease
- Pathogenesis of Disease
- Abnormal Growth Patterns
- Diagnosis
- Chapter Summary
- Interactive Activities
- Quick Self Study

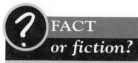
homeostasis
(hō″-mē-ō-stā′-sis)

disease
(di-zēz′)

signs
(sīns)

pallor
(păl′-or)

symptoms
(sim′-tŭms)

syndrome
(sĭn′-drōm)

➤ INTRODUCTION

Changes constantly occur within the body, and yet a steady state called **homeostasis** is generally maintained. A significant disturbance in the homeostasis of the body triggers a variety of responses that often produce **disease.** Disease is a state of functional disequilibrium that may be resolved by recovery or death. Disease produces signs noticeable by laboratory tests or physical examination.

Another important aspect of disease is the way it manifests itself: its signs and symptoms. **Signs** are objective evidence of disease observed on physical examination, such as abnormal pulse or respiratory rate, fever, and **pallor,** or abnormal paleness, whereas **symptoms** are an indication of disease perceived by the patient, such as pain, dizziness, and itching. An attempt will be made throughout this book to relate the signs and symptoms of a disease to the specific malfunctioning caused by the ailment. For example, why does the anemic person feel weak, fatigued, and short of breath? How does a hyperactive thyroid cause weight loss, nervousness, and excessive sweating? Why are the ankles swollen in certain heart conditions? Certain signs and symptoms occur concurrently in some diseases and the combination of symptoms is referred to as a **syndrome.** Down's syndrome is an example of a disease with concurrent signs; the most prominent are mental retardation, an enlarged, protruding tongue, and a characteristic appearance of the eyes.

Diseases can be classified in many ways, but in this book, they will be considered according to the general mechanisms of disease and in the physiologic systems in which they are factors.

on the Practical Side

Maintaining Body Temperature—Preventing Hypothermia
A sudden snow storm causes a driver to become temporarily stranded in the freezing cold. How does the person maintain a normal body temperature in the frigid environment? Superficial blood vessels constrict to prevent heat loss to the environment. Reflex shivering is muscle contraction that produces body heat.

etiology
(ē″-tē-ŏl′-ō-jē)

mutated
(mū-tā-ted)

➤ ETIOLOGY OF DISEASE

An important aspect of any disease is its **etiology,** or cause. Disease often begins at the cellular level. An abnormal gene, acquired through one's heredity or **mutated** (altered) by an environmental factor can start the disease process. Cancer, for example, begins with uncontrolled growth of cells when the genetic information is affected. New research techniques are making it possible to link certain diseases with abnormal gene findings. Many familiar diseases are caused by infectious agents such as bacteria, viruses, fungi, and parasites. The common cold and flu are viral infections, but abscesses and strep throat are caused by bacteria; fungi and parasites are infectious agents that cause athlete's foot and malaria, respectively. Some common bacteria are *Streptococcus, Staphylococcus, Salmonella,* and *E. coli,* which will each be mentioned throughout the text.

Antibiotic-resistant Bacteria
For more than 50 years people have been dependent on antibiotics to treat all kinds of bacterial infections. Some diseases such as tuberculosis were thought to have been erad-

PREVENTION *PLUS!*

Handwashing—A Healthy Habit

Infection can often be prevented by the simple task of thorough handwashing with soap or detergent, rubbing vigorously for at least 10 seconds. Germs tend to accumulate under fingernails and around cuticles so those areas should get special attention. Disease-causing microorganisms may be present on the skin surface, but proper handwashing prevents ingesting them or passing them on to others. Hands should always be washed before handling or eating food, before exiting the bathroom, after playing with pets, and after handling money.

icated through the action of antibiotics. Now, however, new and hardier strains of **bacteria** are developing that can resist the action of antibiotics.

The misuse and overuse of these drugs has caused the problem. Physicians have prescribed antibiotics for colds, flu, and other viral infections, which are untouched by the drugs. Tons of antibiotics are used by food producers to control infections so the environment has become saturated with them. Bacteria have developed immunities to many antibiotics through constant exposure, a condition known as multidrug resistance. To counteract this trend the indiscriminate use of antibiotics must be curtailed. Antibiotic resistance is discussed in more detail in Chapter 3.

bacteria
(băk-tē′-rē-ă)

Disease by the Numbers x + ÷

EPIDEMIOLOGY

There are nearly 62 million cases of the common cold annually. Of these cases, 52.2 million affect Americans under 17 years of age.

➤ PATHOGENESIS OF DISEASE

The source or cause of an illness or abnormal condition, together with its development, is its **pathogenesis.** If the cause of a disease is not known, it is said to be **idiopathic.** **Pathology** is the branch of medicine that studies the characteristics, causes, and effects of disease. The cellular pathologist studies cellular or microscopic changes; the clinical pathologist uses laboratory tests and methods to diagnose disease. A pathologist may specialize in autopsies or surgical findings.

Many diseases are inherited; they are transmitted by a defective gene. Hemophilia, sickle cell anemia, and color blindness are examples of genetic diseases. **Congenital birth defects,** mental or physical, may be due to a developmental error resulting from a maternal infection such as rubella or German measles during pregnancy, the use of certain drugs, or the mother's excessive consumption of alcohol. Some congenital birth defects result from an accident at the time of delivery, such as an interference with oxygen supply.

Environmental factors cause many diseases. Skin cancer, for example, can result from excessive exposure to the ultraviolet light rays of the sun, especially in fair-skinned

pathogenesis
(păth″-ō-jĕn′ĕ-sĭs)
idiopathic
(ĭd″ē-ō-păth′-ĭk)
pathology
(pă-thŏl′-ō-jē)
**congenital birth
defects**
(kŏn-jĕn′-ĭ-tăl bĭrth
dē′-fĕkts)

people. The development of leukemia is an occupational hazard for radiologists and the development of some cancers is linked to asbestos exposure. Many chemicals found in industrial wastes have been found to cause disease.

Malnutrition causes many diseases that are not always due to the unavailability of food, but rather to the inability of the person to use it, which will be explained later. Signs of nutritional deficiency diseases frequently accompany chronic alcoholism.

Stress adversely affects the entire body; it reduces the ability of the immune system to counteract disease. It aggravates some digestive diseases and respiratory ailments—asthma, for example—and other allergic conditions.

on the Practical Side

Fingernails and Health Problems

Clubbing or rounding of the fingertips and nails is often caused by a chronic lack of oxygen. The oxygen deficiency may be due to lung or heart disease. Enlargement in the connective tissue is a compensation for the oxygen deficiency. The nail often separates from the nail bed in psoriasis, fungal infection, and in injury. Dark discoloration may accompany cirrhosis, adult-onset diabetes, cancer, and aging.

➤ ABNORMAL GROWTH PATTERNS

hypertrophy
(hī-pĕr′-trŏ-fē)

Abnormal growth patterns are the cause of many diseases. Enlargement of an organ, **hypertrophy,** will often occur when the organ is required to do extra work. The heart enlarges with prolonged high blood pressure as it must continue to pump blood against great resistance. Heart muscle also hypertrophies when the valves are defective because valves that are either too narrow or too wide require extra pumping action. If one kidney fails, the other enlarges to meet the needs of the body and to compensate for the defective one. When blood flow to the kidneys is inadequate, the kidneys help raise the blood pressure by means of a hormonal secretion. If, however, an organ or body part is not used, it will **atrophy** or, that is, decrease in size or function. Muscles atrophy with a sedentary lifestyle.

atrophy
(ăt′-rō-fē)

hyperplasia
(hī″-pĕr-plā′-zĭ-ă)

hypoplasia
(hī″-pō-plā′-zē-ă)

aplasia
(ă-plā′-zē-ă)

An increased number of cells, **hyperplasia** *(plasia*—formation or development), results in tumor formation (Chapter 4). **Hypoplasia,** on the other hand, is the incomplete development or underdevelopment of an organ or tissue. Developmental failure, **aplasia,** leads to the absence of a structure or tissue. Aplastic anemia (Chapter 7) is such an example. **Metaplasia** is the conversion of normal tissue cells into an abnormal form after chronic stress or injury. **Dysplasia** *(dys*—painful or disordered) is abnormal development, such as a congenital heart defect.

metaplasia
(mĕt″-ă-plā′-zē-ă)

dysplasia
(dĭs-plā′-zē-ă)

functional
(fŭnk′-shŭn-ăl)

A **functional** condition is one in which there is no organic change. Abnormal tissue structure or function is referred to as a **lesion.** A lesion may be the result of a wound, injury, or pathologic condition. Figure 1–1 summarizes abnormal growth patterns.

lesion
(lē′-zhŭn)

➤ DIAGNOSIS

diagnosis
(dī″-ăg-nō′-sĭs)

Diagnosis, the determination of the nature of a disease, is based on many factors, including the signs, symptoms, and, often, laboratory results. Laboratory tests include such familiar procedures as urinalysis, blood chemistry, electrocardiography, and radiography.

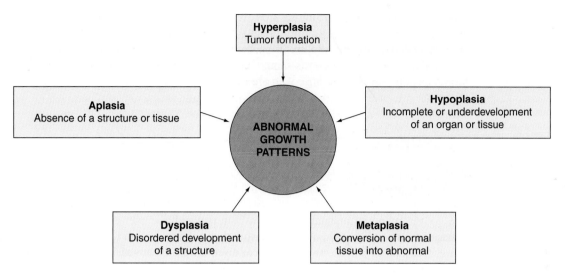

Figure 1–1
Abnormal growth patterns.

Newer diagnostic-imaging techniques such as **computed tomography (CT scan), magnetic resonance imaging (MRI),** ultrasound, and nuclear medicine provide a visualization never before possible. Diagnostic procedures used in determining various diseases are discussed for each system. A physician also derives information for making a diagnosis from a physical examination, from interviewing the patient or a family member, and from a medical history of the patient and family. The physician, having made a diagnosis, may state the possible **prognosis** of the disease, or the predicted course and outcome of the disease.

The treatment considered most effective is prescribed and may include medication, surgery, radiation therapy, or possibly psychological counseling. A patient may be advised to change eating habits, to begin an exercise program, to stop smoking, to control alcohol use, or to manage stress.

The course of a disease varies; it may have a sudden onset and short term, in which case it is an **acute** disease. A disease may begin insidiously and be long-lived, or **chronic.** The term *chronic* is derived from the Greek word *chronos* for time. Diseases that will end in death are called **terminal.** The signs and symptoms of a chronic disease at times subside, during a period known as **remission.** They may recur in all their severity in a period of **exacerbation.** Certain diseases, leukemia and ulcerative colitis, for example, are characterized by periods of remission and exacerbation. A **relapse** occurs when a disease returns weeks or months after its apparent cessation.

Complications frequently occur, meaning that another disease develops in a patient already suffering from a disease. Patients confined to bed with a serious fracture frequently develop pneumonia as a complication of the inactivity. Infection of the testes may be a complication of mumps, particularly after puberty. Anemia generally accompanies leukemia, cancer, and chronic kidney disease. Bacterial infection frequently follows certain predisposing factors such as kidney stones, heart defects, and an enlarged prostate gland. The relationships between the diseases that develop secondarily and the original disease will be discussed in later chapters.

The aftermath of a particular disease is called the **sequela,** a sequel. The permanent damage to the heart after rheumatic fever is an example of a sequela, as is the paral-

**computed
tomography (CT)**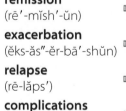
(cŏmpū′-tĕd
to-mŏg′-ră-phe)

**magnetic resonance
imaging (MRI)**
(măg-nĕt′-ĭk
rĕz′-o-năns im′-ăh-jing)

prognosis
(prŏg-nō′-sĭs)

acute
(ă-cūt′)

chronic
(krŏn′-ĭk)

terminal
(tĕr′-mĭ-năl)

remission
(rē′-mĭsh′-ŭn)

exacerbation
(ĕks-ăs″-ĕr-bā′-shŭn)

relapse
(rē-lăps′)

complications
(kōm″-plĭ-ka′-shun)

sequela
(sē-kwē′-lă)

ysis of polio. The sterility resulting from severe inflammation of the fallopian tubes is also a sequela.

An understanding of disease, its cause, the way it affects the body, effective treatments, and its possible prognosis should enable the health professional to alleviate suffering, anxiety, and fear in those who are ill.

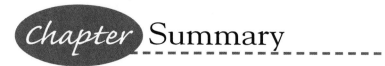

Chapter Summary

The body attempts to maintain homeostasis in the midst of ever-changing conditions. Disease is a state of functional disequilibrium that may be resolved by recovery or death. The etiology, pathogenesis, and diagnosis of disease were discussed. The following chapters of this book will consider the general mechanisms of disease and the physiologic system in which each occurs.

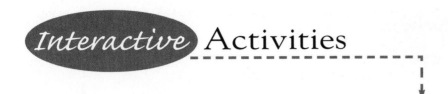

Interactive Activities

CASE FOR CRITICAL THINKING

Athletes develop abnormally high red blood cell counts. Why? In the athlete's case, is this a sign of disease?

MULTIMEDIA EXTENSION ACTIVITIES

www.prenhall.com/mulvihill
Use the above address to access the free, interactive companion Website created for this textbook. Included in the features of this site are chapter specific activities, internet links, and an audio-glossary.

Audio Glossary
Use the CD-ROM disk enclosed with your textbook to hear the pronunciation of the key terms in this chapter.

Quick Self Study

MULTIPLE CHOICE

1. Diagnosis of a disease is based on _____.
   a. signs b. symptoms
   c. laboratory results d. all of the above

2. A(n) _____ disease may have a sudden onset and short terms,
   a(n) _____ disease may begin insidiously and be long-lived.
   a. chronic, acute b. syndrome, acute
   c. acute, chronic d. syndrome, chronic

3. The cause of a disease is _____.
   a. pathogensis b. sign
   c. symptom d. etiology

4. A steady state maintained within the body is called _____.
   a. homeostasis b. trauma
   c. sequela d. syndrome

TRUE/FALSE

_____ 1. A body part that is used excessively will atrophy.

_____ 2. Symptoms are objective evidence of a disease.

_____ 3. Signs may be perceived by the physician.

_____ 4. Exacerbation and remission would characterize a chronic condition.

FILL-INS

1. The predicted outcome of a disease is its _____.
2. If the cause of a disease is not known, it is said to be _____.
3. Return of symptoms after their apparent cessation is _____.
4. The signs and symptoms of a chronic disease at times subside, during a period known as _____.

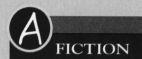

FICTION

The common cold is usually caused by a virus. Antibiotics are ineffective against viruses.

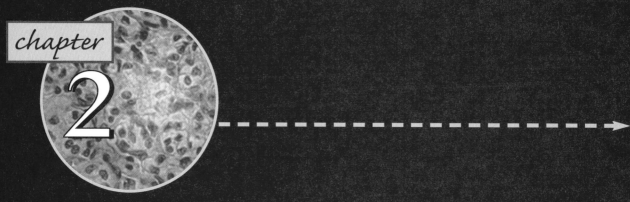

Inflammation, Immunity, and Allergy

Tissues react to local injury, foreign invasion, or irritation by producing an inflammatory response. Although inflammation is painful, it is nature's way of correcting a disorder. Every disease ending in *-itis* is an inflammatory disease, such as appendicitis, bronchitis, and colitis.

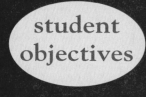

student objectives

After studying this chapter, students should be able to

➤ List and discuss the signs and symptoms of inflammation
➤ Compare and contrast innate and acquired immunity
➤ Explain how the two types of the immune system work together
➤ Describe autoimmunity
➤ Describe HIV's effect on the immune system
➤ Compare and contrast active and passive immunity
➤ Discuss allergy and the immune system

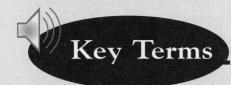

Key Terms

Acquired immunodeficiency syndrome (AIDS)

Activated lymphocytes

Active immunity

Adhesions

Adrenalin

Agglutinate

Allergy

Anaphylaxis

Antibodies

Antigen

Autoimmune diseases

B lymphocytes

Bradykinin

Cell-mediated immunity

Chemotaxis

Chronic fatigue syndrome

Cytotoxic T cells

Dementia

Discoid

Edema

Encephalopathy

Epinephrine

Fibrin

Fibroblasts

Helper T cells

Hemolyze

Heparin

Histamine

Human immunodeficiency virus (HIV)

Humoral immunity

Hyperemia

Hypersensitivity

Immunoglobulins (Ig)

Inflammatory exudate

Keloid

Leukocytes

Leukocytosis

Lymphadenopathy

Lymphatic system

Mast cells

Memory cells

Microliter

Monocytes

Passive immunity

Pathogenic organisms

Phagocytes

Plasma cells

Polymorphs

Pyogenic

Rh factor

Serotonin

SLE

Staphylococci

Streptococci

Suppressor T cells

Suppurative

T lymphocytes

Toxins

Toxoid

Tracheotomy

Vaccine

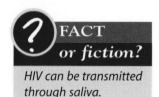

FACT
or fiction?

HIV can be transmitted through saliva.

Read this chapter to find the answer.

pathogenic organisms
(păth″-ō-jĕn′-ĭk or′-găn-ĭsmz)

hyperemia
(hī″-pĕr-ē′-mē-ă)

leukocytes
(loo′-kō-sīts)

polymorphs
(pŏl′-ē-morfs)

histamine
(hĭs′-tă-mĭn)

phagocytes
(făg″-ō-sīts)

chemotaxis
(kē″-mō-tăk′-sĭs)

inflammatory exudate
(ĭn-flăm′-ăh-to″-rē eks′-ū-dāt)

➤ INFLAMMATION AND REPAIR

The cause of the inflammation may be a trauma or injury, such as a sprained ankle or a severe blow. A physical irritant in the tissue—a piece of glass, a wasp sting, or an ingrown toenail—will trigger the response. **Pathogenic organisms**—bacteria, viruses, fungi, or parasites—will do the same. Figure 2–1 shows various agents that are capable of stimulating an inflammatory response.

The chief signs and symptoms of inflammation are redness, swelling, heat, and pain. Inflammation should not be confused with infection. Invading pathogenic organisms are necessary to produce an infection. The invading organisms cause disease by local cellular injury, secretion of a toxin, alteration of DNA by a virus, or by initiating an allergic response. Inflammation, however, is a protective tissue response to injury or invasion by disease-producing organisms.

Vascular changes occur when tissue is traumatized or irritated. Local blood vessels, arterioles, and capillaries dilate, which result in increased blood flow to the injured area. This increased amount of blood, **hyperemia,** causes the heat and redness associated with inflammation. As the blood flow to the site of the injury or infection increases, more and more **leukocytes,** or white blood cells, reach the area. Certain of these white cells, the neutrophils or **polymorphs,** line up within the capillary walls. The polymorphs are specialized to fight against the invading agent or injury.

The damaged tissue releases a substance called **histamine** that causes the capillary walls to become more permeable. This increased permeability enables plasma and neutrophils to move out of the blood vessels into the tissue. Neutrophils are **phagocytes** that have the ability to engulf and digest bacteria and cellular debris. The root word, *phag(o),* means to eat. Figure 2–2 shows the vascular changes that occur with inflammation and the movement of the polymorphs to the infected site. The attraction of the white blood cells to the site of inflammation is called **chemotaxis.**

The plasma and white cells that escape from the capillaries comprise the **inflammatory exudate.** This exudate in the tissues causes the swelling associated with inflammation. The excess of fluid in the tissues puts pressure on sensitive nerve endings, causing pain.

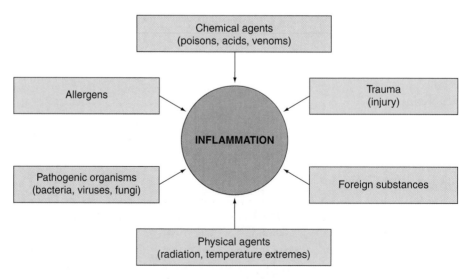

Figure 2–1
Agents capable of stimulating an inflammatory response.

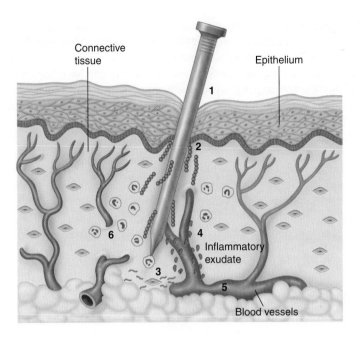

Connective tissue

Epithelium

Inflammatory exudate

Blood vessels

1. Dirty nail punctures skin.

2. Bacteria enter and multiply.

3. Injured cells release histamine.

4. Blood vessels dilate and become permeable, releasing inflammatory exudate.

5. Blood flow to the damaged site increases.

6. Neutrophils (polymorph) move toward bacteria (chemotaxis) and destroy them (phagocytosis).

Figure 2–2
Vascular changes that occur with inflammation.

Bacterial infection may be the cause of an inflammation. Organisms such as **staphylococci** and **streptococci** that produce **toxins** (substances damaging to the tissues) will initiate an inflammatory response. To increase the power of the white cells fighting the infection, the bone marrow and lymph nodes release very large quantities of leukocytes. This increased production of white cells accounts for the elevated white cell count associated with infection. The count may rise to 30,000 or more from the normal range of 7000 to 9000 per cubic **microliter** of blood (μl). The excessive production of white cells is called **leukocytosis.** Leukocytosis is, for example, a sign of appendicitis.

The polymorphs soon die after ingesting bacteria and toxins. Substances are released from the dead cells that liquefy the tissue. This liquefied tissue—dead polymorphs, inflammatory exudate, and bacteria—make up the thick, yellow fluid known as pus. Other phagocytic white cells, the **monocytes** or macrophages, follow the polymorphs in the process of clearing debris. Inflammatory exudate contains a plasma protein, **fibrin,** essential for the blood-clotting mechanism. Fibrin acts in the damaged tissue by forming a clot, thus walling off the infection and preventing its spread.

staphylococci
(stăf″-ĭl-ō-kŏk′-sē)

streptococci
(strĕp″-tō-kŏk′-sī)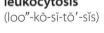

toxins
(tŏk′-sĭns)

microliter
(mī′-krō-lē″-tĕr)

leukocytosis
(loo″-kō-sī-tō′-sĭs)

monocytes
(mŏn′-ō-sīts)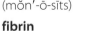

fibrin
(fī′-brĭn)

pyogenic
(pī-ō-jĕn′-ĭk)

suppurative
(sŭp′-ū-rā″-tĭv)

fibroblasts
(fī′-brō-blăsts)

Bacteria that cause pus formation are called **pyogenic** bacteria. An inflammation associated with pus formation is a **suppurative** inflammation. Abscesses, boils, and styes are examples of inflammations with suppuration.

Wound healing and repair can occur only when bacteria have been destroyed. Cut edges of tissue will grow together as connective tissue cells (**fibroblasts**) produce fibers that will close the gap. Figure 2–3 shows the fibroblasts and their fibers healing a skin incision. This is known as scar tissue. Sometimes the connective tissue fibers will an-

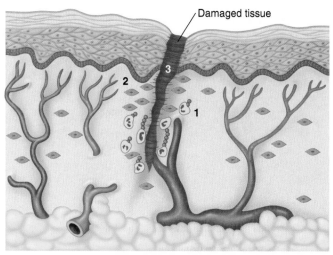

1. Neutrophils phagocytize bacteria.

2. Fibroblasts produce connective tissue fibers.

3. Fibers contract, drawing cut surfaces together.

1. Blood clot forms.

2. Dried clot forms scab.

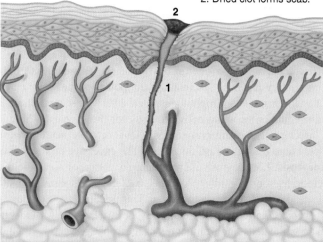

Figure 2–3
Fibroblasts healing a wound.

chor together adjacent structures, causing **adhesions.** The problems associated with adhesions will be explained in later chapters.

A scar after surgery or a severe burn is often raised and hard. This is known as **keloid** healing and is really a benign tumor that is harmless. Surgery to remove such a scar is usually ineffective, as the subsequent incision will have a tendency to heal in the same way.

➤ IMMUNITY

Immunity is the ability of the body to defend itself against infectious agents, foreign cells, and even abnormal body cells, such as cancer cells. The foreign element that triggers the immune response is known as an **antigen.** Immunity includes nonspecific and specific defenses. Nonspecific defenses include inflammation, phagocytosis, physical barriers like the skin, and chemical, defenses such as stomach acid. These defenses are also called *innate* immunity. Specific defenses include humoral and cell-mediated immunity. **Humoral immunity** includes **antibodies** and **cell-mediated immunity** includes **activated lymphocytes.** Antibodies and activated lymphocytes comprise *acquired immunity*. Non-specific defenses fight infections in general, whereas specific defenses target specific pathogenic organisms with antibodies and cells.

An important part of immunity is the body's **lymphatic system.** It consists of a complex network of thin-walled capillaries carrying lymph fluid, nodes, and organs that help to maintain the internal fluid environment of the body. The lymph nodes are small filtering stations that help fight infection. They produce certain white blood cells, lymphocytes, monocytes, and plasma cells that destroy invading organisms. Organs such as the spleen, tonsils, and adenoids are comprised of lymphoid tissue and function in the body's internal defense (Figure 2–4).

How do the tissues of the lymphatic system work with the components of acquired immunity to defend the body against infection? Remember the two basic types of acquired immunity: circulating antibodies or globulin molecules capable of destroying foreign invaders, and activated lymphocytes. The antibodies provide humoral immunity and the activated lymphocytes provide cell-mediated immunity (Figure 2–5). Both types are formed in lymph nodes and lymphoid tissue such as the spleen, bone marrow, tonsils, and adenoids. The lymphoid tissue is placed strategically in the body to intercept invading organisms.

Both humoral and cell-mediated immunity can work together to fight a foreign invader. Both are activated by an antigen, such as *Salmonella* bacteria from an undercooked chicken breast. The antigen will interact with lymphocytes in tissues, in lymph, or in blood.

Two types of lymphocytes provide immunity, the T and B lymphocytes. The lymphocytes responsible for cell-mediated immunity first migrate to and are processed by the thymus gland; hence they are called **T lymphocytes** or activated lymphocytes. The other type of lymphocytes form antibodies and are called **B lymphocytes;** these are responsible for humoral immunity. Antibodies and T lymphocytes are each highly specific for one type of antigen.

B cells can play different roles in humoral immunity. Some B cells interact with antigens and become activated. Some activated B lymphocytes are transformed into **plasma cells** and begin to divide at a rapid rate and produce large numbers of antibodies. These are secreted into the lymph and travel to the blood to be circulated through the body. The antibodies are plasma proteins, gamma globulins called **immunoglobulins (Ig).**

adhesions
(ăd-hē′-zhŭnz)

keloid
(kē′-lŏyd)

antigen
(ăn′-tĭ-jĕn)

humoral immunity
(hū′-mŏr-ăl ĭ-mū′-nĭ-tē)

antibodies
(ăn′-tĭ-bŏd″-ēz)

cell-mediated immunity
(sĕl-mē′-dē-āt″-ĭd ĭm-ū′-nĭ-tē)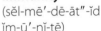

activated lymphocytes
(ăk′-tĭ-vā″-tĭd lĭm′-fō-sīts)

lymphatic system
(lĭm-făt′-ĭk sĭs′-tĕm)

T lymphocytes
(tē lĭm′-fō-sīts)

B lymphocytes
(bē lĭm′-fō-sīts)

plasma cells
(plăz′-mă sĕls)

immunoglobulins (Ig)
(ĭm″-ū-nō-glŏb′-ū-lĭnz)

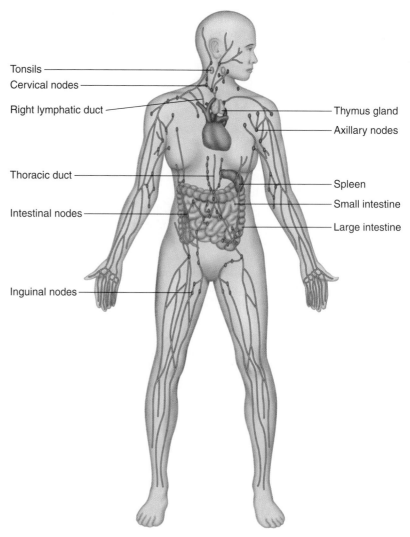

Figure 2–4
The lymphatic system.

Tonsils
Cervical nodes
Right lymphatic duct
Thymus gland
Axillary nodes
Thoracic duct
Spleen
Small intestine
Large intestine
Intestinal nodes
Inguinal nodes

Antibodies bind to antigens and tag the antigen for destruction by the immune system. There are several types of immunoglobulins, each has its own function. See Figure 2–6 for a summary of their functions.

Other B lymphocytes do not become plasma cells and remain dormant until reactivated by the same antigen. These are called **memory cells** and cause a more potent and rapid antibody response. The secondary response begins more rapidly after exposure to the antigen, produces more antibodies, and lasts for a longer time than the initial response. This is the basis for booster shots after vaccination (Figure 2–7).

There are several different kinds of T cells, each with different functions: **cytotoxic T cells, helper T cells** and **suppressor T cells.**

The cytotoxic T cells are often called *killer cells* because they are capable of killing invading organisms. They have on their surfaces receptor proteins that bind tightly to

memory cells
(měm′-ō-rē sěls)

cytotoxic T cells
(sī″-tō-tŏks′-ĭk tē sěls)

helper T cells
(hěl′-pěr T sěls)

suppressor T cells
(sŭ-prěs′-sŏr T sěls)

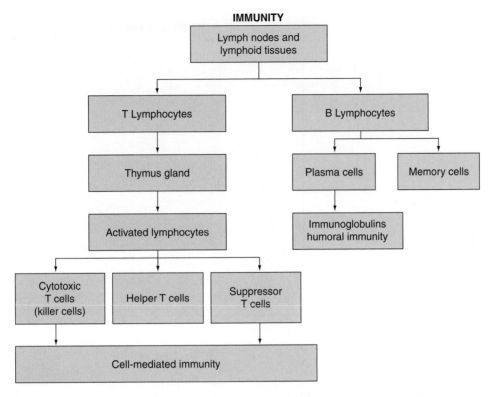

Figure 2–5
Cell-mediated immunity, versus humoral immunity.

IMMUNOGLOBULIN	FUNCTION
IgG	Enhances phagocytosis Neutralizes toxins and viruses Protects newborns
IgE	Allergy
IgA	Localized protection at mucosal surfaces
IgM	First antibody produced Microbe destruction
IgD	Serum function unknown Acts as antigen receptors on B Cell surface

Figure 2–6
There are several types of immunoglobulins; each has its own
function.

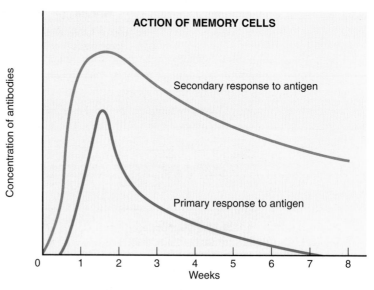

Figure 2–7
Secondary response begins more rapidly after exposure to antigen, produces more antibodies, and lasts for a longer time than initial exposure.

cells or organisms containing a specific antigen. Once bound, the cytotoxic T cells release poisonous substances into the attacked cell. Many organisms can be killed by one killer cell. The cytotoxic cells are important in killing cells that have been invaded by viruses. These T cells also can destroy cancer cells.

The helper T cells get their name from the fact that they help the immune system in many ways. They increase the activity of killer cells, and stimulate B cells to produce more antibodies. Activated helper T cells secrete lymphokines that increase the response of other types of lymphoid cells to the antigen and activate large cells called macrophages to destroy large numbers of invaders by phagocytosis.

➤ AUTOIMMUNITY

autoimmune diseases
(aw″-tō-ĭm-mūn dĭ-zēz′-ĕs)

Suppressor T cells are not well understood. They are thought to be T cells that regulate the immune response by turning it off when the antigen is no longer present. The immune response normally recognizes the difference between the individual's own tissues and those of invaders; this is known as *tolerance*. However, this immune tolerance can fail, and activated T cells and antibodies attack the body's own tissue, causing **autoimmune diseases.** Several of these autoimmune diseases, such as rheumatic fever, glomerulonephritis, myasthenia gravis, and rheumatoid arthritis, are described elsewhere in this book. One very serious autoimmune disease will be considered here, lupus erythematosus.

Systemic Lupus Erythematosus
Systemic lupus erythematosus is a noncontagious inflammatory disease that takes one of two forms: mild or severe. Young women are most frequently affected by systemic

lupus, which may begin suddenly or insidiously. The person experiences a rash, and the skin becomes overly sensitive to sunlight. Joint and muscle pains may be accompanied by fever. The lymph nodes and spleen are frequently found to be enlarged. Periods of exacerbation and remission are characteristic of the disease. The **discoid** form is only a minor disorder in which red, raised, itchy lesions develop. The lesions characteristically form the pattern of a butterfly over the nose and cheeks.

The serious form is **systemic lupus erythematosus (SLE),** which affects not only the skin but also causes the deterioration of collagenous connective tissue. Systemic lupus can affect the glomeruli of the kidney, causing abnormal excretion of albumin and blood, as well as casts (Chapter 10) in the urine. The red cell, white cell, and platelet counts are low. The lining of the heart and the heart valves may deteriorate. Hypersensitivity to an antigen is thought to be the cause of systemic lupus erythematosus. The antigen may be an allergen outside the body or the patient's own tissue to which the patient has become sensitized, an example of autoimmunity.

There is no specific treatment for systemic lupus erythematosus, but, as with many inflammatory diseases, corticosteroids are administered to control the symptoms. The disease may even be fatal, death frequently being the result of kidney or heart failure. The decreased number of leukocytes also reduces resistance to such diseases as pneumonia.

discoid
(dĭs′-koyd)

systemic lupus erythematosus (SLE)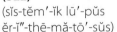
(sĭs-tĕm′-ĭk lū′-pŭs ĕr-ĭ″-thē-mă-tō′-sŭs)

➤ IMMUNE DEFICIENCY

Acquired Immunodeficiency Syndrome (AIDS)

One of the most deadly diseases to affect today's population is **acquired immunodeficiency syndrome (AIDS).** AIDS destroys the individual's immune system, making the person remarkably susceptible to infection. AIDS was first noted among promiscuous homosexual and bisexual men and drug users who shared hypodermic needles. Now, however, the incidence of AIDS is rapidly increasing among heterosexuals.

The causative agent of AIDS is the **human immunodeficiency virus (HIV),** a retrovirus, i.e., it carries its genetic information as RNA rather than DNA. The virus infects certain white blood cells of the body's immune system, namely the helper T-4 lymphocytes, and destroys their ability to fight infection. The virus replicates itself within the lymphocyte, killing it, and spreading to others. These lymphocytes normally activate antibody-producing B-cell lymphocytes, thus the body's immune response is blocked. Kaposi's sarcoma, a rare, slow-growing cancer is also noted more frequently, as are other opportunistic infections, such as *Pneumocystis carinii* pneumonia or *Mycobacterium tuberculosis.*

Signs include unexplained weight loss, generalized **lymphadenopathy** (enlarged lymph nodes), diarrhea, fever, and night sweats in the early stages. **Encephalopathy** (chronic, destructive, or degenerative condition of the brain) and **dementia** (organic loss of intellectual function) occur in a high percentage of AIDS patients with advanced disease.

HIV is transmitted via contaminated body fluids including blood, semen, vaginal secretions, and breast milk. Therefore, HIV is transmitted during unprotected anal, oral, or vaginal intercourse, birth, breastfeeding, and the sharing of needles. HIV is found in saliva, but in such small concentrations that it is estimated a person would have to ingest a bucket of saliva to actually get the virus from saliva.

In some cases, recipients of blood transfusions before blood screening was done developed AIDS. Reliable tests for the presence of the virus now minimize the risk of

acquired immunodeficiency syndrome (AIDS)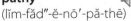
(ă-kwīrd′ ĭm″-ū-nō-dĕ-fĭsh′-ĕn-sē sĭn-drōm)

human immunodeficiency virus (HIV)
(hū′-măn ĭm″-ū-nō-dĕ-fĭsh′-ĕn-sē vī′-rĭs)

lymphadenopathy
(lĭm-făd″-ĕ-nō′-pă-thē)

encephalopathy
(ĕn-sĕf″-ă-lŏp′-ă-thē)

dementia
(dē-mĕn′-shē-ă)

contracting it through contaminated blood transfusion. Blood donors do not contract the virus from giving blood because a new needle is used each time.

HIV Infection

Even before full-blown AIDS develops, the virus is destroying the immune system of the HIV-positive individual. Studies have shown that large amounts of the virus can be present during the asymptomatic stage of the disease. The virus resides in high concentration in lymph nodes where it continues to increase. Anonymous testing for HIV antibodies is available for free at local health departments. Antibodies may take up to ninety days to form.

There is a long and variable latent period of 2 to 8 years between HIV infection and the development of full-blown AIDS. An individual who tests positive for HIV may manifest some of the signs of AIDS, such as flulike symptoms when first infected, but may recover and be symptom-free for some period of time. The long latent period increases the risk of spreading the infection because individuals are not aware they have the disease. Once infected, the patient is infected for life. Eventually a threshold is crossed and the HIV-infected person develops AIDS. One must have one of twenty-three indicator diseases to be diagnosed with AIDS, and have a T_4 (or CD4) cell count of less than 200.

Disease by the Numbers x + ÷

EPIDEMIOLOGY

As of the end of 1999, an estimated 33.6 million people worldwide—32.4 million adults and 1.2 million children under age 15—were living with HIV/AIDS. More than 69% of these people (23.3 million) live in Subsaharan Africa; another 18% (6.0 million) live in South and Southeast Asia. Worldwide, approximately 1 in every 100 adults age 15–49 years is infected with HIV. In 1999, more than 15,000 new infections occurred every day. More than 80% of all adult HIV infections have resulted from heterosexual intercourse.

Precautions for Healthcare Professionals

Healthcare professionals must exercise great precautions when handling blood or bodily secretions of AIDS patients. Several workers have contracted the virus by accidental sticks. The best protection against HIV exposure is consistent adherence to the standard recommendations of the Centers for Disease Control and Prevention (CDCP) and the guidelines required by the Occupational Safety and Health Administration (OSHA), which are as follows.

OSHA requires employers to train employees who are at risk of exposure to blood-borne pathogens; training must be held during work hours and at no cost to employees. Appropriate instruction on handwashing, the use of gloves, gowns, and protective eye covering, and the proper disposal of sharps must be provided. Information must be given on the facility's Exposure Control Plan, blood-borne disease symptoms and modes of transmission, and use and limitations of risk-reduction methods. Employees must be informed of hepatitis B vaccination availability (Chapter 12), actions to take in case of emergencies, and procedures to follow if exposure incidents occur.

BIOHAZARD

Figure 2–8
Required warning on potentially
hazardous material.

Warning labels bearing the biohazard symbol (Figure 2–8) in fluorescent orange or orange-red must be part of, or securely affixed to, containers used to store, transport, or dispose of potentially infectious material. Refrigerators and freezers used for such material must also be labeled. Red bags or red containers may be substituted for labels on containers of infectious wastes.

Treatment

Development of a vaccine to prevent the spread of AIDS has not yet been possible. The genetic makeup of the AIDS virus varies greatly from strain to strain, which complicates the attempt to develop an AIDS vaccine. HIV tends to mutate frequently, which adds to the difficulty of producing a vaccine.

Researchers around the world are working toward designing drugs to effect a cure for AIDS. There is no cure for AIDS, but a cocktail of drugs has stopped HIV replication to such an extent that the viral load becomes undetectable in some individuals. A combination of two drug types is used, nucleotide analogs and protease inhibitors. The well-publicized AZT and several others are nucleotide analogs. These drugs stop viral DNA production. Protease inhibitors stop the assembly of viruses. A common cocktail contains two analogs such as AZT and 3TC plus a protease inhibitor. It is important to realize that these drugs are very expensive, cause side effects, and the regimen of pill taking throughout the day is very demanding. If the drugs are not taken as prescribed or if the therapy is stopped, resistance may occur. The sooner drug therapy begins after infection, the better the chances are that the immune system will not be destroyed by HIV.

Chronic Fatigue Syndrome

Chronic fatigue syndrome is a peculiar disease that affects primarily young professionals in the prime of life. It has been dubbed "yuppie flu" because of the class of individuals affected. The flulike symptoms include severe and persistent fatigue, muscle and joint pain, and fever. The person experiences trouble with concentration and memory.

The cause and cure are unknown although much research has been done on the disease. It was thought at first to be psychosomatic or the result of depression, but changes have been found in the patient's immune system. No particular virus has been proven to be the cause, but blood tests have shown an immune response consistent with a viral

**chronic fatigue
syndrome**
(krŏn'-ĭk fă-tēg'
sĭn'-drōm)

infection. Some, but not all, individuals have antibodies to Epstein-Barr virus. Other evidence points to herpes virus b.

➤ VACCINATION

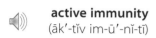

active immunity
(āk´-tĭv im-ū´-nĭ-tī)

vaccine
(văk´-sēn´)

toxoid
(tŏks´-oyd)

Two types of artificial immunity can be administered, active and passive immunity. In **active immunity,** the person is given a vaccine or a toxoid as the antigen, and he or she forms antibodies to counteract it. A **vaccine** consists of a low dose of dead or deactivated bacteria or viruses. Because the organisms have been specially treated to deactivate them, they cannot cause disease. As protein foreign to the body, these antigens do trigger antibody production against them. A **toxoid** works similarly. It consists of a chemically altered toxin, the poisonous material produced by a pathogenic organism. Having been treated chemically, the toxin will not cause disease. It will, however, stimulate the immune response.

This type of immunity, in which cells are exposed to an antigen and begin to form the corresponding antibodies, is long-lived. This kind of protection is given to prevent diseases such as polio and diphtheria. Time is required to build up immunity, and a booster shot is frequently given for a stronger effect. Once cells have been sensitized to these viruses, bacteria, or toxins, they will continue to produce antibodies against them.

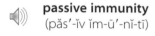

passive immunity
(păs´-ĭv ĭm-ū´-nĭ-tī)

What if a person is exposed to a serious disease such as hepatitis, tetanus, or rabies and has no immunity against it? It takes time to build antibodies and time is limited. In this case, the person is given **passive immunity,** doses of preformed antibodies from immune serum of an animal, usually a horse. This type of immunity is short-lived but acts immediately. Figure 2–9 contrasts active and passive immunity.

PREVENTION *PLUS!*

Disease Prevention through Vaccination

Today, children are needlessly catching dangerous illnesses like measles, whooping cough, hepatitis, and meningitis. Without immunization at the right times, children can get any one of these very serious or even fatal diseases. Vaccines are both effective and cost-effective. "Effective" does not mean that every individual who has been vaccinated is 100% protected. No vaccine can accomplish that kind of guarantee. Effective means that most vaccinated people will be protected, particularly when a high proportion of people in a population are immunized. Reactions to the vaccines may occur, but they are usually mild. Serious reactions are very rare but may occur. Remember, the risks from these potentially dangerous childhood illnesses are far greater than the risk of a serious reaction from an immunization. The list below includes childhood immunization recommendations from the American Academy of Pediatrics.

Hepatitis B	Polio
Diphtheria	Measles
Tetanus	Mumps
Pertussis	Rubella
H. influenza	Varicella

ACTIVE IMMUNITY	PASSIVE IMMUNITY
Person forms antibodies	Preformed anitbodies received
Vaccine (deactivated bacteria or virus)	Immune horse serum
or	or
Toxoid (chemically altered toxin)	Antibodies, cells in breast milk
Long-lived immunity Requires time to act	Short-lived immunity Acts immediately

Figure 2–9
Differences between active and passive immunity.

➤ HYPERSENSITIVITY—ALLERGIES

Closely related to the concept of immunity is **allergy,** or **hypersensitivity.** Some diseases are actually the result of an individual's immune response, which causes tissue damage and disordered function rather than immunity. The immune phenomena are destructive rather than defensive in the individual who is hypersensitive or allergic (atopic) to an antigen. Hypersensitivity diseases or allergic diseases may manifest themselves locally or systemically.

allergy
(ăl'-ĕr-jē)
hypersensitivity
(hī"-pĕr-sĕn"-sĭ-tiv'-ĭ-tē)

The abnormal sensitivity to pollens, dust, dog hair, and certain foods or chemicals is the result of overproduction of IgE. IgE has an affinity for certain cells, basophils and **mast cells,** and attaches to them. Mast cells are in connective tissue and contain **heparin, serotonin, bradykinin,** and histamine. As the antigen attaches to the antibody, the mast cells break down and release the above-named chemicals. Histamine causes the dilation of the blood vessels and makes them susceptible to plasma leakage. The leakage of plasma into the tissues causes **edema,** or swelling, which when localized in the nasal passages results in the familiar congestion and irritation of hay fever. If the tissue damage and edema are near the skin, the welts and itching of hives may appear. Antihistamines are quite effective in the treatment of hives but less so for hay fever. A typical allergic reaction is illustrated in Figure 2–10.

mast cells
(măst sĕls)
heparin
(hĕp'-ă-rĭn)
serotonin
(sĕr"-ō-tōn'-ĭn)
bradykinin
(brăd"-ē-kī'-nĭn)
edema
(ĕ-dē'-mă)

Allergy shots can desensitize the hypersensitive person. Small amounts of the offending antigen are administered, and concentrations are gradually increased. Desensitization inoculations for such people depend on their ability to produce IgG and work by causing an increase of IgG in the bloodstream. The IgG binds to the allergen in the blood before it binds to IgE in the tissues, subsequently reducing the amount of tissue damage. Local (atopic) allergies are as simple as development of a stuffy nose after inhaling pollen, while systemic (anaphylactic shock) allergy reponses are life-threatening. Both result from activation of mast cells bound to IgE. That is, large amounts of antibody (IgE) are attached to mast cells, but in systemic **anaphylaxis** these are activated throughout the body, releasing massive amounts of histamine and other powerful chemicals.

anaphylaxis
(ăn"-ă-fĭ-lăk'-sĭs)

The mechanisms of the systemic anaphylactic reaction are the same as in the local response. There is a generalized change in capillary permeability leading to hypotension,

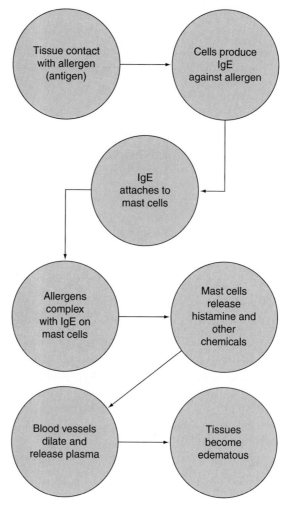

Figure 2–10
Typical allergic reaction.

low blood pressure, and shock. Smooth muscle contraction in the respiratory tract causes respiratory distress resembling asthma. Fluid in the larynx may threaten to obstruct the airways and necessitate a **tracheotomy,** creation of an opening into the trachea to facilitate passage of air or evacuation of secretions.

Less severe signs may include skin flush, hives, swelling of lips or tongue, wheezing, and abdominal cramps. Life-threatening signs include weakness and collapse due to low blood pressure, inability to breathe, and seizures.

The most vital therapy is prompt intramuscular injection of **epinephrine (adrenalin).** Certain allergic individuals have to carry epinephrine with them, which can be self-injected in an emergency.

Type I hypersensitivities are labeled anaphylactic and involve excess IgE bound to mast cells and activated by allergens to produce either local severe inflammation (atopic allergy) or systemic severe inflammation (anaphylactic shock) (see Figure 2–11). These are produced by bee venom, foods, or pollen. Type II hypersensitivities are labeled

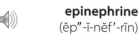
tracheotomy
(trā″-kē-ŏt′-ō-mē)

epinephrine
(ĕp″-ĭ-nĕf′-rĭn)

adrenalin
(ă-drĕn′-ă-lĭn)

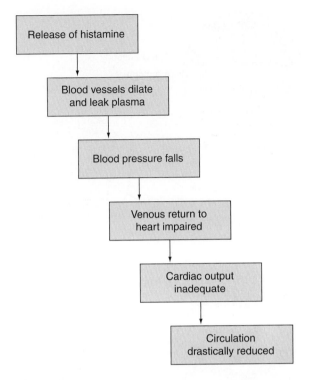

Figure 2–11
Sequence of vascular events in anaphylactic shock.

on the Practical Side

Medical Alert Bracelets
A life may be saved in an emergency by providing medical personnel with vital information. Bracelets, necklaces, and/or wallet cards can alert caregivers to severe allergies such
as to penicillin, bee or wasp stings, or certain foods. Insulin-dependent diabetics can be
identified if encountered while in a coma or insulin shock and unable to speak for themselves.

cytotoxic or cytolytic, and involve IgM or IgG interacting with foreign cells to cause
their destruction. An example of this is an incompatible blood transfusion.

A person with type A blood has A antigens on the red cells and antibodies against
type B blood in the serum. If such a person receives a type B transfusion, the antigens
and antibodies will interact. The red blood cells will **agglutinate,** or clump together, and
hemolyze (rupture). Massive hemolysis occurs. (see Figure 2–12).

Another example of the cytolytic allergic response would be an Rh positive (Rh^+)
blood transfusion to an Rh negative (Rh^-) recipient. Rh^- blood means that the Rh antigen or factor is not present. This transfusion would cause no trouble, but in the transfusion the Rh^- recipient is exposed or sensitized to the **Rh factor** and begins to form antibodies against this foreign protein. Subsequent Rh^+ transfusions would cause clumping
and rupture of red blood cells. Rh incompatibility during pregnancy is also a delayed

agglutinate
(ă-gloo″-tĭ-nāt)

hemolyze
(hē′-mŏ-līz)

Rh factor
(R-h făc′-tŏr)

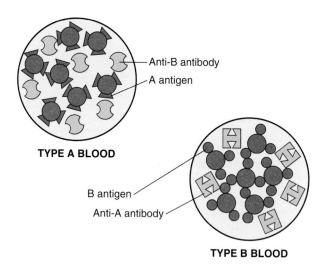

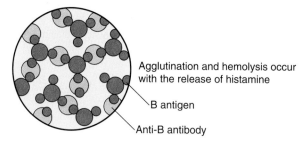

Figure 2–12
Cytotoxic allergy (incompatible blood transfusion).

allergic reaction. An Rh$^-$ mother can become sensitized by the fetus' Rh$^+$ blood and make antibodies that destroy the fetal red blood cells. This does not generally occur during the first pregnancy, as the mother has not yet become sensitized. Rh incompatibility is examined more closely in Chapter 7.

Figure 2–12 shows this sequence of events. There is a type III hypersensitivity involving deposition of antibody-antigen complexes in tissues such as the kidney (causing glomerulonephritis triggered after a streptococcal infection) or the lung (causing farmer's lung, triggered by mold spore inhalation). The complexes may cause tissue destruction. Types I, II, and III are all immediate hypersensitivities; they develop within about a half-hour or sooner.

Another type of allergic reaction can occur in anyone but is a delayed reaction. Initial exposure to an antigen results in activation of a T-cell-mediated immune response, which is slow to develop (delayed). For example, the first time one contacts poison ivy there will be no reaction. However, T cells may become sensitized to it. On the next exposure, the typical rash and irritation, caused by T-cell secretion of cytokines (toxic substances) that damage the tissues where the ivy oil has been absorbed, will develop. This is the type of reaction in contact dermatitis and the tuberculin test. Tissue and organ rejections are also examples of delayed hypersensitivity reactions.

Chapter Summary

The immune reaction provides the body with a strong defense against invading organisms. The body recognizes foreign antigens and responds to counteract them with antibodies and activated lymphocytes. Antibodies produce humoral immunity; activated lymphocytes produce cell-mediated immunity. B cells produce the different types of immunoglobulins involved in humoral immunity. Several types of T cells including killer cells, helper cells, and suppressor cells are involved in cell-mediated immunity. An abnormality in the immune system can cause disease when the body becomes hypersensitive to its own tissue and destroys it. This is known as autoimmunity. Systemic lupus erythematosus is such a disease. The most serious failure in the immune system is acquired immune deficiency syndrome, or AIDS. Artificial immunity can be provided by vaccination. In active immunity the individual is given a vaccine or a toxoid and actively makes antibodies to counteract it. Preformed antibodies are given in passive immunity. Allergies can be considered a side effect of immunity. Allergic diseases are the result of an immune response that causes tissue damage and disordered function rather than immunity. Hypersensitivity to harmless substances is the result of abnormally formed immunoglobulins in the allergic person. Allergies range in severity from local tissue damage, as in hay fever and hives, to a systemic anaphylactic reaction that can be life-threatening.

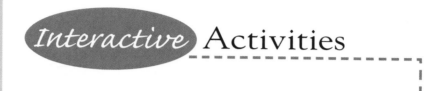

Interactive Activities

CASE FOR CRITICAL THINKING

Tetanus is caused by bacteria that enter the body through wounds in the skin. The bacteria produce a toxin that causes spastic muscle contraction. Death often results from failure of the respiratory muscles. A patient comes to the emergency room after stepping on a nail. If the patient has been vaccinated against tetanus, he is given a tetanus booster shot, which consists of the toxin altered so that it is harmless. If the patient has never been vaccinated against tetanus, he is given an antiserum shot against tetanus. Explain the rationale for this treatment.

MULTIMEDIA EXTENSION ACTIVITIES

www.prenhall.com/mulvihill
Use the above address to access the free, interactive companion Website created for this textbook. Included in the features of this site are chapter specific activities, internet links, and an audio-glossary.

Audio Glossary
Use the CD-ROM disk enclosed with your textbook to hear the pronunciation of the key terms in this chapter.

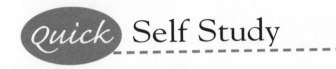

Quick Self Study

MULTIPLE CHOICE

1. What are the signs and symptoms of inflammation?
   a. redness
   b. swelling
   c. heat
   d. pain
   e. all of the above

2. Excess fluid in the tissues is _____.
   a. adhesion
   b. keloid
   c. edema
   d. suppurative

3. _____ cells produce antibodies.
   a. T
   b. B

4. Resistance of the skin to invading organisms is _____.
   a. innate immunity
   b. acquired immunity

TRUE/FALSE

_____ 1. Activated lymphocytes provide humoral immunity.

_____ 2. Antibodies and T cells are specific for one antigen.

_____ 3. People immediately test positive for HIV antibodies.

_____ 4. Adrenalin is used to treat severe allergic reactions.

FILL-INS

1. The virus responsible for AIDS causes severe immunodeficiency of
   _____ cells.

2. Ig _____ plays a role in allergy.

3. Some B cells remain dormant until reactivation by the same antigen. These are called
   _____.

4. _____ T cells can kill invading organisms.

FICTION

HIV cannot be transmitted through saliva. You would have to ingest a bucket of saliva!

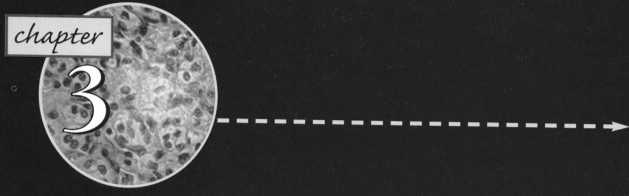

Infectious Diseases

What is the impact of infectious disease on human health? According to the World Health Organization, of 52 million recent deaths occurring worldwide each year, about 17 million are caused by infectious diseases. Of course, many more than 17 million people become ill each year with an infectious disease, and that suffering remains uncounted. As the world population grows, infectious disease will continue to grow in importance, especially among the expanding young and elderly populations.

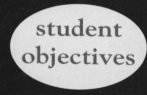

student objectives

After studying this chapter, students should be able to

➤ Define infectious diseases

➤ Describe and compare the characteristics of bacteria, viruses, fungi, helminths, and arthropod vectors

➤ Explain the chief ways that infectious diseases are transmitted

➤ Explain the kinds of treatment for bacterial, viral, fungal, and parasitic infectious diseases

➤ Describe how vaccines work and the names and uses of common vaccines

➤ Understand the appropriate use of antibiotics and explain the problem of antibiotic resistance

➤ Describe examples and the causes of re-emerging infectious diseases

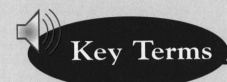

Key Terms

Amoeboids

Antibiotic resistance

Antibiotics

Bacilli

Binary fission

Capsid

Cell walls

Ciliates

Cocci

Communicable

Contagious

Disinfection

Endemic

Endospores

Endotoxin

Epidemic

Flagellates

Flatworms

Gram stain

Horizontal transmission

Incidence

Infectious diseases

Infestations

Isolation

Latent infection

Lyse

Mycelia

Noncommunicable

Outbreak

Pandemic

Pathogens

Prevalence

Quarantine

Reportable diseases

Reservoirs

Roundworms

Spirilla

Spirochetes

Spores

Sporozoans

Standard precautions

Vectors

Vertical transmission

Vibrios

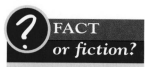

infectious diseases
(ĭn-fĕk′-shus dĭ-zēz′-ĕz)

contagious
(kŏn-tā′-jŭs)

communicable
(kŏ-mū′-nĭ-kă-b′l)

noncommunicable
(nŏn-kŏ-mū′-nĭ-kā-b′l)

pathogens
(păth′-ō-jĕns)

cell walls
(sĕl wawls)

cocci
(kŏk′-sī)

bacilli
(bă-sĭl-ī)

spirilla
(spī-rĭl′-ă)

spirochetes
(spī′-rō-kēts)

vibrios
(vĭb′-rē-ōs)

gram stain
(grăm stāns)

binary fission
(bī′-nār-ē fĭsh′-ŭn)

➤ INTRODUCTION TO INFECTIOUS DISEASES

Some infectious diseases described in this book have been in existence for a long time, whereas others have emerged as new pathology. It is important to have a framework for understanding the infectious diseases described. This chapter will describe the nature of infectious diseases, survey the types of microorganisms responsible for infections, explain their transmission, and outline treatment and control strategies.

Infectious diseases are those diseases caused by pathogenic microorganisms. These diseases may be transmitted to humans by other humans or by some other element in the environment. Those diseases transmitted from human to human are said to be **contagious** or **communicable.** Measles and influenza are well-known contagious diseases. Infectious diseases are classified as **noncommunicable** if not transmitted directly by humans. For example, rabies can be transmitted by the bite of a rabid raccoon, and cholera is transmitted by consumption of feces-contaminated water. In any case, some type of pathogenic microorganism causes these diseases.

➤ PATHOGENIC MICROORGANISMS

Most microorganisms do not cause disease. Those that do cause disease are called **pathogens.** Humans can be infected by a variety of pathogens, ranging from tiny single-celled bacteria to macroscopic complex worms (Figure 3–1).

Bacteria

Bacteria are microscopic single-celled organisms. A simple structure (no nucleus or membranous organelles) and small size (1 to 10 μm) are key characteristics that differentiate bacteria from other single-celled organisms. Although often described as simple, they are far from primitive, for they have adapted to a wide variety of habitats and have evolved complex strategies for infecting and surviving in the human body.

Bacteria have **cell walls,** a rigid layer of organic material surrounding their delicate cell membranes. These walls give bacteria their characteristic shapes. Bacteria may have spherical, round cells called **cocci,** rod-shaped cells called **bacilli,** spiral-shaped cells called **spirilla,** corkscrew-shaped cells called **spirochetes,** and comma-shaped cells called **vibrios.** Figure 3–1 shows the cell structure of a rod-shaped bacterium. The walls protect these cells; should walls be disrupted, cells are susceptible to bursting. This is the action of the antibiotic penicillin. This antibiotic interferes with correct cell wall construction of certain types of bacteria. The bacteria cell walls may be thick, thin, or absent. The thickness of the cell wall accounts for the way certain cells stain during the gram stain procedure. During the **gram stain,** thick-walled cells turn purple and thin-walled cells become red and, thus, bacteria can be identified using this technique. Identification is critical to obtain an accurate diagnosis and effective treatment of an infection. Table 3–1 lists common gram-positive and gram-negative pathogens and the diseases associated with them. Other bacteria that do not fit into the above categories of shape and gram stain properties include the chlamydias and rickettsias, which are intracellular parasites. Arthropod vectors transmit many of these.

Bacteria grow rapidly and reproduce by splitting in half, a process known as **binary fission.** Under favorable conditions, this process may take only 30 minutes. So, a small number of cells may increase to a very large number in a relatively short time. The reproduction of a cell and its genetic material occurs with very few errors or mutations. Still, this rapid growth rate virtually guarantees that mutations will arise, and some of these will favor survival of the bacteria under certain conditions.

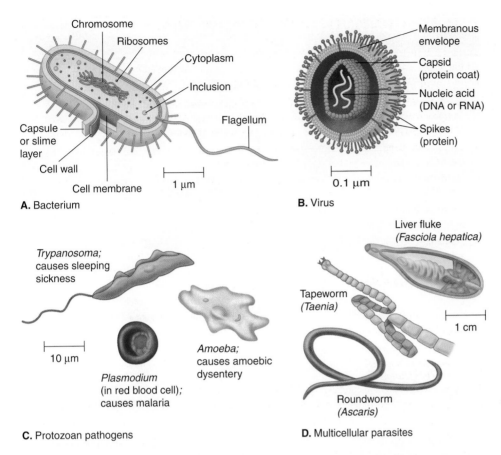

Chromosome
Ribosomes
Cytoplasm
Inclusion
Flagellum
Capsule
or slime
layer
Cell wall
Cell membrane
1 μm
A. Bacterium

Membranous
envelope
Capsid
(protein coat)
Nucleic acid
(DNA or RNA)
Spikes
(protein)
0.1 μm
B. Virus

Trypanosoma;
causes sleeping
sickness
10 μm
Plasmodium
(in red blood cell);
causes malaria
Amoeba;
causes amoebic
dysentery
C. Protozoan pathogens

Liver fluke
(Fasciola hepatica)
Tapeworm
(Taenia)
1 cm
Roundworm
(Ascaris)
D. Multicellular parasites

Figure 3–1
Types of pathogenic organisms include bacteria (A), viruses (B), protozoa (C), and helminths, or worms (D).

Some bacteria produce **endospores,** commonly called spores. Endospores are structures formed to cope with harsh environmental conditions. The endospore contains the genetic material of the cell packaged in a tough outer coat that is resistant to desication, acid, extreme temperature, and even radiation. Endospores germinate and form growing cells when conditions are correct. Certain diseases, like tetanus and botulism, can be caused by endospores that contaminate food, water, or wounds.

Bacteria cause illness in humans in a variety of ways. Some bacteria produce toxins that interfere with normal physiology. For example, tetanus is caused by the toxin produced by the bacterium *Clostridium tetani.* The tetanus toxin interferes with the ability of muscle cells to relax, resulting in frozen, rigid muscles characteristic of the disease. Other toxins are enzymes that enable the bacteria to spread through tissues and to obtain nutrients. A particularly potent toxin called **endotoxin** causes life-threatening shock. This toxin is released into tissues when gram-negative cells die. Some signs and symptoms of bacterial infection are not generated by the bacteria themselves but rather by the immune response to the infection. Common characteristics of certain bacterial infections include swelling, redness, pain, fever, and pus.

endospores
(en′-dō-spōrz)

endotoxin
(ĕn″-dō-tŏk′-sĭn)

TABLE 3–1. COMMON BACTERIAL PATHOGENS AND ASSOCIATED DISEASES

BACTERIAL PATHOGENS	DISEASE(S)
Gram-positive cocci	
Staphylococcus aureus	Skin infections, food poisoning
Streptococcus pyogenes	Pharyngitis (strep throat)
Streptococcus pneumoniae	Lobar pneumonia
Gram-positive bacilli	
Clostridium tetani	Tetanus
Clostridium botulinum	Botulism
Bacillus anthracis	Anthrax
Gram-negative cocci	
Neisseria gonorrhoeae	Gonorrhea
Gram-negative bacilli	
Salmonella typhimurium	Salmonellosis
Legionella pneumophila	Legionellosis (Legionnaire's disease)
Pseudomonas aeurginosa	Urinary tract infections, burn infections
Spirilla	
Campylobacter jejuni	Acute enteritis, diarrhea
Helicobacter pylori	Gastritis, peptic ulcer
Spirochetes	
Treponema pallidum	Syphilis
Borrelia burgdorferi	Lyme disease
Vibrios	
Vibrio cholerae	Cholera
Chlamydias and rickettsias	
Chlamydia trachomatis	Trachoma, sexually transmitted chlamydia
Rickettsia prowazekii	Typhus
Rickettsia rickettsii	Rocky Mountain Spotted Fever

Viruses

capsid
(kăp′-sĭd)

Viruses are infectious particles made of a core of genetic material (either RNA or DNA) wrapped in a protein coat **(capsid).** Some viruses also have a lipid membrane surrounding their capsid. Viruses are not considered living organisms because they do not independently grow, metabolize, or reproduce. Viruses must carry out their life processes by entering cells and directing the cells' energy, materials, and organelles for these purposes.

Certain viruses infect and grow in only certain types of human cells. Some viruses, like cold viruses, target only cells of the respiratory epithelium. Others, like herpes viruses, reproduce in nervous tissue. Signs and symptoms of infection result from the way these viruses reproduce in cells or from the way the immune system responds to

lyse
(līz)

latent infection
(lā′-tĕnt
ĭn-fĕk′-shun)

viral infection. Some viruses cause the cells they infect to **lyse,** or rupture. This is the case when HIV infects and reproduces within T cells. The resultant T-cell deficiency leads to the immunodeficiency in AIDS. Other viruses sustain a **latent infection,** whereby the viruses insert themselves in cells and do not reproduce. At this time no symptoms may be present. Later, something triggers the viruses to become active, and symptoms of the disease manifest themselves. This pattern is seen in the waxing and waning of herpes infections. Other viruses cause abnormal cell growth because the viral genetic material interferes with the cell's growth-control genes. The result may be cancer. Human papillomavirus infection is linked to cervical cancer. Table 3–2 lists examples of viruses and their associated diseases.

Protozoa

Protozoa are single-celled eukaryotic microorganisms. They are much larger than bacteria and have complex internal structures, including a nucleus and membranous organelles. Protozoa are found in nearly every habitat and most do not cause disease. Protozoa are classified as **amoeboids, flagellates, ciliates,** and **sporozoans.**

    Amoeboids move by means of cell membrane extensions called pseudopodia. These extensions may be familiar in another context—in human phagocytic leukocytes, which use pseudopodia to crawl about and ingest particles. An amoeba of great health concern is *Entamoeba histolytica,* the cause of amoebic dysentery. The flagellates swim by using one or more whiplike appendages called flagella. Pathogens in this group include *Trypanosoma,* the cause of African sleeping sickness, and *Giardia,* the cause of giardiasis, an intestinal infection. Ciliates move by means of numerous short hairlike projections called cilia. There are few pathogens among the ciliates. Sporozoans are not mobile. *Plasmodium* is the most notorious among them because it causes malaria. This diverse group of microorganisms causes disease in a variety of ways. Protozoa may invade and destroy certain tissues, or they may provoke damaging inflammatory responses.

amoeboids
(ă-mē′-boydz)

flagellates
(flăj′-ĕ-lāts)

ciliates
(sĭl″-ē-āts)

sporozoans
(spor″-ō-zō″-ăns)

Fungi

Fungi are single-celled or multicelled organisms. Fungal cell walls contain a special polysaccharide called chitin. Fungi have filaments called **mycelia** specialized for absorption of nutrients. They also have reproductive structures bearing **spores,** which are known allergens. Healthy human tissue is relatively resistant to fungal infections but may be susceptible under certain circumstances. Fungi can more easily infect damaged tissue than intact healthy tissue. Also, immunocompromised hosts may be unable to resist fungal infections. Fungi cause disease by producing toxins, interfering with normal organ structure or function, or by inducing inflammation or allergy. Some common fungal diseases include candidiasis, an infection of skin or mucous membranes caused by the yeast *Candida.* Histoplasmosis is a respiratory infection caused by *Histoplasma,*

mycelia
(mī-sē′-lē-ă)

spores
(spōrz)

TABLE 3–2. VIRAL PATHOGENS AND THEIR DISEASES	
VIRUSES	**DISEASES**
DNA viruses	
Herpesviruses	
Herpes simplex 1	Cold sores and fever blisters
Herpes simplex 2	Genital herpes
Varicella-Zoster	Chicken pox and shingles
Hepatitis B	Hepatitis ("serum hepatitis")
Epstein-Barr	Infectious mononucleosis
RNA viruses	
Influenza A, B, C	Influenza ("flu")
Hepatitis A, C, D, E, G	Infectious hepatitis
Rhinovirus	Common cold
Human Immunodeficiency Virus	HIV infection/AIDS

which is inhaled in dust from soil contaminated with bird droppings. *Microsporum* and *Trichophyton* cause a variety of ringworm infections of the skin, hair, and nails.

Helminths

The wormlike animals, which include roundworms and flatworms, are called helminths. Like other animals, helminths are complex multicellular motile organisms. They often have well-developed reproductive systems capable of producing large numbers of off-spring. Many helminths have also evolved complex life cycles and strategies for infecting new hosts. Infections with these organisms are often called **infestations.**

Roundworms are relatively round in cross-section. They include filarial (thread-like) worms that infect the lymphatic system, like *Wucheria,* the cause of elephantiasis. The large human roundworm *Ascaris* infects the intestines whereas the pinworm *Enterobius* infects the large intestine.

Flatworms, as the name suggests, have flattened bodies. *Schistosoma,* a type of helminth called a fluke, causes schistosomiasis, an infection of blood vessels. This infection is found in Southeast Asia, Africa, and parts of South America. Tapeworms like *Taenia* infect the intestines.

In some cases, transmission of helminths is relatively straightforward: *Ascaris* eggs can be swallowed in feces-contaminated food or water. In other cases, many pieces of a complex life cycle need to be in place to sustain infections. For example, although the juvenile *Schistosoma* can infect a person simply by swimming to a human foot and bur-rowing through the skin, the complete life cycle of *Schistosoma* depends on a particular snail as an intermediate host for development of other immature stages of the worm. The water in which the snails grow needs to be still and needs also to be contaminated with infested human urine or feces. Certain helminths are transmitted by arthropod vectors, which will be discussed later in this chapter.

Helminths cause disease by using the host's nutrients, as pinworms and tapeworms do when they infest the intestines. Others feed on blood, causing anemia. *Ascaris* can block or perforate the intestines when infestations become large, or the eggs or worms themselves can induce severe inflammatory responses.

Arthropod Vectors

Animals with jointed legs and a hard exoskeleton are called arthropods. These include ticks, mites, lice, flies, mosquitoes, and fleas. Some arthropods act as disease **vectors.** That is, the animals transmit pathogenic microorganisms to humans. An arthropod may transmit a pathogen when biting and feeding on human blood. The *Anopheles* mosquito transmits *Plasmodium* when it feeds on an infected human and carries the malaria parasite to another human. Some arthropods simply carry pathogens on their bodies. The housefly *Musca* can carry bacteria on its feet. In many cases, the arthropod is an essential part of the pathogen's life cycle. Humans will not get infected with the pathogen unless the appropriate arthropod vector is present. Therefore, it is very important to identify these arthropods and to understand their lives if the diseases they carry are to be understood.

Other animals are also important for infectious diseases. Some animals act as **reservoirs** of infection, acting as sources of the pathogen and potential sources of disease. Certain hoofed animals and domestic cattle are reservoirs for African sleeping sickness. Deer and mice can carry the spirochete and harbor the tick that transmits Lyme disease. Still other animals are the only means by which a disease is transmitted. Rabies viruses are transmitted by the bite of infected raccoons, foxes, bats, and domestic dogs.

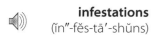

infestations
(ĭn″-fĕs-tā′-shŭns)

roundworms
(rownd′-wĕrms)

flatworms
(flăt′-wĕrms)

vectors
(vĕk′-tors)

reservoirs
(rēz′-ĕr-vwors)

➤ INFECTION PREVENTION AND CONTROL

Effective prevention and control of infectious diseases requires knowledge of the nature of the pathogens and their means of transmission.

Transmission and Epidemiology

Epidemiology is the study of the transmission, occurrence, distribution, and control of disease. Infectious diseases can be transmitted directly from an infected human to a susceptible human. This route is called **horizontal transmission.** Influenza, gonorrhea, measles, and many other diseases described elsewhere in this book are transmitted this way. Other infectious diseases are transmitted from one generation to the next, as when syphilis, HIV/AIDS, or ophthalmia neonatorum are transmitted to newborns from infected mothers. This route is called **vertical transmission.**

Humans transmit pathogens in respiratory droplets, blood, semen, feces, urine, and through direct physical contact. Measles, pneumonia, tuberculosis, and influenza are well-known diseases transmitted in respiratory droplets generated by coughing and sneezing. HIV and hepatitis B and C are viruses transmitted in blood and blood products. Sexually transmitted diseases like gonorrhea, chlamydia, and HIV are transmitted in semen and vaginal secretions. Food poisoning and dysentery are transmitted by consumption of feces-contaminated food and water.

In some cases, humans are not involved in direct transmission of a disease. For example, an effective campaign to control malaria would require control of its mosquito vector.

Study of the distribution and frequency of diseases can help predict and prevent disease. The number of new cases of a disease in a population is its **incidence.** The incidence of some diseases follows a pattern, as when influenza incidence increases in winter and subsides in summer, or when Lyme disease increases in summer and subsides in winter. The number of existing cases of the disease is known as its **prevalence,** and this information can tell how significant the disease is to a certain population. When a disease always occurs at low levels in a population, it is said to be **endemic.** If a disease occurs in unusually large numbers over a specific area, it is said to be **epidemic.** Influenza occurs as epidemics. When an epidemic has spread to include several large areas worldwide, it is said to be **pandemic.** AIDS is considered to be pandemic. When a disease suddenly occurs in unexpected numbers in a limited area and then subsides, this is described as an **outbreak.**

Certain diseases are under constant surveillance in the United States. Such diseases are called **reportable diseases.** Physicians are required to report the occurrence of these diseases to the Centers for Disease Control and Prevention. This ensures tracking and identification of disease occurrence and patterns. Chlamydia infections were not reportable before 1998. After these infections became reportable, it was discovered that the number of chlamydial infections surpassed gonorrhea.

Control of infectious diseases can be achieved by preventing transmission and by treating infected persons. **Isolation** of infected persons in hospitals or self-imposed isolation, such as when a person with influenza remains home in bed, can be effective. **Quarantine** is the separation of persons who may or may not be infected from healthy people until the period of infectious risk is passed. **Disinfection** of potentially infectious materials is necessary to prevent transmission. Medical and dental implements need disinfection to remove human pathogens after use. **Standard precautions** are required of medical personnel when handling patients or bodily fluids. These precautions are used

horizontal transmission
(hŏr″-ă-zŏn′-tăl trăns-mĭsh-ŭn)

vertical transmission
(vĕr′-tĭ-kăl trăns-mĭsh′-ŭn)

incidence
(ĭn′-sĭ-dĕns)

prevalence
(prĕv′-ă-lĕns)

endemic
(ĕn-dĕm′-ĭk)

epidemic
(ĕp″-ĭ-dĕm′-ĭk)

pandemic
(păn-dĕm′-ĭk)

outbreak
(owt′-brāk)

reportable diseases
(rē-pōrt′-ă-b′l dĭ-zēz′-ēz)

isolation
(ī-sō-lā′-shŭn)

quarantine
(kwor′-ăn-tēn″)

disinfection
(dĭs″-ĭn-fĕk′-shŭn)

standard precautions
(stăn′-dārd prĭ-kaw′-shŭns)

in all situations, whether a patient is infected or not, and include the use of gloves, correct disposal of bodily fluids, needles, and other waste. Sanitation techniques that remove infectious sewage from drinking and bathing water and prevent sewage from contaminating food can dramatically reduce the incidence of cholera and dysentery. The treatment of infected persons is a critical component of prevention.

Treatment of Infectious Disease

The effective treatment of a particular infectious disease depends on the type of pathogen. Bacterial infections can be treated with a variety of **antibiotics.** The target of some antibiotics is the unique bacterial cell wall. Penicillin and related drugs act on the cell wall, and they are especially useful in controlling gram-positive bacteria. Other antibiotics target the protein synthesis machinery of the cell. This is effective because the ribosomes and enzymes involved in bacterial protein synthesis are sufficiently different from those in human cells. Other antibiotics interfere with bacterial metabolism or with DNA and RNA synthesis. Antibiotic resistance plays an important role in the increased incidence of bacterial infections.

Correct use of antibiotics can prevent the development of **antibiotic resistance.** Resistance arises when bacteria adapt to antibiotics and the adaptation becomes common in the bacterial population, soon rendering the antibiotics ineffective. An antibiotic should be used only for bacterial infections. A number of infections, like influenza and the common cold, are viral and are not treatable with antibiotics. Some viral ailments closely mimic bacterial infections. For example, it turns out that group A streptococci cause only 15% of pharyngitis cases, so only a small proportion of sore throats are really strep throat. Most sore throats are really caused by viral infections, some of which closely mimic strep throat because the symptoms include swelling and exudate. If antibiotics are used for many of these viral infections, bacterial populations will more likely evolve resistance to those antibiotics. The Centers for Disease Control and Prevention has asked physicians to perform the rapid strep antigen test to confirm the presence of group A streptococci before prescribing antibiotics. The appropriate antibiotic should be prescribed. Guidelines are shared and updated for physicians so that the most effective types and dosages are used for certain infections. Patients need to follow through on the prescription. Patients should use the antibiotics for the entire time prescribed, should not end treatment early, and should not save antibiotics.

Viruses do not have the cell walls of bacteria nor do they have metabolic or protein synthesis machinery. Viruses are not susceptible to antibiotics. Viruses need human cells to reproduce and decode their genetic material. Some antiviral drugs interfere with this process by acting as nucleic acid analogues, substances that mimic the correct DNA or RNA bases. These analogues are used to manufacture the viral genetic material but, in fact, do not function as the normal DNA or RNA bases. Viruses are not replicated correctly and are eventually reduced in number or eliminated. Other antiviral drugs interfere with the assembly of new virus particles inside cells or interfere with the attachment of viruses to host cells and, thus, prevent infection before disease begins.

Fungi present a special problem, because their cells are so similar to human cells. Antifungal drugs are targeted against fungal walls and membranes but can affect human cells as well, leading to serious toxic side effects.

Protozoa are treated with drugs that interfere with protein synthesis and metabolism. Certain antibiotics may be used to treat protozoal infections.

Helminths are susceptible to drugs that paralyze their muscles or interfere with their carbohydrate metabolism.

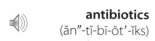

antibiotics
(ăn″-tĭ-bī-ŏt′-ĭks)

antibiotic resistance
(ăn″-tĭ-bī-ŏt′-ĭk rĭ-zĭs′-tăns)

TABLE 3–3. UNIVERSALLY RECOMMENDED VACCINATIONS

POPULATION	VACCINES
All young children	Measles, mumps, and rubella Diphtheria-tetanus toxoid and pertussis Poliomyelitis *Haemophilus influenzae* type B Hepatitis B Varicella
Previously unvaccinated or partially vaccinated adolescents	Hepatitis B Varicella Measles, mumps, and rubella Tetanus-diphtheria toxoid
All adults	Tetanus-diphtheria toxoid
All adults aged >65 years	Influenza Pneumococcal

Although effective treatments have been discovered and used for many important infections, certain problems remain. One complication is that resistant microorganisms can evolve, rendering existing treatments useless. Another difficulty is that some treatments are accompanied by unacceptable toxic side effects. For these reasons, preventive measures are the best choice for long-term control of certain diseases.

Vaccination

Vaccination is the presentation of antigens from a microorganism to provoke an immune response and, thus, to prevent future infection by that microorganism. Natural immunity occurs when a person is infected by or exposed to a microorganism. The individual's immune system responds and produces memory cells that are primed to protect the person from future encounters with that microorganism. The initial infection can cause a great deal of discomfort and major complications, including death. Preventive vaccination is recommended and practiced. Vaccines may contain dead bacteria, extracted antigens, inactivated toxins, virus particles, or genetically engineered proteins.

Because they are designed to prevent disease, vaccines have been used to help eliminate certain diseases. Smallpox has been eliminated by thorough vaccination of susceptible populations. Polio may be the next major infectious disease to be eliminated through vaccination. Administration of a series of vaccines in infancy and childhood has controlled many serious childhood diseases. Diphtheria, whooping cough, measles, and other contagious and potentially serious infections are now much less common. Vaccines can protect healthcare workers from hepatitis B and other pathogens. Table 3–3 describes the recommendations of the Centers for Disease Control and Prevention for vaccinations for various populations.

➤ RE-EMERGING INFECTIOUS DISEASES

Infections still account for a significant amount of morbidity and mortality in the United States. Recent data from the Centers for Disease Control and Prevention show that infectious disease mortality has increased significantly between 1980 and 1996 from about 42/100,000 to about 66/100,000. Moreover, certain infections that were once considered under control have re-emerged as important health threats.

The factors behind the re-emergence of tuberculosis are described in Chapter 13. One of the factors is increased antibiotic resistance of the tuberculosis pathogen. Antibiotic resistance plays an important role in the increased incidence of other bacterial infections. In addition to antibiotic resistance, changes in climate, urbanization, increased crowding, fast world travel, and disruption of social and governmental structure are responsible for the emergence of new pathology or re-emergence of old infectious diseases.

Climate changes can alter the breeding ranges of arthropod vectors like mosquitoes and flies. Malaria, Dengue fever, yellow fever—all mosquito-borne infections—show sensitivity to climate. Even in areas where malaria is endemic, it occurs with less frequency in higher and cooler elevations. In 1987, when the temperature averaged 1° higher than the previous year in Rwanda, the incidence of malaria increased 337% because higher, cooler, drier areas became favorable for the malarial mosquitoes.

After increased urbanization brought humans and deer in close proximity, Lyme disease became prominent in northeastern United States in recent years. Much of that area was cleared for farms, driving out deer and their predators. Forest and deer have reclaimed the farmland, but the predators have not returned. As urban centers grow, the human and deer populations inevitably come in contact with more frequency, giving the Lyme disease ticks ample opportunity to attach to humans and their pets.

Recently, the population of the world has reached six billion people. Most of the growth has occurred and will continue to occur in the most densely populated and poorest cities. In the next few years, the World Health Organization projects that, of the top 15 or so most populous cities, only Tokyo will be in a so-called industrialized nation. Crowding, malnutrition, and lack of medical resources will become critical. Infectious diseases thrive on these conditions.

Scientists need to continue basic research into the cause, transmission, prevention, and treatment of infectious diseases for future generations.

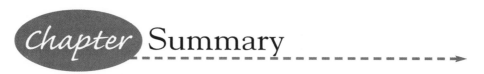

Chapter Summary

Infectious diseases remain a significant cause of morbidity and mortality in the United States and throughout the world. The diseases are caused by a variety of pathogenic microorganisms, viruses, helminths, and arthropod vectors. The characteristics of each are important to understand to implement effective prevention and treatment. As human populations grow, pathogens will evolve, and infectious diseases likely will remain a threat to human life.

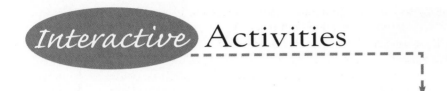

Interactive Activities

CASE FOR CRITICAL THINKING

Based upon what you learned about transmission and control of infectious diseases, compare how one would approach the control of influenza with the control of malaria. Explain which methods would be useful for each disease.

MULTIMEDIA EXTENSION ACTIVITIES

www.prenhall.com/mulvihill
Use the above address to access the free, interactive companion Website created for this textbook. Included in the features of this site are chapter specific activities, internet links, and an audio-glossary.

Audio Glossary
Use the CD-ROM disk enclosed with your textbook to hear the pronunciation of the key terms in this chapter.

Quick Self Study

MULTIPLE CHOICE

1. A strain of cholera has appeared in unusual amounts in south Asia, South America, and even in North America. The occurrence of this cholera strain can be described as _____.
   a. endemic
   b. pandemic
   c. epidemic
   d. outbreak

2. Viruses are different from bacteria in that viruses _____.
   a. can not grow on their own
   b. have cell membranes
   c. have genetic material
   d. are single-celled organisms

3. Malaria is caused by _____.
   a. a mosquito
   b. *Plasmodium*
   c. *Trypanosoma*
   d. varicella virus

TRUE/FALSE

_____ 1. Most microorganisms cause disease.

_____ 2. Viruses are not considered living organisms because they do not independently grow, metabolize, or reproduce.

_____ 3. When an infectious disease is transmitted directly from an infected human to a susceptible human, it is known as a horizontal transmission.

_____ 4. One of the factors behind the re-emergence of tuberculosis is increased antibiotic resistance of the tuberculosis pathogen.

FILL-INS

1. Infectious diseases are those diseases caused by _____ _____.

2. _____ is the presentation of antigens from a microorganism to provoke an immune response and, thus, prevent future infection by that microorganism.

3. Animals with jointed legs and a hard exoskeleton are called _____.

4. _____ is the study of the transmission, occurrence, distribution, and control of disease.

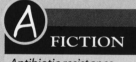

FICTION

Antibiotic resistance and other factors are responsible for the re-emergence of many infectious diseases.

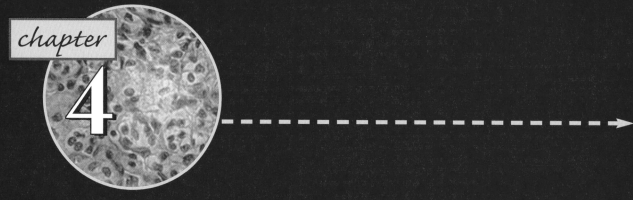

chapter

4

Neoplasms

The discovery of a lump or a mass can be a frightening experience as one's first thought often is the possibility of cancer. The swelling or tumor may indicate a serious condition, or it may be relatively harmless.

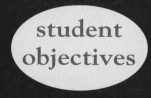

student
objectives

After studying this chapter, students should be able to
➤ Identify risk factors in cancer
➤ List the warning signs of cancer
➤ Compare and contrast benign and malignant tumors
➤ Discuss diagnosis and treatment options for cancer
➤ Discuss prevention and cancer

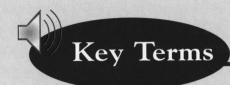

Key Terms

Adenocarcinomas

Adenoma

Anaplasia

Angioma

Anorexia

Benign

Biopsied

Cachexia

Carcinogenesis

Carcinogens

Carcinoma

Cyst

Dysphagia

Epidermoid carcinomas

Exfoliative cytology

Human Papillomavirus (HPV)

Initiation

Leiomyomas

Leukopenia

Lipoma

Malignant

Malignant melanoma

Metastasis

Metastasize

Mutagens

Myoma

Neoplasm

Nevus

Oncogene

Pap

Papilloma

Progression

Promotion

Sarcoma

Teratoma

Tumor

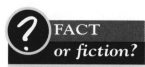

FACT
or fiction?

The use of tanning
booths decreases your
risk of skin cancer.

*Read this chapter to find the
answer.*

 neoplasm
(nē′-ō-plăsm)

 tumor
(tū′-mŏr)

 malignant
(mă-lĭg′-nănt)

 benign
(bĕ-nīn′)

➤ INTRODUCTION TO CANCER

Cancer is the second leading cause of death in the United States. Uncontrolled cell division is the hallmark feature of cancer. A **neoplasm** or **tumor** is a mass of new cells that grows in a haphazard fashion with no control and no useful function. As the tumor continues to grow, normal cells are destroyed. As the tumor grows, it can protrude into normally open space and obstruct that space; it can also exert pressure and cause pain.

Neoplasms are divided into two classes: **malignant** and **benign.** A malignant neoplasm tends to spread and possibly causes death whereas a benign neoplasm is noncancerous. There is a great difference in the growth rate of various tumors. At times, there may be a period of remission when the progress of the growth seems to be temporarily halted. Remission can occur spontaneously or may follow a type of therapy.

Disease by the Numbers   x + ÷

EPIDEMIOLOGY

In the year 2000, about 552,200 Americans will die of cancer, more than 1,500 people each day. Cancer is the second leading cause of death in the U.S. In the U.S. one in four deaths is from cancer. The following list shows the top ten cancers in the United States.

Lung	Non-Hodgkin's lymphoma
Colon and rectum	Leukemia
Female breast	Ovarian
Prostate	Brain
Pancreatic	Stomach

Causes of Cancer

What are some of the possible causes of cancer? Environmental causes probably account for well over half of all cancer cases. Various chemicals (benzene, asbestos, vinyl chloride, arsenic) show definite evidence of human carcinogenicity. Other chemicals (chloroforms, DDT, formaldehyde, PCBs) are probable human **carcinogens,** based on evidence from animal experiments. Exposure to ultraviolet light is the major risk factor in skin cancer. Exposure to ionizing radiation (x-rays, radon, atomic bombs) can increase the risk of leukemia and thyroid cancer.

About one-third of all cases of cancer in the United States are directly attributable to cigarette smoking. The price of smoking a pack of cigarettes is $3\frac{1}{2}$ hours of one's life. Cigarette smoking introduces powerful **mutagens** to the lungs. These mutagens cause considerable damage to genes in the lung cells. When these genes are damaged, lung cancer results.

Some tumors seem to result from viral infection. Viruses can be isolated from certain tumors, and these viruses cause virus-containing tumors to develop in other individuals. About 15% of human cancers are associated with viruses. Viruses invade cells and may alter the genetic material of the cell.

Genetics may also play a role in cancer. Any gene having the potential to induce a cancerous transformation is called an **oncogene.** Oncogenes have been implicated in cancers including breast, lung, leukemia, and colon cancer.

Nutrition may be a risk factor in cancer. About one-third of cancer deaths in the United States every year are due to dietary factors. The types of food, preparation, por-

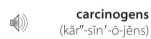 **carcinogens**
(kăr″-sĭn′-ō-jĕns)

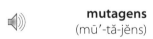 **mutagens**
(mū′-tă-jĕns)

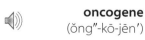 **oncogene**
(ŏng″-kō-jēn′)

on the Practical Side

Sun Screens and Tanning Spas

A deeply tanned body is considered by many to be beautiful, but the sunlight that produced the tan has already done its damage. Prolonged exposure to the ultraviolet (UV) light rays of the sun causes premature aging of the skin, wrinkles, liver spots, and a leathery texture. Most importantly, it causes premalignant lesions, warty growths called keratoses, and skin cancer. Fair-skinned individuals are the most susceptible, but no one is exempt from the danger. Sunscreens, lotions with an SPF (sun protection factor) of at least 15, should be used when exposure to the sun is necessary.

Popular tanning spas that provide a year-round tan also provide a great risk for developing skin cancer. Some people think that tanning indoors is safer than tanning outdoors. The beds in tanning salons use unfiltered, long UV rays, the main cause of photoaging (wrinkling) of the skin. The extra exposure to UV light in tanning booths may seriously increase the risk of getting skin cancer.

tion size, variety, and caloric balance can play a role. Possible causes of cancer are summarized in Figure 4–1.

Hormones are related to certain forms of cancer. At times, hormones may stimulate the growth of the cancer. In other cancers, hormones are used for treatment. A noncancerous mole never becomes cancerous before puberty, the time when the sex hormone level increases. Cancer of the prostate gland in stimulated by the male hormone testosterone,

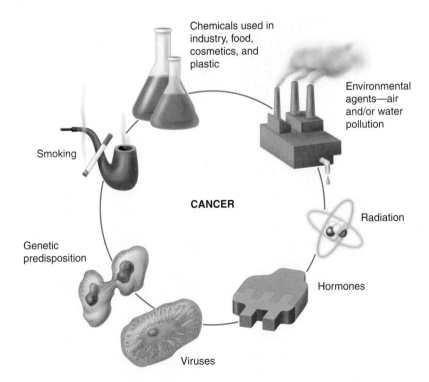

Figure 4–1
Possible causes of cancer.

but its growth is inhibited by estrogen therapy. The ovaries are sometimes removed after breast cancer surgery to prevent estrogen stimulation of other tumors. Many cancers are more common in either men or women, which seems to indicate a hormonal relationship.

Development of Cancer

Because of extensive research, cancer is now a highly curable chronic disease and one that is potentially preventable. Development of cancer (**carcinogenesis**) requires a long period of time, often decades, from the initial exposure to the carcinogen, the cause of the cancer, to the malignancy. In other words, there is a latent period.

Cancer development includes three stages, **initiation, promotion,** and **progression.** Initiation is the stage in which there is a genetic change in a cell, an altering of the DNA by some agent, chemical, radiation, or an oncogenic virus, a virus capable of causing cancer. During the promotion stage, these altered cells proliferate and resemble benign neoplasms, which can either regress to normal-appearing tissue or evolve into cancer. Sometimes the individual's own immune system can reverse carcinogenesis. Removing or avoiding the causative agent at this stage can prevent the development of cancer. The third stage, progression, includes a change from a precancerous to a malignant lesion, at which time growth rate increases and the malignancy can invade and metastasize. These devastating aspects of cancer occur late in the process of carcinogenesis. Figure 4–2 illustrates the steps in carcinogenesis.

Signs and Symptoms of Cancer

Signs and symptoms of cancer vary with the site of the tumor. Pain is usually not an early symptom of cancer. It is only when the mass has grown, causing an obstruction or putting pressure on nerve endings, that pain is experienced. Infection frequently accompanies cancer and may cause pain.

There are certain warning signs that a cancerous tumor might be present. Abnormal bleeding or discharge from a natural body opening such as the rectum or vagina may be an indication of a tumor. Blood in the urine, sputum, or vomitus should be investigated. This bleeding may not be caused by cancer at all, but it is a precautionary measure to have it checked.

A thickening or lump, particularly in the breast, indicates a tumor or a cyst. A **cyst** is a sac or capsule containing fluid and is usually harmless. The tumor might well be benign, but the possibility of a malignancy exists, and it should be examined by a physi-

carcinogenesis
(kăr″-sĭ-nō-jĕn′-ĕ-sĭs)

initiation
(ĭn-ĭsh″-ī-ā′-shŭn)

promotion
(prō-mō′-shŭn)

progression
(prō-grĕsh′-ŭn)

cyst
(sĭst)

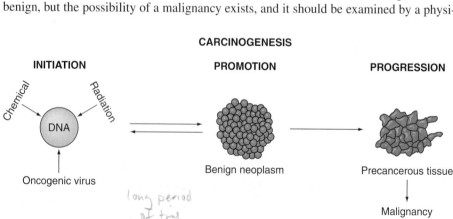

Figure 4–2
Development of cancer.

The American Cancer Society lists several signs of cancer, the first letter of each word spelling the acronym, **CAUTION.**

Change in bowel or bladder habits
A sore that does not heal
Unusual bleeding or discharge
Thickening or lump in breast or elsewhere
Indigestion or difficulty in swallowing
Obvious change in wart or mole
Nagging cough or hoarseness

Figure 4–3
Warning signs of cancer.

cian. The American Cancer Society urges women to perform monthly self-examinations of each breast and to have mammography on a regular basis. Men should perform a testicular self-examination every month and have their prostate gland checked by a physician at regular check-ups.

Another sign of a possible cancer is a persistent cough or hoarseness. A growth in the respiratory tract, or one pressing on it, acts as an irritant in stimulating the cough reflex.

A change in bowel activity, intermittent constipation and diarrhea, may indicate an obstruction in the colon. Difficulties in urination such as urgency, burning sensations, and the inability to start the stream of urine may signal a tumor in the urinary system. In men, it may signal a tumor of the prostate gland.

Normally the body has excellent healing ability. If a sore or an ulceration fails to heal after a period of time, there is some reason for it, and the lesion should be examined. A mole may change color, darken, enlarge, or become itchy. This can signal a transition from a benign growth to one that is malignant.

A person experiencing difficulty in swallowing (**dysphagia**) or loss of appetite (**anorexia**) may have some kind of obstruction in the upper gastrointestinal tract. These symptoms, particularly if accompanied by rapid weight loss, are significant.

A severe anemia may indicate internal bleeding from a malignant lesion or malfunctioning of the bone marrow caused by replacement of normal tissue by cancerous cells. Chemotherapy and/or radiation also affect the blood-clotting mechanism. Excessive production of a hormone can signal a tumor, benign or malignant, of an endocrine gland. Figure 4–3 lists warning signs that may indicate a malignancy. The first letter of each word spells the acronym, CAUTION.

➤ TYPES OF CANCER

There are two major types of cancer, carcinoma and sarcoma; the suffix *oma* means a tumor. **Carcinoma** is the more common form, affecting epithelial tissues, skin, and mucous membranes lining body cavities. Tumors of the skin are called **epidermoid carcinomas.** Carcinoma is also the malignancy of glandular tissue such as the breast, liver, and pancreas. Cancerous glandular tumors are known as **adenocarcinomas;** the prefix *adeno* always refers to a gland. Although these tumors develop in either epithelial or

dysphagia
(dĭs-fā′-jĭ-ă)

anorexia
(ăn″-ō-rĕk′-sē-ă)

carcinoma
(kăr″-sĭ-nō′-mă)

epidermoid carcinomas
(ĕp″-ĭ-dĕr′-moyd kăr″-sĭ-nō′-măs)

adenocarcinomas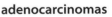
(ăd″-ĕ-nō-kăr″-sĭn-ō′-măs)

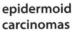

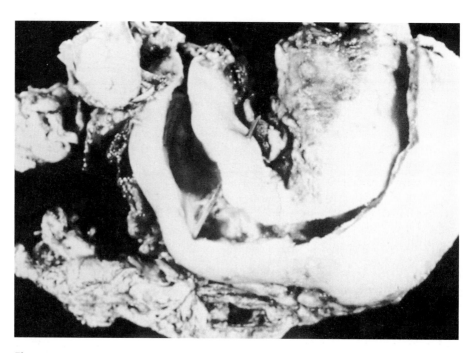

Figure 4–4
Adenocarcinoma of the stomach. White area is the greatly thickened stomach wall. (*Courtesy of Dr. David R. Duffell.*)

glandular tissue, they invade deeper and surround tissues. Cancer of the mouth, lung, and stomach are examples of carcinoma. Figure 4–4 shows an adenocarcinoma of the stomach.

sarcoma
(săr-kō′-mă)

anaplasia
(ăn″-ă-plā′-zĭ-ă)

Sarcoma is the less common cancer, but it spreads more rapidly and is highly malignant. Connective tissue tumors, such as those of bone, muscle, and cartilage, are sarcomas. Rapidly growing tumors show little differentiation, and this lack of form is referred to as **anaplasia,** the prefix *an* meaning without and *plasia,* meaning form. These rapidly growing, undifferentiated tumors are the most responsive to radiation treatment. Figure 4–5 contrasts carcinoma and sarcoma.

	CARCINOMA	SARCOMA
Affects	Epithelial and glandular tissue	Connective tissue
Examples	Skin, breast, and liver cancer	Cancer of bone, muscle, and cartilage
Incidence	More common	Less common
Growth rate	Slower	Faster
Metastasis	Principally through lymph vessels	Principally through the blood

Figure 4–5
Distinctions between carcinoma and sarcoma.

➤ BENIGN TUMORS

Benign tumors are different from malignant tumors. Benign growths are generally encapsulated with clearly defined edges, which makes their removal from surrounding tissue relatively easy. Benign tumors do not metastasize nor do they recur after surgical removal. Only rarely do these tumors ulcerate and bleed. A benign tumor differentiates somewhat in its development and resembles the structure from which it grew.

This does not mean that benign tumors pose no threat. A tumor on the brain or in the spinal cord, even if it is benign, puts pressure on nerves and seriously affects the functioning of the nervous system. Any tumor can obstruct a passageway such as the trachea, shutting off the air supply, or the esophagus, making it impossible to swallow. A benign tumor of a gland can cause oversecretion of its hormone with very serious effects. If a tumor of the anterior pituitary gland develops before puberty, the increased secretion of growth hormone leads to the development of a giant. An adrenal gland tumor produces an oversecretion of androgens (male sex hormones) and causes masculinization of females.

Types of Benign Tumors

Tumors are classified according to the tissue in which they develop. A common benign tumor is the **lipoma,** a soft, fatty tumor that develops in adipose (fat) tissue. As it grows, it pushes normal tissue aside. Lipomas are commonly found on the neck, back, and buttocks—anyplace where there is fat.

lipoma
(lĭ-pō′-mă)

A **myoma** is a tumor of the muscle; the prefix *myo* refers to muscle. These tumors are rare in voluntary muscle but do develop in smooth or involuntary muscle. Myomas are the tumors of the uterus referred to as *fibroids.* Fibroid tumors are also called **leiomyomas,** specifying a tumor of smooth muscle. Leiomyomas are the tumors most commonly found in women. If the tumors are small they may cause no symptoms, but if they become large they can cause menstrual problems or difficulties, even spontaneous abortion, during a pregnancy.

myoma
(mī-ō′-mă)

leiomyomas
(lī″-ō-mī-ō′-măs)

The typical red birthmark, or "port-wine" stain, is another type of benign tumor. It is an **angioma,** a tumor composed of blood vessels. Lymph vessels can also comprise an angioma, but because lymph is colorless a tumor of this type is colorless. An angioma is one type of benign tumor that is not encapsulated. Advanced laser technology is now being used effectively to gradually erase port-wine stains.

angioma
(ăn″-jĭ-ō′-mă)

The common mole is a benign tumor called a **nevus** and, like the angioma, it is not encapsulated. This tumor of the skin contains a black pigment called *melanin* and is sometimes called a *melanoma.* There is also a cancerous condition known as **malignant melanoma** so the name nevus is better used when the tumor is benign. The nevus is congenital but may not be apparent until later in life; it usually enlarges at puberty. This benign tumor can change to a malignant melanoma. An increase in size and pigmentation, bleeding, or itchiness may indicate this transformation to the malignant type.

nevus
(nē′-vŭs)

malignant melanoma
(mă-lĭg′-nănt mĕl″-ă-nō′-mă)

An epithelial tumor that grows as a projecting mass on the skin, or from an inner mucous membrane, is a **papilloma** or polyp. The common wart is an example of a papilloma. This tumor has a fixed base with a stalk growing from it. A growth of this type in the intestinal tract or uterus can be moved back and forth on the stalk and become irritated.

papilloma
(păp-ĭ-lō′-mă)

A benign tumor of glandular tissue is an **adenoma.** It often develops in the breast, thyroid gland, or in mucous glands of the intestinal tract. The adenoma is an example of a benign tumor that resembles the structure from which it develops. Glands and ducts

adenoma
(ăd″-ĕ-nō′-mă)

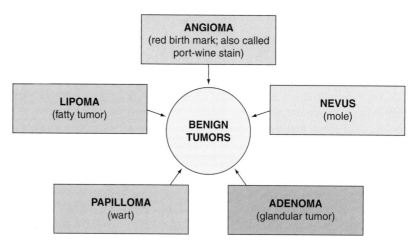

Figure 4–6
Examples of benign tumors.

are found within the tumor, and it may be secretory. Various benign tumors are summarized in Figure 4–6.

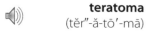
teratoma
(tĕr″-ă-tō′-mă)

A unique benign tumor of the ovary is the **teratoma** or dermoid cyst. Lining the cyst is epidermis, skin with its usual appendages: hair, oil and sweat glands, even teeth. The cyst contains oily material from the sebaceous (oil) glands. The teratoma probably stems from some primitive cell that has the potential of developing in several directions. When these cysts develop on a long pedicle, or stalk, twisting may occur and cause acute abdominal pain; surgical removal is then necessary.

Differences Between Malignant and Benign Tumors

Malignant tumors are usually larger and more irregular in shape than benign tumors. Benign tumors are generally encapsulated, whereas malignant ones are not. A malignancy is invasive and penetrating, destroying underlying tissue; this is not characteristic of benign tumors. Malignant tumors grow at a faster rate than benign tumors and metastasize, setting up new colonies of cells at distant sites. Benign tumors resemble the tissue in which they developed, but malignant tumors lack form.

➤ MALIGNANT TUMORS

The key features of malignant tumors are their uncontrolled growth and tendency to **metastasize,** to spread to other sites.

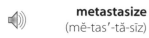
metastasize
(mĕ-tas′-tă-sīz)

The rapid growth of the malignant tumor uses up the body's nutrients, its supply of glucose, and amino acids, which, coupled with the patient's inability to eat, cause severe weight loss. The patient becomes weak and emaciated in appearance; this condition is referred to as **cachexia.**

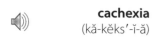
cachexia
(kă-kĕks′-ĭ-ă)

Types of Malignant Tumors

Malignant melanoma is cancer of the melanocytes, the cells that produce skin pigment. It accounts for only a small percentage of skin cancers, but its incidence is increasing rap-

on the Practical Side

Do a skin self-examination once a month. Stand in front of a mirror and carefully examine your skin. Use the ABCD skin rule to help you see differences.

A = Asymmetry, one half of a mole does not match the other half

B = Border irregularity, the edges are irregular

C = Color, not the same all over

D = Diameter, larger than a pencil eraser or is growing larger

idly and it is often deadly. Melanoma can begin wherever there is pigment; most melanomas appear spontaneously, but some develop from pigmented moles. Melanoma usually appears as a spreading brown to black patch that metastasizes rapidly (Figure 4–7). The chance for survival is about 50%, and early detection helps. The American Cancer Society suggests that everyone should do a skin examination and apply the ABCD rule for recognizing melanoma.

Malignant mesothelioma is fairly rare. This disease is linked to asbestos workers, miners, and ship builders. The main cause of this cancer is contact with asbestos. This type of cancer begins in the tissue that surrounds different organs inside the body. This tissue, called mesothelium, protects organs by making a special fluid that allows the organs to move. Most malignant mesotheliomonas start in the chest cavity or abdomen. It is a serious disease and it is often advanced before symptoms appear, so the prognosis is not as good as it is for cancers that are detected earlier.

Metastasis

Unfortunately, when a malignant tumor develops in an organ such as the breast or prostate gland, it tends to spread to other parts of the body. This spread of the cancer to distant sites is known as **metastasis.**

metastasis
(mĕ-tas′-tă-sĭs)

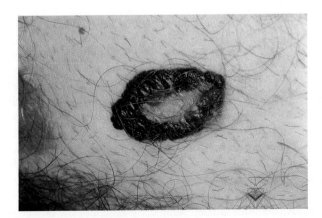

Figure 4–7
Melanoma. (*Courtesy of Jason L. Smith, MD.*)

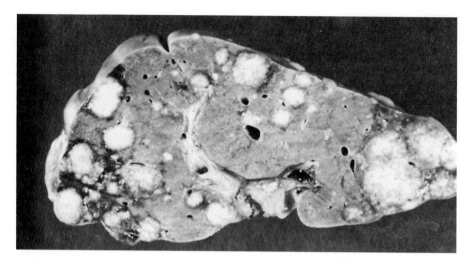

Figure 4–8
Malignant tumors of the liver that have metastasized from other sites (*Courtesy of Dr. David R. Duffell.*)

Carcinoma spreads principally through the lymph vessels, affecting the lymph nodes. This is the reason for removal of the axillary lymph nodes in a radical mastectomy (removal of the breast). Regional lymph nodes are removed in surgical operations for malignant tumors of the colon. Carcinoma can also spread through the bloodstream. Malignant tumors of the liver that have developed through metastases are seen in Figure 4–8.

The metastasis of sarcoma is generally through the blood vessels. Clusters of cancer cells can break off from the primary sites and travel as emboli to the liver, lungs, brain, or other organs. Frequently, it is a secondary site of cancer that is discovered first.

➤ DIAGNOSIS AND TREATMENT

Diagnosis of Cancer

X-ray techniques, particularly those using contrast dyes, can show the site of a mass or tumor. The tumor can only be diagnosed as malignant through microscopic examination of the cells and tissue. All tumors removed surgically must be sent to a pathology department for this study. When a suspected tumor is **biopsied,** a small sample is removed and examined microscopically for abnormalities. A technique known as the *frozen section* enables the pathologist to determine immediately whether the sample is malignant. This is extremely helpful during surgery. A sample of the tissue is sent to the laboratory, the surgeon waits for the result, and then determines the extent of the surgery required based on the report. Further examination of the tissue generally follows.

Another means of obtaining cells for microscopic examination is through scrapings, washings, and secretions from suspected areas. This is called **exfoliative cytology.** It takes advantage of the fact that cancer cells in the early stages tend to be cast off or shed. This technique is helpful in diagnosing early cancer of the bronchus and uterus. It is the principle of the Pap smear, which was named for its originator, Dr. George N. Papanicolaou. Fine-needle aspiration is also used to suction cells from a tumor for microscopic examination.

biopsied
(bī'-ŏp-sēd)

exfoliative cytology
(ĕks-fō'-le-ă-tĭv sī-tŏl'-ō-jē)

GRADE	APPEARANCE	SURVIVAL RATE
TABLE 4–1. TUMOR GRADES		
1	Tumor cells differentiated and closely resemble parent tissue	High
2 & 3	Tumor cells moderately or poorly differentiated	Moderate
4	Tumor cells so undifferentiated that tissue origin cannot be readily recognized	Low

There are different stages of cancer development. The preinvasive stage means that the tumor has not yet penetrated into underlying tissues. If cancer of the cervix can be determined at this stage through the Pap smear, surgical removal offers good prognosis.

Once the cancer has become invasive its total removal is very difficult. The edges of the malignant tumor are poorly defined and, if it is not entirely removed, the cancer will recur. If the tumor has metastasized, surgery is of little benefit.

Pathologists grade tumors by the microscopic appearance of the suspected cells. Grading is helpful in determining proper treatment. Table 4–1 shows how tumors are graded.

Staging neoplasms is a means of estimating how much the tumor has spread. A system has been developed by which tumors are staged according to their size and extent, number of lymph nodes involved, and metastases of the primary tumor.

Treatment of Cancer

Surgery and radiation therapy are very effective in the early stages of breast and uterine cancer and other cancers that are readily accessible. Fast-growing, undifferentiated tumors respond best to radiation therapy; radiation has a greater destructive action on fast-growing cells than on normal cells. Leukemia and Hodgkin's disease, a malignancy of the lymph nodes and lymphoid tissue, respond well to radiation and chemotherapy. Hormonal therapy, a type of chemotherapy, is used to treat cancer of the prostate, either by removal of the androgen sources, which stimulate the tumor growth, or by administration of estrogens, which inhibit it. Chemotherapy, the use of antineoplastic agents that are metabolic inhibitors and cell-killing chemicals, is effective in treating leukemia and many other cancers. Side effects from the potent chemicals include gastrointestinal dis-

on the Practical Side

Hair Loss with Chemotherapy

The chemicals used in treating cancer destroy rapidly dividing cells of the tumor. The chemicals, however, affect not only malignant cells, but all rapidly dividing cells. This includes the epidermal cells of the hair follicle that give rise to hair. As these cells are killed by the chemotherapy, hair is lost. Hair growth usually resumes after treatment as previously dormant epidermal cells become active.

leukopenia
(loo″-kō-pe′-nē-ă)

turbances, loss of hair, and reduced immunity. The latter is due to an abnormal decrease in the number of circulating white blood cells, **leukopenia.**

➤ PREVENTION

Prevention includes measures that stop cancer from developing. Early detection includes exams and tests intended to find cancer as early as possible, when it can be treated most effectively with the fewest side effects. Early detection can save lives and reduce suffering from cancers of the breast, colon, rectum, cervix, prostate, testes, oral cavity, and skin. Some of these cancers can be found early by self-examination (breast, skin, testes), physical examination (prostate, colon), x-rays (mammogram), or lab tests (Pap smear).

The sites most responsible for cancer deaths are lungs, breast, and colon, and many of these cancers can be prevented by changes in lifestyle. Cigarette smoking and use of tobacco products cause about 30% of all cancers. Cigarette smoking is considered the single most preventable cause not only of cancer but also of diseases such as heart disease, chronic bronchitis, and emphysema. Diet and nutrition also play a significant role in reducing the risk of cancer. Reduction of fat intake and the inclusion in the diet of fruits, vegetables, and fiber have been found to reduce the risk of breast and colon cancer. Vitamin A in the diet, specifically carotene-containing foods, has a protective effect against lung cancer.

Early detection of a potential malignancy is extremely significant in preventing carcinogenesis. Widespread use of the Papanicolaou **(Pap)** smear has greatly decreased the incidence and mortality from invasive cervical cancer. The use of mammography has led to early detection of breast cancer, which can be cured.

The association between sex and cervical cancer has been known for many years. Studies show that early sexual activity and multiple partners increase the incidence of cervical cancer. A high rate of sexually transmitted infections, multiple pregnancies, and early age at first pregnancy are often linked to this cancer. The **human papillomavirus** (HPV) responsible for genital warts (Chapter 15) seems to be the causative agent in uterine cervical carcinoma.

Risk factors including lifestyle choices such as smoking, sun exposure, use of tanning salons, diet, or alcohol abuse can be modified. Other risk factors like age, race, or genetics cannot be changed. An ounce of prevention is worth a pound of cure (Figures 4–9 and 4–10).

pap
(păp)

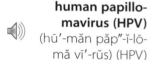

**human papillo-
mavirus (HPV)**
(hū′-măn păp″-ĭ-lō-
mă vī′-rŭs) (HPV)

PREVENTION *PLUS!*

Cancer Prevention through Nutrition

Here are some recommendations to help you reduce your risk of cancer:

1. Eat five or more servings of fruit and vegetables each day.

2. Choose foods low in fat.

3. Limit consumption of meats, especially high-fat meats.

4. Limit your consumption of alcoholic beverages, if you drink at all.

5. Stay within your healthy weight range.

Breast Self-Examination (BSE)

Step 1 Observe breasts in front of a mirror and
in good lighting in four positions:
  With arms relaxed and at sides
  With arms lifted over head
  With hands pressed against hips
  With hands pressed together at waist, leaning forward

Look at each breast individually, and compare them.
Look for any visible abnormalities, such as lumps, dimpling,
deviation, recent nipple retraction, irregular shape, edema,
discharge, or asymmetry.

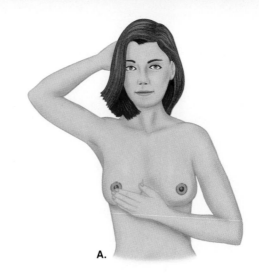

A.

Step 2 Palpate both breasts while standing or sitting, with
one hand behind head (Figure A). Palpation in the shower with
water and soap makes the skin slippery and easier to palpate.
Use the pads of fingers to palpate all areas of the breast, using
the concentric circles technique (Figure B). Press the breast tissue
gently against the chest wall, and be sure to palpate the axillary tail.

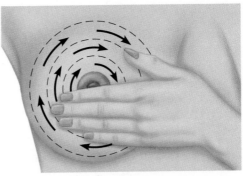

B.

Step 3 Palpate breasts again while lying down, as described
in Step 2. Place a folded towel under the shoulder and back on
the side to be palpated. The arm on the examining side should
be over the head, with the hand under the head (Figure C).

Step 4 Palpate the areola and nipples next.
Compress the nipple to check for discharge
(Figure D).

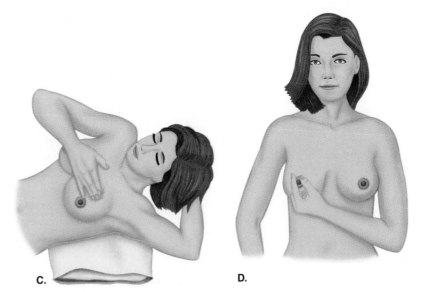

Step 5 Use a calendar to keep a record
of BSE. Perform BSE at the same time
each month, usually 5 days after the
onset of menses, when there is less
hormonal influence on tissues.

C.

D.

Figure 4–9
Procedure for Breast Self-Examination (BSE).

Testicular Self-Examination

- Examine testicles while taking a warm shower or bath, or just after if using a mirror to compare size.

- The scrotum, testicles, and hands should be soapy to allow easy manipulation of the tissue.

- Gently roll each testicle between the thumb and fingers of each hand. If one testicle is substantially larger than the other, or if any hard lumps are detected, consult a physician immediately.

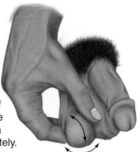

- Normal scrotal contents may be confusing. Just above and behind the testicle is the epididymis. It feels soft and tender overall, although parts of it may be rather firm. This is normal. The spermatic cord, a small, round, moveable tube, extends up from the epididymis. It feels firm and smooth. Of greatest concern is any hard lump felt directly on the testicle, even if it is painless.

- Choose a day out of each month on which to examine yourself. Most men choose an easy day to remember, such as the first or last day of the month.

Figure 4–10
Procedure for Testicular Self-Examination.

Chapter Summary

Cancer is the second leading cause of death in the United States. Uncontrolled cell division is the hallmark feature of cancer. The development of cancer is a slow process that includes three stages: initiation, promotion, and progression. Causes of cancer include the environment, chemicals, ultraviolet light, lifestyle, viruses, genetics, hormones, and exposure to ionizing radiation. Carcinoma is the more common type of cancer. It affects epithelial tissues and glands and spreads principally through the lymph system. Sarcoma affects bone, muscle, and cartilage and spreads rapidly through the blood. Neoplasms or tumors are divided into two classes: malignant and benign. Malignant tumors are invasive and spread by metastasis. Benign tumors are generally encapsulated, and they neither metastasize nor recur after surgical removal. Early detection and treatment of cancer can often lead to a cure. Detection can include self examinations, examination by a physician, and laboratory tests and x-rays. Cancer is treated by surgery, radiation, and chemotherapy, depending on the type and the location. Cancer prevention includes a healthful diet and lifestyle.

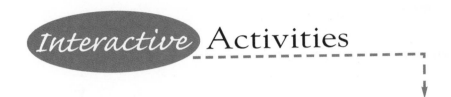

Interactive Activities

CASE FOR CRITICAL THINKING

Tumor cells can often grow in culture, so that researchers can observe their response to experimental drugs. How might such a procedure benefit a cancer patient?

MULTIMEDIA EXTENSION ACTIVITIES

www.prenhall.com/mulvihill
Use the above address to access the free, interactive companion Website created for this textbook. Included in the features of this site are chapter specific activities, internet links, and an audio-glossary.

Audio Glossary
Use the CD-ROM disk enclosed with your textbook to hear the pronunciation of the key terms in this chapter.

Quick Self Study

MULTIPLE CHOICE

1. Which of these lists the 3 stages of cancer development in their proper order?
   a. promotion, progression, initiation
   b. progression, promotion, initiation
   c. initiation, progression, promotion
   d. initiation, promotion, progression

2. Cancer cells are sensitive to radiation therapy and chemotherapy because they are constantly _____.
   a. dying
   b. shriveling
   c. dividing
   d. rupturing

3. A woman should do a breast self-exam _____.
   a. once a week
   b. once a month
   c. once a year
   d. twice a year

4. The spread of cancer to distant sites is called _____.
   a. benign
   b. malignant
   c. metastasis
   d. lipoma

TRUE/FALSE

_____ 1. Benign tumors do not metastasize.

_____ 2. A carcinogen is a cancer-causing agent.

_____ 3. The environment is not a risk factor for some types of cancer.

_____ 4. Cancer is the number 5 cause of death in the United States.

FILL-INS

1. You should apply a sunscreen with an SPF of at least _____.

2. A _____ is a sac or capsule containing fluid and is usually harmless.

3. CAUTION stands for _____.

4. A _____ is when a small sample is removed and examined microscopically for abnormalities.

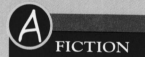

FICTION

Tanning salons do not decrease your risk of skin cancer.

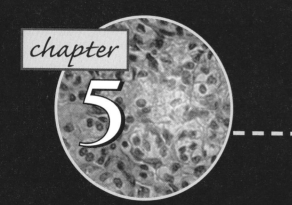

Hereditary Diseases

Have you ever been startled by observing a particularly strong family resemblance? How is this similarity between brothers and sisters, children and parents, and even between cousins explained? You can say, "It's because of their genes," which is true, but what about two brothers of the same parents who do not resemble each other at all? How does this phenomenon called inheritance work?

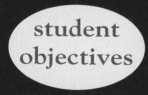

student objectives

After studying this chapter, students should be able to

➤ Understand DNA's role in heredity
➤ Describe mechanisms of transmission of hereditary diseases and give examples
➤ Discuss abnormal chromosome diseases
➤ Describe genetic diseases involving the sex chromosomes
➤ Describe congenital diseases

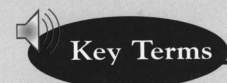

Key Terms

Achondroplasia

Achondroplastic dwarfism

Alleles

Atresia

Autosomes

Chromosomes

Congenital diseases

Deoxyribonucleic acid (DNA)

Dominant

Down's syndrome

Fragile X syndrome

Galactosemia

Genes

Hermaphrodites

Heterozygous

Homozygous

Infarcts

Karyotype

Klinefelter's syndrome

Nondisjunction

Phenylketonuria

Polydactyly

Pyloric stenosis

Recessive

Sex-linked inheritance

Sickle cell anemia

Tay-Sachs

Trisomy 21

Turner's syndrome

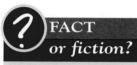

FACT *or fiction?*

There is no treatment for red-green colorblindness.

Read this chapter to find the answer.

➤ INTRODUCTION TO HEREDITY

All genetic information is contained in the nucleus of each cell, and each time the cell divides, in growth and repair, the information is passed on to the daughter cells. The vehicle of transmission is the DNA molecule, which duplicates itself when a cell is about to divide, providing an exact copy for each daughter cell.

on the Practical Side

Identification by Fingerprints

The value of fingerprints and footprints has increased greatly not only at crime scenes, but in the identification of abducted infants and children. No two sets of fingerprints are identical. The dermis, or true skin, projects upward into the epidermis in curving parallel ridges forming the pattern of fingerprints and footprints. In this age of biotechnology, "genetic fingerprints" are used for identification in criminal and paternity cases.

deoxyribonucleic acid (DNA)
(dē-ŏk″-sē-rī″-bō-nū-klē′-ĭk ăs′-ĭd)

chromosomes
(krō′-mō-sōms)

genes
(jēns)

autosomes
(au′-tō-sōms)

karyotype
(kăr′-ē-ō-tīp)

alleles
(ă-lēls′)

homozygous
(hōm″-ō-zī′-gŭs)

heterozygous
(hĕt″-ēr-ō-zī′-gŭs)

dominant
(dŏm′-ĭ-nănt)

recessive
(rē-sĕs′-ĭv)

DNA, which stands for **deoxyribonucleic acid,** is the blueprint for protein synthesis within the cell. At the time of cell division, the DNA is assembled into units called **chromosomes.** Each human cell contains 46 chromosomes divided into 23 pairs. Half of the chromosomes were inherited from each parent. The chromosomes contain thousands of **genes,** each of which is responsible for the synthesis of one protein. Forty-four of the chromosomes are called **autosomes,** and two are called the X and Y (or sex) chromosomes, the ones that determine the gender of the person. A combination of XY chromosomes results in a male, and XX chromosomes result in a female. This chromosomal composition of the nucleus is called the **karyotype** of the cell. The karyotype can be visualized microscopically and photographed to determine chromosomal abnormalities.

The genes inherited from each parent for a particular trait, such as eye color, hair color, and hair type, occupy a particular site on a chromosome. **Alleles** are alternative forms of a gene. If the pair of alleles are similar, the person is **homozygous** for that trait. If the alleles are different, one for dark and one for light hair, for example, the person is **heterozygous.** Some alleles always produce an effect and are said to be **dominant.** The result of the dominant allele is the same whether a person is homozygous or heterozygous. The allele for brown eyes, for example, is dominant to that for blue eyes. Other alleles are **recessive** and only manifest themselves when the person is homozygous for the trait. This is significant in many hereditary diseases.

Certain factors may cause a deviation from the basic principles of inheritance that have been described. Some alleles are codominant, so that both are expressed. An example of codominant alleles is found in blood type AB. The allele for the A factor is inherited from one parent and that for the B factor from the other, but both alleles are expressed. At times, a dominant allele is not fully expressed, a condition known as reduced penetrance.

➤ TRANSMISSION OF HEREDITARY DISEASES

Many of the diseases described throughout this book are called *hereditary* or *familial diseases.* In this chapter, the mechanism of transmission will be explained. Some diseases are inherited from a single autosomal dominant allele. One such defective gene causes Huntington's chorea, a disease described in Chapter 16, and another causes polydactyly, explained later in this Chapter. Other diseases are inherited as autosomal recessives, with one defective allele being inherited from each parent, making the person homozygous for that trait. Cystic fibrosis is such a disease. A third type of inheritance is sex-linked, with the defective allele on the X chromosome. Red-green color blindness and hemophilia are examples of sex-linked inherited diseases.

Autosomal Dominant

A defective dominant allele is usually transmitted from a parent who is heterozygous for the trait. If the other parent is normal for the particular condition, each child has a 50% chance of being affected and manifesting the genetic defect. This is illustrated in Figure 5–1. The disease appears in every generation, with males and females being equally affected. Exceptions to the rule are minimal.

Polydactyly, extra fingers or toes, is an example of an autosomal dominant disorder. A boy or girl inheriting the defective allele from either parent will have the abnormality. **Achondroplasia** is another disorder resulting from one defective dominant allele (Figure 5–2). The prefix *a* means a lack, *chondro* refers to cartilage, and *plasia* to formation. In this disease, cartilage formation in the fetus is defective. Normally, the fetal skeleton develops as cartilage that is gradually replaced by bone. In achondroplasia, the defective cartilage formation results in improper bone development and **achondroplastic dwarfism.** The long bones of the arms and legs are short, the trunk of the body is normal in size, the head is large, and the forehead very prominent. The person develops sexually, has normal intelligence, and is muscular and agile.

Autosomal Recessive

These diseases manifest themselves only when a person is homozygous for the defective allele. Two parents who are both carriers of the recessive allele are themselves heterozygous for the trait and do not have the disease. Each child has a 25% chance of

polydactyly
(pŏl″-ē-dak′-tĭ-lē)

achondroplasia
(ă-kŏn″-drō-plā′-sĭ-ă)

achondroplastic dwarfism
(ă-kŏn″-drō-plăs′-tĭk dwarf′-ĭzm)

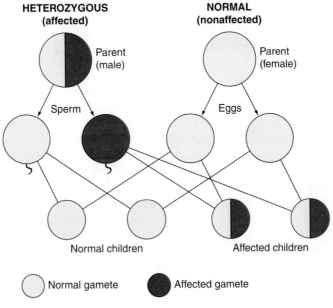

Figure 5–1
Transmission of autosomal dominant disorders (50% chance for an affected child).

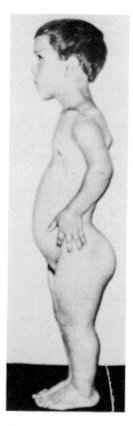
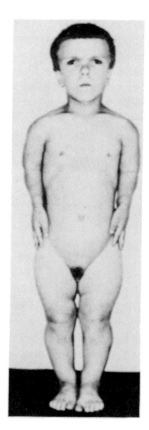

Figure 5–2
A 12-year-old achondroplastic dwarf. Note the disproportion of
the limbs to the trunk, the curvature of the spine, and the
prominent buttocks.

being affected. This is shown in Figure 5–3. The recessive allele appears more frequently
in a family, and close intermarriage, as between first cousins, increases the risk of the
particular disease.

phenylketonuria
(fĕn″-ĭl-
kē″-tō-nū′-rē-ă)

   Phenylketonuria, also called PKU, is caused by an autosomal recessive allele.
Persons with PKU lack a specific enzyme that converts one amino acid, phenylalanine,
to another, tyrosine. This mechanism is illustrated in Figure 5–4. As a result, high levels of phenylalanine and its derivatives build up in the blood and are toxic to the brain,
interfering with normal brain development. If the condition is not diagnosed and treated
early, severe mental retardation results. Physical development proceeds normally, but the
child is very light in color. Production of the pigment melanin is impeded because of inadequate tyrosine, a result of the missing enzyme. The child may manifest disorders of
the nervous system, such as a lack of balance, and may possibly suffer convulsions.

   To prevent the serious mental retardation that accompanies PKU, newborn babies
are routinely screened for the disease. If it is found, a synthetic diet is prescribed that
eliminates phenylalanine. Good results have been achieved with this treatment. The diet
is unpleasant, and controversy exists as to the length of time the diet must be maintained.
To begin treatment immediately, by excluding phenylalanine during the earliest years of
life, seems to be the most critical factor in preventing mental retardation.

galactosemia
(gă-lăk″-tō-sē′-mē-ă)

   Galactosemia is another example of an inborn error of metabolism resulting from
autosomal recessive inheritance. The person with this disease lacks the enzyme neces-

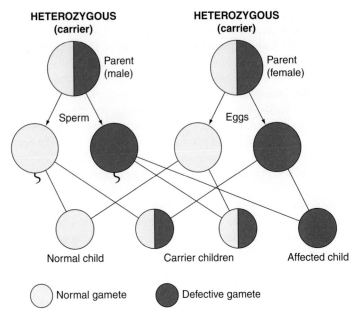

Figure 5–3
Transmission of recessive disorders (25% chance for an affected child).

sary to convert galactose, a sugar derived from lactose in milk, to glucose. Galactose accumulates in the blood and interferes with development of the brain, liver, and eyes. If untreated, mental retardation develops. The liver becomes enlarged and cirrhotic, and ascites fluid (see Chapter 12) accumulates in the abdominal cavity. Intestinal distress results in vomiting and diarrhea. Early diagnosis and treatment of galactosemia can prevent these signs, and development will then proceed normally. The treatment consists of eliminating lactose from the diet.

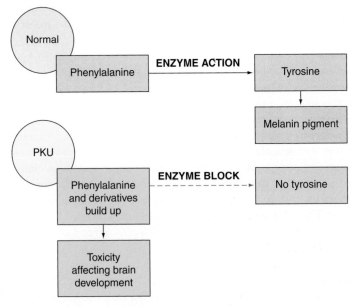

Figure 5–4
Enzyme block in phenylketonuria (PKU).

Sickle cell anemia
(sĭk'-l sĕl
ă-nē'-mē-ă)

infarcts
(ĭn'-fărkts)

Sickle cell anemia, a severe anemia generally confined to blacks, will be described in Chapter 7. Sickle cell anemia is an autosomal recessive disorder, in which the hemoglobin is abnormal, resulting in deformed red blood cells. The improperly formed cells become lodged in capillaries and block circulation, causing necrosis and **infarcts,** death of tissues. The sickle-shaped red blood cells rupture easily, and they are removed from the circulation by the spleen. The depletion of red blood cells results in severe anemia.

The person with sickle cell anemia is homozygous for the trait by inheriting one defective allele from each parent. A person who is heterozygous for sickle cell has both normal and abnormal hemoglobin and possesses the sickle cell trait. The person is mildly anemic, but the one defective allele provides an advantage. The person with sickle cell trait has an increased resistance to malaria that is significant in tropical climates where malaria abounds.

Tay-sachs
(tă-săks')

Tay-Sachs is an autosomal recessive condition that primarily affects families of Eastern Jewish origin. An enzyme deficiency causes abnormal lipid metabolism in the brain, which results in progressive mental and physical retardation. Symptoms appear by 6 months of age when no new skills are learned, convulsions occur, and blindness may develop. A cherry-red spot may be seen on each retina. Children usually die between 2 and 4 years of age. There is no specific therapy for the condition so care treats the symptoms.

Sex-linked Inheritance

Diseases of sex-linked inheritance generally result from defective genes on the X chromosome, because the Y chromosome is small and carries very few genes. A defective recessive gene on the single X chromosome of a male is unmasked, and the trait is expressed. A female may be heterozygous for the gene, having a defective recessive allele on the one X chromosome but a normal allele on the other X. That female is then a carrier of the disease, and she has a 50% chance of transmitting the allele to her sons and daughters. An affected male transmits the disease only to his daughters, inasmuch as they receive his X chromosome. His sons are unaffected, as the Y chromosome is normal. This is illustrated in Figure 5–5. The abnormalities of **sex-linked inheritance** are generally confined to the male and are transmitted by the female. In a rare case, the female may have the sex-linked disease if she is homozygous for the recessive gene.

**sex-linked
inheritance**
(sĕks-līnkt
ĭn-hĕr'-ĭ-tăns)

Color Blindness Red-green color blindness, the inability to distinguish between certain colors, is a disorder of sex-linked inheritance. It is generally confined to males, although it is possible for a female to be color-blind if she receives the recessive allele from each parent, which is rare.

The allele for color blindness is on the X chromosome, but the allele for normal vision is dominant to it. A male with the recessive allele on his one X chromosome will express the trait and be color-blind.

The defect that causes color blindness is apparently in certain specialized receptors of the retina called cones. There are three types of receptors that are stimulated by wavelengths of the primary colors: red, green, and blue. Impulses are then sent to the brain and interpreted. The color-blind person is most frequently unable to distinguish reds and greens. Corrective lenses are now available which may offer some treatment for red-green color blindness.

Hemophilia People with hemophilia do not bleed more profusely or bleed faster than normal; they bleed for a longer period of time. There have been significant advances in treating hemophilia in the last decade. A new genetically engineered clotting protein is

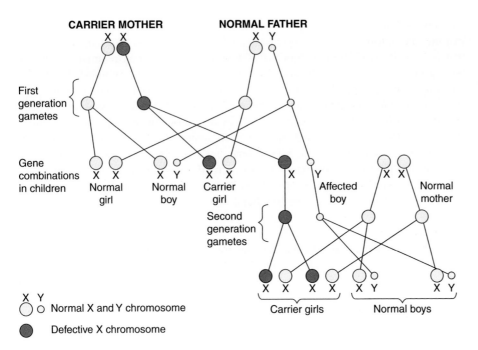

Figure 5–5
Transmission of sex-linked disorders.

now used for treatment. Research is also actively underway to develop gene therapy for the disease. The therapy will replace the missing or deficient gene with one that has the instructions for producing the clotting factor. Gene therapy has been successful in treating mice with hemophilia B.

Disease by the Numbers   X + ÷

EPIDEMIOLOGY

In the United States, 20,000 patients have Hemophilia A or B; 859% of them have Hemophilia A.

Fragile X Syndrome   **Fragile X syndrome** is a genetic condition associated with mental retardation. It is identified by a break, or weakness, on the long arm of the X chromosome. Because this is an abnormality of a sex chromosome, it is often refered to as X-linked. Mothers are the carriers and their sons are at risk of being affected, whereas daughters are at risk of being carriers and sometimes are mildly affected. Estimates on the prevalence of fragile X is about 1 in 1,000 males. The prevalence of carriers in the population is 1 in 600. Fragile X may account for up to 10% of mental retardation. It is the most common inherited cause of mental retardation known. The gene responsible for fragile X has been identified (FMR-1), so fragile X is diagnosed by DNA testing.

   The physical features associated with fragile X syndrome include a long narrow face, prominent ears, jaw, and forehead. Enlarged testicles are another physical characteristic. Loose joints, particularly in the finger joints, are also quite common in childhood. Physical features are often more subtle in females. About 80% of boys with fragile X

Fragile X syndrome
(fră'-jĭl ĕks sĭn'-drōm)

have mental impairment ranging from severe retardation to low-normal intelligence. The majority are mildly to moderately retarded. Girls are much less affected, with estimates that about 30% with the condition have some degree of mental retardation. Men and boys with fragile X are usually socially engaging, but they have an unusual style of interacting with other people. They tend to avoid direct eye contact during conversation, and hand-flapping or hand-biting is common. They may have an unusual speech pattern characterized by a fast and fluctuating rate of repetitions of sound, words, or phrases. They also may have a decreased attention span, hyperactivity, and motor delays.

There is no cure for fragile X syndrome, but medical intervention can improve the problems in attention and hyperactivity. A variety of medications can treat attention span, hyperactivity, and other behavior problems. In addition, speech and physical therapy as well as vocational training can be beneficial.

Familial Diseases

Some diseases appear in families, but the means of inheritance are not understood. Examples of diseases with a higher incidence in certain families are epilepsy, diabetes, cardiovascular problems and allergies and familial polyposis. The cause of these diseases does not seem to be a single gene but the effect of several genes working together.

➤ ABNORMAL CHROMOSOME DISEASES

The hereditary diseases that have been described so far result from a defective gene. Abnormalities in the chromosomes, either in their number or structure, cause other disorders. At times, chromosomes fail to separate properly during cell division, causing one daughter cell to be deficient and one to have an extra chromosome. The loss of an autosomal chromosome is usually incompatible with life because each autosome contains a large number of essential genes. A fetus affected by this condition is generally spontaneously aborted. The loss of a sex chromosome or the presence of an extra one is less serious, but many abnormalities accompany the condition.

Down's Syndrome

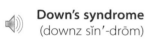

Down's syndrome
(downz sĭn′-drōm)

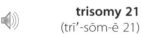

trisomy 21
(trī′-sōm-ē 21)

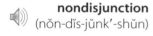

nondisjunction
(nŏn-dĭs-jŭnk′-shŭn)

Down's syndrome is an example of a disorder caused by the presence of an extra autosomal chromosome. Chromosome 21 is in triplicate, which is called **trisomy 21.** The extra chromosome results from **nondisjunction,** the failure of two chromosomes to separate as the gametes, either the egg or the sperm, are being formed.

The Down's syndrome child is always mentally retarded. The excessive enzyme production from the extra genes may have a toxic effect on the brain. The child can be taught simple tasks and is generally very affectionate.

The life expectancy of a child with Down's syndrome is relatively short because of complications that accompany the condition. Congenital heart diseases are common, and there is a greater susceptibility to respiratory tract infections, including pneumonia. There is also a higher incidence of leukemia than in a normal child.

The Down's syndrome child has a very characteristic appearance. The eyes appear slanted because of an extra fold of skin at the upper, medial corner of the eye; the tongue is coarse and often protrudes; and the nose is short and flat. The child is usually of short stature, and the sex organs are underdeveloped. A straight crease extends across the palm of the hand, and the little finger is often shorter than normal (Figure 5–6).

The incidence of Down's syndrome is higher in mothers over age 35 than in younger women and the risk increases with age.

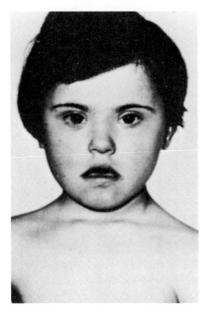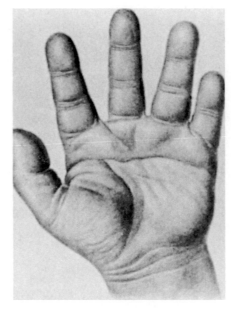

Figure 5–6
Left. Face of a 5-year-old girl with Down's syndrome. Note widely set eyes, underdeveloped bridge of the nose, partially open mouth, and protruding tongue. **Right.** Short, broad hand of a 9-year-old Down's syndrome patient, showing shortened fifth finger and transverse crease across palm.

➤ SEX ANOMALIES

Turner's Syndrome

One of the sex chromosomes is missing in **Turner's syndrome,** resulting in a karyotype of 45, XO. Such a karyotype indicates that the person has forty-five chromosomes, with only one X chromosome. The person appears to be female, but the ovaries do not develop; thus, there is no ovulation or menstruation, and the person is sterile. The nipples are widely spaced, the breasts do not develop, and the person is short of stature and has a stocky build. Congenital heart disease, particularly coarctation of the aorta (described in Chapter 8), frequently accompanies Turner's syndrome. Facial deformities are often present. Figure 5–7 shows a patient with Turner's syndrome.

Turner's syndrome
(tŭr'-nĕrz sĭn'-drōm)

Klinefelter's Syndrome

An extra sex chromosome is present in **Klinefelter's syndrome,** and the person's karyotype is 47, XXY. This person has forty-seven chromosomes, including two X and one Y chromosome. This person appears to be a male but has small testes that fail to mature and produce no sperm. At puberty, with the development of secondary sex characteristics, the breasts enlarge and a female distribution of hair develops. There is little facial hair, and the general appearance is that of a eunuch. The person is tall (with abnormally long legs), is mentally deficient, and is sterile (Figure 5–8).

Klinefelter's syndrome
(klīn'-fĕl-tĕrs sĭn'-drōm)

Hermaphrodites

The number of true **hermaphrodites** who have both testes and ovaries is small. Pseudohermaphrodites do develop, and they have either testes or ovaries, usually nonfunctional, but the remainder of the anatomy is mixed. This condition is referred to as sex reversal, in which the chromosomal sex is different from the anatomic sex. Sex

hermaphrodites
(hĕr-măf'-rō-dīts)
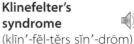

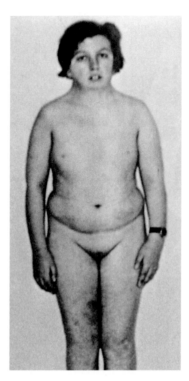

Figure 5–7
A 21-year-old patient with Turner's
syndrome. The chest is broad and the
nipples are small and pale. Pubic hair
is totally lacking.

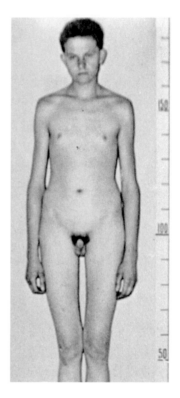

Figure 5–8
A 19-year-old patient with
Klinefelter's syndrome. Extremities
are excessively long, pubic hair
is scanty, and genitals are
underdeveloped. Body proportions
resemble those of a eunuch.

reversal occurs during fetal life. The sex glands are neutral during the first few weeks
after conception, but the male gonads differentiate at about the sixth week under the influence of masculinizing hormone. In the absence of an adequate amount of this hormone, ovaries develop, and the individual is anatomically female but chromosomally
male (XY).

Some cases of pseudohermaphroditism result from excessive production of sex hormones from the adrenal cortex. An affected female develops male secondary sexual characteristics at a very early age. The external genitalia of pseudohermaphrodites resembles that of both males and females. A pseudohermaphrodite is shown in Figure 5–9.

➤ CONGENITAL DISEASES

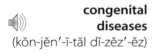

**congenital
diseases**
(kŏn-jĕn′-ĭ-tăl dĭ-zĕz′-ĕz)

Congenital diseases are those appearing at birth or shortly after, but they are not caused
by genetic or chromosomal abnormalities. Congenital defects usually result from some
failure in development during the embryonic stage, or in the first 2 months of pregnancy.
Congenital diseases cannot be transmitted to offspring.

Various factors—inadequate oxygen, maternal infection, drugs, malnutrition, and
radiation—can interfere with normal development. Rubella, or German measles, con-

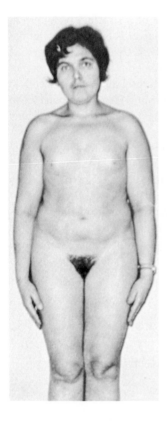

Figure 5–9
A 22-year-old patient with pseudohermaphroditism, reared as a girl because of ambiguous genitalia. Surgery and tissue studies showed the gonads to be testes.

tracted by the mother during the first trimester of pregnancy, can produce serious birth defects. The rubella virus is able to cross the placental barrier and affect the central nervous system of the embryo, causing mental retardation, blindness, and deafness. Cerebral palsy and hydrocephalus can develop as a result of the viral infection.

PREVENTION *PLUS!*

Rubella infection when a woman is pregnant can harm the fetus. The best way to prevent rubella during pregnancy is to get vaccinated before even **thinking** about getting pregnant. Pregnant women should not get the rubella vaccine. Wait 3 months after vaccination before becoming pregnant.

Syphilis can be transmitted to a developing fetus and cause multiple anomalies—structural deformities, blindness, deafness, and paralysis; children with congenital syphilis may become insane. Syphilitic infection of a fetus frequently results in spontaneous abortion or a stillbirth. A mother with syphilis should be treated for it before the fifth month of pregnancy to prevent fetal infection. A child born with syphilis should be treated immediately with penicillin, but considerable irreversible damage may have already occurred.

The tragic effect of the drug thalidomide, used during pregnancy many years ago, alerted the public to the danger of drugs to the developing embryo. Babies who had been exposed to thalidomide before birth were born without limbs or had flipperlike appendages.

Many congenital defects result from improper closure of a structure or failure of parts to unite. Congenital heart diseases are discussed in Chapter 8. Spina bifida, an improper union of parts of the vertebral column, is explained in Chapter 16. Congenital defects of the alimentary tract include various types of obstructions. The absence or closure of a normal body opening or tubular structure is called **atresia.** Atresia occurs in various parts of the gastrointestinal tract. The lack of an opening from the esophagus to the stomach is esophageal atresia; it is frequently accompanied by an abnormal opening between the esophagus and the trachea.

Intestinal atresia is a complete obstruction of the intestine, resulting in vomiting, dehydration, scanty stool production, and distention of the abdomen. The bile ducts are blocked in biliary atresia, and the inability to secrete bile into the duodenum causes severe jaundice to develop. The liver and spleen become greatly enlarged. Another congenital obstruction of the intestinal tract is **pyloric stenosis,** in which the circular sphincter muscle is hypertrophied, closing the opening between the stomach and the duodenum. Symptoms include projectile vomiting, dehydration, constipation, and weight loss. Corrective surgery has been very effective in removing these congenital obstructions of the intestinal tract, just as it has been for congenital heart disease.

atresia
(ă-trē′-zē-ă)

pyloric stenosis
(pĭ-lōr′-ĭk stĕ-nō′-sĭs)

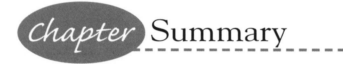

Chapter Summary

Genetic information is encoded in the DNA molecule, which duplicates itself when a cell is about to divide. DNA provides a blueprint from protein synthesis in the daughter cells and comprises the genes that are arranged on the chromosomes. Some genes are dominant and are always expressed, whereas others are recessive and require two similar genes for the expression of a trait. One pair of chromosomes, the X and Y chromosomes, determines the gender of the fetus. The other forty-four chromosomes are called autosomes.

Some diseases develop if only a single dominant autosomal gene is received. An example of this is Huntington's chorea, a devastating disease of the central nervous system. Other diseases develop only if a recessive gene is received from each parent, as is the case in phenylketonuria. Other diseases are sex-linked, affecting primarily males but being transmitted through females. This is the inheritance pattern in color blindness, hemophilia, and fragile X syndrome. Some diseases are found within families but are not attributable to a particular gene. The action of several genes seems to be responsible. Epilepsy, diabetes, and allergies are thought to be caused in this way.

In addition to diseases inherited by specific genes, gross chromosomal abnormalities result in other disorders. Down's syndrome is caused by chromosome 21 being in triplicate (trisomy 21). A missing or extra sex chromosome produces sex anomalies and usually mental retardation.

Certain conditions are apparent at birth or soon after, but they are not the result of genetic or chromosomal abnormalities. These are congenital diseases caused by various factors during early development. Certain heart malformations, absence of a natural body opening, or failure of a structure to close are examples of congenital diseases. Congenital diseases are not passed on to offspring.

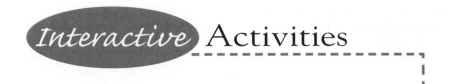

Interactive Activities

CASE FOR CRITICAL THINKING

What is the reason that Turner's and Klinefelter's syndromes can occur as a result of nondisjunction in either the sperm or egg, but XYY can occur only as a result of nondisjunction in the sperm?

MULTIMEDIA EXTENSION ACTIVITIES

www.prenhall.com/mulvihill
Use the above address to access the free, interactive companion Website created for this textbook. Included in the features of this site are chapter specific activities, internet links, and an audio-glossary.

Audio Glossary
Use the CD-ROM disk enclosed with your textbook to hear the pronunciation of the key terms in this chapter.

Quick Self Study

MULTIPLE CHOICE

1. The sex chromosomes of a normal male are _____.
   - a. XX
   - b. YY
   - c. XY
   - d. XYY

2. Humans have _____ chromosomes.
   - a. 23
   - b. 46
   - c. 96
   - d. 21

3. _____ alleles only manifest themselves when the person is homozygous for the trait.
   - a. recessive
   - b. dominant
   - c. homozygous
   - d. heterozygous

4. Sex-linked diseases affect men more than women because _____.
   - a. men have two X chromosomes
   - b. men have two Y chromosomes
   - c. men have one X chromosome
   - d. men have no Y chromosomes

TRUE/FALSE

___T___ 1. DNA contains genetic information.

___T___ 2. The incidence of Down's syndrome increases with the mother's age.

___F___ 3. Fragile X syndrome is found equally in men and women.

___F___ 4. A patient with Turner's syndrome has an extra sex chromosome.

FILL-INS

1. _____ diseases are those appearing at birth or shortly after, but they are not caused by genetic or chromosomal abnormalities.

2. _____ have both functional testes and ovaries.

3. _____ is an example of a familial disease.

4. A female carrier of a sex-linked trait has a _____% chance of transmitting the allele to her offspring.

FICTION

There are lens available to treat some forms of colorblindness.

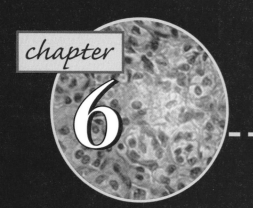

6

Dietary Deficiencies and Excesses: Malnutrition, Obesity, and Alcoholism

Disease can result from a dietary deficiency, such as malnutrition, or from excess, as in obesity and alcoholism. Psychoneurotic diseases, anorexia, and bulimia, are examples of diseases involving dietary deficiency or excess.

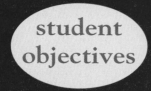

student objectives

After studying this chapter, students should be able to
➤ Know the function and importance of vitamins and minerals in the diet
➤ Compare nutrients to food and metabolism
➤ Identify the causes and manifestations of malnutrition
➤ Relate obesity to (other) body systems and their functioning
➤ Identify manifestations of alcoholism
➤ Know criteria/characteristics of fetal alcohol syndrome (FAS)

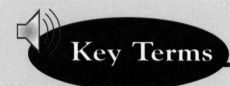

Key Terms

Amenorrhea

Amphetamines

Anorexia nervosa

Arrhythmia

Bulimia

Carotene

Collagen

Conjunctiva

Delirium tremens

Ecchymoses

Epistaxis

Esophageal varices

Glycogen

Gynecomastia

Hepatic coma

Hypercalcemia

Hypervitaminosis

Nystagmus

Obesity

Osteomalacia

Pancreatitis

Prothrombin

Rhodopsin

Rickets

Thrombis

Wernicke's
encephalopathy

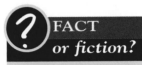

FACT or fiction?

In addition to tasting great, beans, nuts, and seeds are excellent sources of dietary fiber and low in fat.

Read this chapter to find the answer.

➤ NUTRIENTS

Ever heard the phrase "We are what we eat"? Certainly it makes sense to be aware of diet along with food preferences when it comes to healthful living. After all, the body is made of basically the same chemicals consumed as food. Therefore, to understand nutritional problems, it seems appropriate to become acquainted with the fundamental aspects of nutrition.

➤ METABOLISM

Food intake in some form is necessary to start the digestive process that will enable nutrients to provide the necessary maintenance of the body. After ingestion of a meal, the food (chemicals) must be metabolized or processed by a complex series of biochemical reactions involving all cells in the body. Metabolism involves mixing chemicals (food) in small molecular forms with oxygen in order to burn them. In this complex arrangement, another biological fuel is produced—ATP. This compound is then used directly to push cellular activities, which includes muscle contractions and nerve impulses. As ATP is constructed from food sources, waste products of H_2O and CO_2 are released along with heat. Heat, of course, helps maintain proper body temperature (37°C).

Nutrients are sorted or selected portions of food that provide the energy link necessary to make ATP and heat. Excess food is metabolized into fat or glycogen and stored as a reserve fuel.

More specifically, nutrients include carbohydrates (sugar types), proteins and lipids/fats, plus vitamins (e.g., A, B, C), minerals like calcium and potassium, and water. The overall value of these nutrients is to promote growth, especially in the early years; cell and tissue repair; and a broad balancing of body systems. As nutrients play their role, they assist in maintaining the physiologic balance called homeostasis.

Now consider the diseases or situations whereby the body is unable to use nutrients properly or when the individual consumes food excessively. In either case, the person is not maintaining a healthy state. The results of malnutrition or obesity require considerable attention. The effort to control the situation functionally is sometimes beyond the control of the individual. The reader may find it useful to refer occasionally to Figure 6–1 to see the impact of nutritional problems.

➤ MALNUTRITION

Diseases that may be classified as nutritional diseases stem from a wide range of causes. Malnutrition caused by lack of resources, lack of knowledge, or the unavailability of proper foods comprises one end of the spectrum; obesity, hypervitaminosis, or alcoholism is at the other extreme.

The concept of malnutrition is generally associated with an inadequate availability of food, but one can suffer nutritional deficiencies in the midst of plenty. Several diseases that will be discussed in this book are actually nutritional diseases in that they deprive the body of essential dietary elements.

Various malfunctionings of the gastrointestinal system (Chapter 11) prevent the use of nutrients in the diet. The absence of gastric, intestinal, or pancreatic enzymes to digest proteins, carbohydrates, and lipids can deprive the body of these nutrients. Pancreatitis (Chapter 12), for example, may interfere with digestion when the diseased pancreas is unable to function properly. Digestive disturbances that cause persistent vomiting or diarrhea also may result in malnutrition, by prematurely eliminating nutrients.

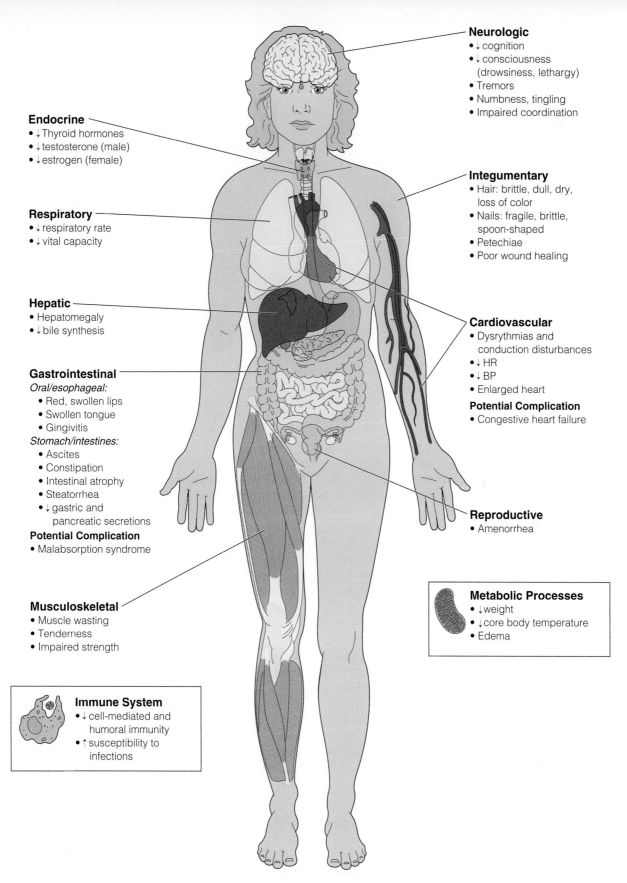

Neurologic
- ↓ cognition
- ↓ consciousness (drowsiness, lethargy)
- Tremors
- Numbness, tingling
- Impaired coordination

Endocrine
- ↓ Thyroid hormones
- ↓ testosterone (male)
- ↓ estrogen (female)

Integumentary
- Hair: brittle, dull, dry, loss of color
- Nails: fragile, brittle, spoon-shaped
- Petechiae
- Poor wound healing

Respiratory
- ↓ respiratory rate
- ↓ vital capacity

Hepatic
- Hepatomegaly
- ↓ bile synthesis

Cardiovascular
- Dysrythmias and conduction disturbances
- ↓ HR
- ↓ BP
- Enlarged heart

Potential Complication
- Congestive heart failure

Gastrointestinal
Oral/esophageal:
- Red, swollen lips
- Swollen tongue
- Gingivitis

Stomach/intestines:
- Ascites
- Constipation
- Intestinal atrophy
- Steatorrhea
- ↓ gastric and pancreatic secretions

Potential Complication
- Malabsorption syndrome

Reproductive
- Amenorrhea

Musculoskeletal
- Muscle wasting
- Tenderness
- Impaired strength

Metabolic Processes
- ↓ weight
- ↓ core body temperature
- Edema

Immune System
- ↓ cell-mediated and humoral immunity
- ↑ susceptibility to infections

Figure 6–1
Some effects of undernutrition.

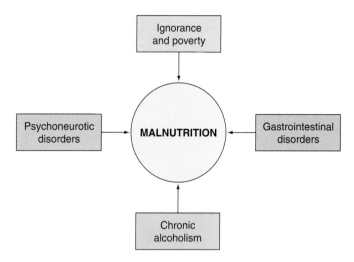

Figure 6–2
Possible causes of malnutrition.

Not only is the digestion of foodstuffs essential for proper nourishment, but the products of digestion must be absorbed through the intestinal wall. Bile secretion, essential for the absorption of lipids, including the fat-soluble vitamins A, D, E, and K, may be inadequate for reasons such as liver dysfunction, a diseased gallbladder, or obstruction of the bile ducts. The malabsorption syndrome (Chapter 11) causes the loss of essential nutrients in the stools. Pernicious anemia (Chapter 7) develops in the absence of gastric intrinsic factor needed for absorption of vitamin B_{12} from the digestive tract. This condition occurs even if vitamin B_{12} is present in the diet.

Impaired blood circulation through the liver because of cirrhosis or severe hepatitis (Chapter 12) deprives the body of proteins normally synthesized by the liver. The storage of nutrients in the liver is also diminished when the organ is severely damaged. The liver, which normally stores glucose (as **glycogen**), vitamins, and iron also produces bile.

glycogen
(glī′-kŏ-jĕn)

Diabetes mellitus (Chapter 14) is a metabolic disease in which glucose cannot enter the cells to be used in the absence of insulin. Glucose is lost in the urine, and the untreated diabetic metabolizes fat reserves and even tissue protein.

In addition to the diseases already described that can result in malnutrition, the failure to eat properly is associated with other problems that will be discussed in this chapter. For example, disease of psychoneurotic origin in which willful starvation leads to total emaciation and even death, will be explained.

The effect on the body of excessive food intake that leads to obesity, and of toxicity that results from hypervitaminosis, will be discussed. The medical aspects of alcoholism, many of which are related to malnutrition, will also be explained. Figure 6–2 summarizes causes of malnutrition.

➤ VITAMIN DEFICIENCIES

The importance of vitamins included in a healthful diet will be discussed in Chapter 20 on Wellness. The following vitamin deficiencies result in various disorders and are summarized in Figure 6–3.

DEFICIENT VITAMIN	DISEASE	MANIFESTATIONS	TREATMENT AND/OR PREVENTION
Thiamine	Beriberi	Nervous and cardiovascular disorders	Thiamine and thiamine-enriched foodstuffs
Niacin	Pellagra	Dermatitis, diarrhea, and dementia	Niacin supplements, diet including meat and whole grain cereals
Riboflavin		Similar to niacin	Balanced diet and riboflavin supplement
Vitamin C	Scurvy	Bleeding gums and hemorrhages into tissues	Supplemental doses of vitamin C, citrus fruits, and greens
Vitamin A	Night blindness	Poor vision in dim light; dry, cracked mucous membranes	Diet including dairy products, egg yolks, and vegetables
Vitamin D	Rickets, osteomalacia	Weak, deformed bones	Vitamin D supplements, vitamin D fortified milk, and exposure to sunlight
Vitamin K		Tendency to hemorrhage	Normal diet

Figure 6–3
Summary of vitamin deficiencies.

Vitamin A Deficiency

Vitamin A is essential for vision because it is an essential component of **rhodopsin,** the pigment that absorbs light in the rods of the retina. A lack of vitamin A results in an inability to see in dim light, a condition known as night blindness.

It is thought that vitamin A contributes to the integrity of mucous membranes—those membranes that line the respiratory, gastrointestinal, and urogenital tracts. In the absence of vitamin A, the membranes become dry and susceptible to cracking, permitting the entrance of infectious organisms. The **conjunctiva,** the membrane that lines the eyelids and covers the eyeball, also becomes dry and cracked, making it a target for infection.

Vitamin A deficiencies are most commonly seen in parts of India and China where the diet is limited. The condition also exists when vitamin A is present in the diet but cannot be used because of malabsorption (Chapter 11).

Vitamin A is derived from a plant pigment, **carotene,** which is converted into vitamin A by the liver. Dairy products, egg yolks, and vegetables, (yellow and green), like carrots, are good sources of vitamin A.

Vitamin D Deficiency (Rickets)

Rickets is a bone disease in children in which calcification is impaired, resulting in weak, deformed bones (Chapter 17). Vitamin D is essential for the absorption of calcium from the gastrointestinal tract. Rickets develops when vitamin D is deficient in

rhodopsin
(rō-dŏp′-sĭn)

conjunctiva
(kŏn″-jŭnk-tī′-vă)

carotene
(kăr′-ō-ten)

rickets
(rĭk′-ĕts)

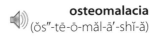

osteomalacia
(ŏs″-tē-ō-măl-ā′-shĭ-ă)

the diet. The lack of vitamin D in adults results in a softening of the bones, a disease known as **osteomalacia** (Chapter 17).

Rickets and osteomalacia can be prevented by a diet that includes vitamin D-fortified milk. Exposure to sunlight also provides a source of vitamin D, as ultraviolet light converts a substance in the skin (sterol) to vitamin D. Rickets and osteomalacia can be treated by administering vitamin D concentrate and improving the diet, and by exposure to sunlight.

Disease by the Numbers x + ÷

It is now recognized that a deficiency of folic acid in the diet may lead to nearly 40% of the heart attacks in American men. Dozens of studies show that just 0.4 mg/day of folate is enough to reduce homocysteine—an amino acid, associated with higher risk of heart attack and stroke. Taking a one-a-day multiple vitamin is an inexpensive measure to add days, weeks, or years to a healthier life.

Vitamin K Deficiency

prothrombin
(prō-thrŏm′-bĭn)

Vitamin K is essential to the blood-clotting mechanism and is made in the intestine by bacterial action. The liver synthesizes an enzyme, **prothrombin,** with the aid of vitamin K. Prothrombin initiates the chain reaction in the blood coagulation process. In the absence of prothrombin, hemorrhaging occurs. Excessive use of antibiotics can destroy the normal flora (naturally occurring bacteria) of the intestine and, thus, prevent the production of vitamin K. Green leafy vegetables and liver are good sources of vitamin K. Attempting to balance medications and diet may result in unforeseen complications.

Vitamin C (Ascorbic Acid) Deficiency

A lack of vitamin C prevents proper formation of the cementing substance that holds epithelial cells together. This causes capillary walls to be weak and to rupture easily, resulting in hemorrhage into surrounding tissues. Small black-and-blue spots appear all over the body as a result of the rupture of blood vessels. Anemia may develop over a period of time and manifest itself by weakness, palpitation, and breathing difficulties.

The gums are particularly affected, and they bleed easily. The open lesions provide an entry for bacteria, and, as the gum tissue becomes necrotic, the teeth loosen and fall out. Synthesis of **collagen,** a fibrous protein in connective tissue, is impaired, causing wounds to heal poorly. Such a disease condition is called scurvy.

collagen
(kŏl′-ă-jĕn)

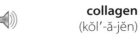

PREVENTION *PLUS!*

It is well-established that vitamin E is an antioxidant or free radical fighter. However, in addition to being a cancer fighter, vitamin E appears able to prevent strokes and heart attack.

In mice studies, vitamin E given in megadoses causes an anticoagulant-type effect. Actually, the natural vitamin E, quinone, seems to be even more potent once it combines with oxygen. Apparently vitamin E, quinone, competes with a major clotting factor—vitamin K. So, by taking vitamin E, a person may be getting more ammunition against the number one killer as well as protection from cancer.

A vitamin C deficiency can be prevented by a diet that includes fresh fruits and vegetables, particularly tomatoes, citrus fruits, and greens. The activity of the vitamin is lost by heating and drying.

It was reported in the 18th century that sailors in the British Navy suffered from scurvy. After various diet trials were conducted by the naval surgeon (James Lind) using fruits and vegetables, a daily portion of lime juice was administered to ward off the disease. Thereafter, the British, especially military personnel, are affectionately called "Limey."

➤ HYPERVITAMINOSIS

An excess of vitamins, particularly of vitamins A and D, can be harmful because the excess produces a toxicity **(hypervitaminosis).** Children can become very ill after swallowing a large number of vitamin pills, and they can experience gastrointestinal disturbances and drowsiness. A generalized edema develops that even increases intracranial pressure. The affected child is irritable and fails to gain weight. The symptoms are reversible once the toxicity has subsided.

Excessive vitamin D causes too much calcium to be absorbed from the gastrointestinal tract. **Hypercalcemia** results in deposits of calcium in organs such as the kidney, heart, lungs, and the walls of the stomach. The digestive system is affected, and excessive thirst and polyuria develop. Some of the damage to the tissues may be irreversible. Consult Figure 6–1 for reference.

hypervitaminosis
(hī″-pěr-vī″-tă-min-o′-sĭs)

hypercalcemia
(hī″-pěr-kăl-sē′-mē-ă)

➤ MINERAL DEFICIENCIES

Minerals are only required in minute amounts, but a lack of them has serious consequences. An inadequate level of calcium prevents proper bone formation and maintenance, as described in Chapter 17. A calcium deficiency also interferes with the blood-clotting mechanism. One type of anemia develops in the absence of the iron needed to form hemoglobin. One type of goiter (endemic) results from insufficient iodine.

Potassium may be adequate in the diet but missing from the body under certain conditions. An excessive secretion of aldosterone from adrenal cortex causes a loss of potassium through the kidneys. A prolonged loss of fluid through vomiting or diarrhea removes potassium, as will the action of certain diuretics. The muscles are weak in a potassium deficiency, and the heart muscle is particularly affected.

Sodium is usually adequate in the diet but may be lacking in Addison's disease (Chapter 14), in which aldosterone is not secreted by the adrenal cortex. Sodium is essential for the transmission of nerve impulses and muscle contraction. The principal functions of minerals are summarized in Figure 6–4.

➤ ANOREXIA NERVOSA

Anorexia nervosa is a disease of psychoneurotic origin in which the aversion to food leads to emaciation and malnutrition. Anorexia nervosa is most common in teenage girls, and the incidence of the disease has greatly increased in recent years. The nation's obsession with thinness is now even affecting preteens. The disease is rare in males and older age groups. The desire to be thin and the patient's misconception of her own body size underlie the onset of the disease. The individual may have been socially normal before the initial dieting or may have shown some social maladjustments.

anorexia nervosa
(ăn″-ō-rĕks′-ĭ-ă
nĕr-vō′-să)

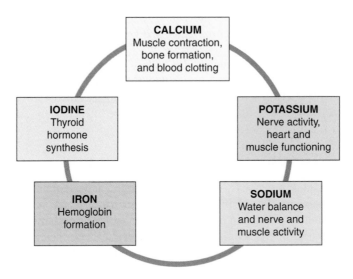

Figure 6–4
Minerals and their principal functions.

Anorexics actually starve themselves, yet deny that they are not eating adequately. Personality changes are noticeable inasmuch as they become irritable, full of anxiety, and depressed. They may become hostile toward their parents who encourage proper eating habits.

Anorexia nervosa is not an accurate name for this disease. *Anorexia* means loss of appetite, but the individual with this disease experiences hunger and may be obsessed with food. They may elaborately prepare food for others but not for themselves. Counting calories and weighing food becomes ritualistic. The individual often prepares food—consisting primarily of fruits, vegetables, and cheese—when alone and sure that no one is giving him or her extra calories. At least they do not suffer from a vitamin deficiency, but they will avoid all carbohydrates.

Hunger may cause occasional orgies of overeating, after which the individual then induces vomiting and uses laxatives excessively. They exercise strenuously, increasing the weight loss, becoming absolutely emaciated in appearance. The face is gaunt with protruding bones, yet the person denies being thin, and even perceives herself or himself as fat. An anorexia nervosa patient is seen in Figure 6–5.

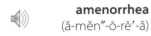

amenorrhea
(ă-mĕn″-ō-rē′-ă)

Amenorrhea, the absence of menstruation, always accompanies anorexia nervosa. The ovaries stop producing estrogen and gonadotropins are not secreted by the anterior pituitary. Amenorrhea occurs early in the disease, so it is not considered a result of malnutrition. A possible hypothalamic disturbance is indicated in which releasing factors for the gonadotropins are not being secreted. In rare cases of males with anorexia nervosa, the levels of gonadotropic hormones and testosterone are also decreased.

The person with anorexia nervosa rejects the suggestion to see a physician. If the person can be persuaded to be examined, the findings include low blood pressure, decreased heart rate, and anemia. Dehydration caused by the induced vomiting and excessive use of laxatives results in a depletion of potassium. This deficiency causes muscular weakness and heart abnormalities. A lowered resistance because of malnutrition makes the person susceptible to infections.

Treatment is directed toward correcting the malnutrition and the abnormal psychological state. Hospitalization is usually required to assure close observation of eating and

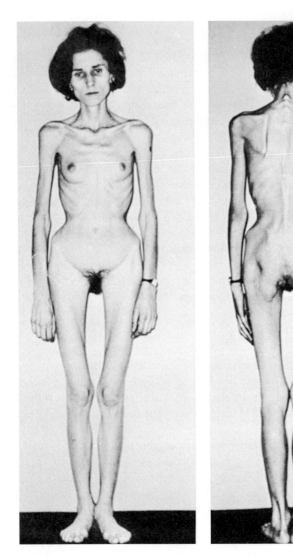

Figure 6–5
A 19-year-old patient with anorexia nervosa shows emaciation and
premature aging. Note protruding bones, muscle atrophy, and sunken
abdomen. Patient is about 5'6" tall and weighs 66 pounds.

bathroom habits. The patient may resist eating the required diet, for fear of becoming
fat. The therapist must assure the patient that the weight gained will help make for a
more attractive and improved health. Cooperation between the patient and therapist is
essential to recovery.

The psychological problems that underlie the disease must be uncovered and proper
psychotherapy given as the condition of anorexia nervosa is extremely serious. The patient can actually starve to death, and a depressed state may result in suicide. Even after an apparent recovery, close supervision is required as relapses of the disease are common and the mortality rate is quite high.

➤ BULIMIA

bulimia
(bū-lĭm′-ĭ-ă)

Bulimia, a gorge–purge syndrome, is the opposite of, yet similar to, anorexia nervosa. Teenage girls and women in their early twenties are the usual victims of this condition. As in anorexia nervosa, the goal of the person is to avoid weight gain. Bulimics may be of average weight or obese, and therefore, the disease may not be detected. Food-eating binges followed by induced vomiting and the use of laxatives and diuretics are the manifestations of this condition.

The detrimental long-term effects include tooth decay, constant sore throat, and swollen salivary glands from the abnormal acidity of the induced vomiting. Dehydration and electrolyte imbalance cause serious disturbances, and liver damage is common. Sudden death from heart failure or stomach rupture is possible.

Bulimia, like anorexia nervosa, is linked to a psychoneurotic condition, such as depression. The patient is therefore treated with antidepressants and psychological counseling. The condition may persist through much of the bulimic's life, and management, rather than cure, is often the ultimate goal.

The reader may be aware of a friend, a family member, or a famous personality who has struggled with anorexia nervosa or bulimia.

➤ OBESITY

obesity
(ō-bē′-sĭ-tē)

The problem of **obesity** affects many people in our mechanized, modern society. Machines, appliances, and modes of transportation reduce the need for expending energy to obtain food. High-calorie foods that are attractively packaged are readily available and easy to prepare. Life-styles that include TV snacks, eating late at night, and a diet of "fast foods" contribute to the high incidence of obesity in the country.

Obesity is a nutritional disorder in which an abnormal amount of fat accumulates in adipose tissue. Adipose tissue is found under the skin, around organs such as the kidney, and in the omentum and mesentery of the peritoneal cavity. Adipose tissue acts as a reserve energy supply and as an insulating material against body heat loss. An excess of fat tissue is harmful, putting an undue strain on the heart and interfering with the contraction of muscles.

A person is considered obese if his or her weight is 15% to 20% more than the ideal weight given in standard life insurance height-weight tables. These tables give the proper weight ranges for men and women of light, medium, and heavy frames. A person is overweight if the upper limit of the appropriate range is exceeded.

Obesity develops when an excess (of calories) is consumed for the energy expended by a person. Too much food or too little exercise causes the deposition of fat. The rate of fat synthesis is faster than the mobilization of fat to active muscles for the production of energy.

on the Practical Side

Artificial Sweeteners
The popular artificial sweetener, Nutra Sweet (aspartame) is used in many soft drinks, foods, and for table use. Very small quantities of Nutra Sweet are required compared to table sugar (sucrose) because of its intense sweetness. This robust sweetness greatly reduces caloric intake.

The distribution of fat varies in males and females and may be genetically determined. Men accumulate fat in the upper trunk and not in the arms and legs, but women store fat in the lower trunk and in the arms and legs. Women also have more subcutaneous fat than men, which is probably an effect of the female sex hormones. Estrogen in birth control pills, for example, often causes a weight gain, primarily from water.

Causes of Obesity

Obesity generally results from overeating high-calorie foods—refined sugar and fats— and from insufficient exercise. Genetic factors are probably involved, as obese children tend to have parents who are overweight. Obesity that develops in children is due to the formation of an increased number of adipose cells, the number of which may be genetically determined.

Culture and environment also play a part in the obesity of children. Excessive intake of food may be encouraged, and, too often, good behavior is rewarded with foods such as cookies and candy. This overfeeding of children sets a regulatory system of the hypothalamus at a level that will maintain the habit of overeating.

The central nervous system regulates food intake. An area of the hypothalamus contains the "satiety center," which has an inhibiting effect on the "feeding center." The satiety center senses when enough food has been eaten, and it inhibits the feeding center from stimulating further food intake. Eating should be directed toward relieving genuine hunger. The obese person tends to eat because food is available, tastes good, or looks attractive.

Adult-onset obesity tends to result from an enlargement of already existing adipose cells rather than from an increase in their number. The number of adipose cells formed in childhood is irreversible and, for this reason, a child's diet should be carefully controlled to prevent excessive weight gain throughout life. Rarely is obesity caused by a hypoactive thyroid, a popular misconception. Excessive water retention is not a cause of obesity. Adipose cells, which are filled with fat, contain very little water.

Psychological factors can cause obesity if a person's reaction to stress often precipitates a desire for food as a means of satisfaction.

Diseases Aggravated by Obesity

Excessive weight poses many problems, both psychological and physical. The obese person feels unattractive and may become withdrawn. Children who are obese have difficulty participating in sports, are often teased about their weight, and are ridiculed by their peers.

Cardiovascular problems accompany obesity, and the death rate because of these ailments is significantly higher among the obese than among those who are not. Atherosclerosis develops as a result of the high level of serum lipids. Excessive fat deposits in heart muscle interfere with its contractions, the heart is overworked as it pumps blood through the extensive vascularity of the adipose tissue, and the left ventricle enlarges. Hypertension is often a complication of obesity.

Respiratory difficulties of hypoventilation with carbon dioxide retention occur when the chest wall cannot be moved adequately. Fat deposits interfere with contraction of the diaphragm and the other respiratory muscles. Inadequate oxygenation of the brain results in lethargy or somnolence.

Osteoarthritis, a degenerative joint disease, is aggravated by excessive weight. As will be explained in Chapter 17, osteoarthritis affects primarily weight-bearing joints: the knees, hips, and lower spine. Flat feet also worsen because of obesity.

Varicose veins frequently develop in the obese, as the excessive adipose tissue interferes with the return of blood from the legs. Diaphragmatic hernias and gallbladder disease are also more common in overweight people.

Adult-onset or Type II diabetes occurs far more often in those who are obese than in those who are not. A habit of excessive carbohydrate intake overtaxes the beta cells, the insulin-producing cells of the pancreas, and they cease functioning. One of the most serious complications of diabetes is atherosclerosis, to which obese people are already prone.

The liver is an important organ for the metabolism of fat, but when fat is in excess, metabolic disturbances occur, and fat accumulates in the liver. The fatty infiltration severely injures the liver cells, so they are no longer able to function. This condition is known as "fatty liver" and occurs in chronic alcoholism as well as in obesity. The complications of obesity are summarized in Figure 6–6.

Diagnosis and Treatment of Obesity

Comparison of a person's weight with the standard height-weight tables mentioned previously is the best way to diagnose obesity. Another mechanism to measure the thickness of subcutaneous fat is with an instrument called a skin-fold caliper. The percentage of body fat can then be determined using a special chart.

amphetamines
(ăm-fĕt′-ă-mēns)

Obesity is treated with diet, exercise programs, and drugs, but the most efficient method is diet. Appetite depressants, **amphetamines** and related compounds, may be prescribed at the beginning of a diet regimen while the patient is establishing new eating habits. The use of amphetamines must be carefully controlled to prevent side effects and possible addiction. These drugs can cause excessive nervousness, restlessness, insomnia, dry mouth, and constipation.

A good diet should be nutritionally balanced and include protein, some unsaturated fat, enough carbohydrate to provide glucose to the cells and to minimize the feeling of hunger, and vitamins and minerals. Reduction diets that consider the patient's size, sex, physical activity, and desired speed of weight loss are the most satisfactory. Women usually lose weight on a diet of 1000 to 1200 calories per day, and men lose on a diet of 1500 to 2000 calories.

Fad diets or crash diets are rarely successful and may even be harmful by causing malnutrition or metabolic disturbances. These diets do not help the obese person to change eating habits or train the appetite; weight lost on fad diets is generally regained.

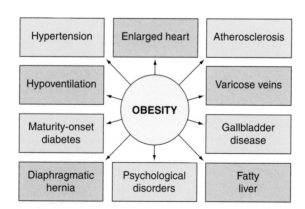

Figure 6–6
Complications of obesity.

The adipose cells are not destroyed with weight loss, but only shrink in size and readily increase in size with fat when the diet is stopped. An exercise program should accompany the reducing diet; the strenuousness of the exercise depends on the physical condition of the person. Moderate exertion is required to burn up calories, but even a regular program of walking can increase muscle tone.

Obesity is easier to prevent than to overcome. By establishing proper eating habits in childhood, an excessive number of adipose cells will not be formed if the diet is nutritionally high but calorically low. Control of diet is particularly important if a child has a genetic tendency toward obesity.

Excessive weight gain can occur during certain periods of childhood, infancy, early school age, and puberty. In women, pregnancy and the menopause are times when weight is easily gained, and special care should be taken to avoid excessive caloric intake. The avoidance of sugar in the form of pastries and soft drinks, and fat in cream, fried foods, gravy, and salad dressing will limit caloric intake and subsequent weight gain. Alcohol is also very high in calories—100 calories per ounce—and has no nutritional value.

Weight reduction in the overweight person dramatically improves the physical ailments associated with obesity. Blood pressure is reduced, the level of circulating lipids that cause atherosclerosis is lowered, and the distress of osteoarthritis is lessened. Diabetes is more easily controlled when excessive weight is lost. The self-image of the obese person who successfully loses weight is greatly improved, and the psychological change makes the effort worthwhile.

Nutrition and dieting seem to be of major importance in our high-tech, fast-paced world. Many energetic, highly driven individuals rigidly watch their diet, work out, jog, bike, and strive to be fit. However, in the U.S. there is also a culture of obesity, a culture of couch potatoes. Many of the obese start as babies or youngsters and continue that profile as adults. Consider the following facts.

"Obesity is epidemic in the U.S.," declares the Centers for Disease Control and Prevention in a recent survey. The Centers for Disease Control and Prevention defines obesity as having body mass 30% greater than the ideal body weight. Their data show that in the U.S. in 1991 about 1 in 8 persons were considered obese (12%). Data for 1998 show almost 1 in 5 are obese (17.9%). This change reflects a 50% increase in only 7 years and researchers are at a loss to explain it fully.

Yet, dieting is a typical New Year's resolution for many determined to shed extra pounds. Thousands of pounds need to be lost in order to have a healthier population. Sadly, for many in the U.S. and the world abundant calories are not accompanied by sufficient nutrients.

Malnutrition and starvation lead to many illnesses, both physical and mental and are a major cause of human suffering. Dietary deficiencies weaken, cripple, and kill youngsters and adults alike. If health care is inadequate for these individuals, many lives are lost. Malnourished populations become more vulnerable in times of internal political strife, cultural disputes, or war. Such turmoil in turn causes further breakdown of society that leads to more starvation and malnutrition. These problems tend to cross national borders, affecting many nations politically and economically. Nutrition is complicated indeed.

➤ ALCOHOLISM

Alcoholism is a serious disease with far-reaching consequences. It disrupts marriages, adversely affects children, and threatens job security. Physical damage to the alcoholic person is extensive, affecting the nervous system, the cardiovascular system, and the gastrointestinal tract particularly. The American Medical Association supports the following definition of alcoholism: "Alcoholism is an illness characterized by significant impairment that is directly associated with persistent and excessive use of alcohol. Impairment may involve physiological, psychological, or social dysfunction."

The alcoholic is totally dependent on the drug (alcohol) and centers life around it, making sure of an adequate supply and opportunity to drink. The use of other drugs with alcohol frequently compounds the problem. Most authorities agree that there is no single cause of alcoholism but that a combination of factors contribute to its onset and progression. There is no conclusive evidence that it is caused by a genetic factor.

Many psychological problems have been proposed as the cause of alcoholism: emotional disturbances during childhood, a feeling of insecurity, hostility, depression, and countless others. Although any of these factors may play a part in the complex etiology of alcoholism, none is considered the sole cause.

The sociological setting may be a factor in the development of the disease. In some circles, heavy drinking is considered a socially sanctioned behavior. Parties are not considered complete without alcohol, and often the host or hostess will encourage the guests to have "one more drink" when they have already had too much. The effects of alcohol on the nervous system include a feeling of relaxation and a release from anxieties, tension, and fears. As this experience is repeated through heavy drinking, alcohol becomes the habitual response to the problems of life.

Signs and Symptoms of Alcoholism

Alcoholism can have an insidious and gradual onset. The alcoholic generally experiences feelings of guilt and denies that drinking has become a problem. He or she begins to drink surreptitiously, drinks early in the day, and gulps down drinks when the opportunity arises. Periods of intoxication becomes regular and more serious, and blackouts are common, with periods of complete amnesia. Behavior becomes irresponsible, resulting in arrest for drunken driving, frequent absenteeism from work, and family problems. The alcoholic resents any discussion about drinking and generally resists treatment.

A physician may suspect alcoholism in a patient whose face is flushed and who shows a tremor about the mouth and tongue. Coarse tremors of the hands are observed, the patient may appear nervous and complain of digestive or motor disturbances. Further examination of the patient reveals other complications of alcohol abuse. Long-term abuse of alcohol takes its toll on the digestive system, the cardiovascular system, and the brain. Malnutrition often accompanies alcoholism depriving the patient of essential nutrients such as vitamins for cellular activity.

Effects of Excessive Alcohol on the Central Nervous System   Alcohol is a depressant on the central nervous system. Large quantities of alcohol interfere with the transmission of nerve impulses in the brain and affect coordination, speech, and judgment. A very high concentration of alcohol in the blood can even suppress the respiratory, cardiac, and vasomotor centers of the brain, causing shock and death.

The effect of alcohol on the central nervous system depends on the amount and the time span in which it was consumed. Alcohol is rapidly absorbed from the gastrointestinal tract into the blood. Some alcohol is absorbed from the stomach, but most is absorbed from the duodenum. Drinking "on an empty stomach" is not only irritating to the gastric mucosa, but the alcohol is more rapidly absorbed by the blood when there is nothing in the duodenum to delay gastric emptying.

Alcohol is carried to the liver through the portal vein and is then circulated through the body. Most metabolism and detoxification of alcohol actually occurs in the liver, but the rate of the reaction is limited. Enzymes convert alcohol to acetaldehyde and other fragments that are burned to produce energy. About one ounce of alcohol is metabolized per hour by the liver.

The effect of excessive alcohol ingestion wears off when it has been metabolized. This causes a period of nerve excitability, a release from the depressive effect, that accounts for the "morning-after" tremors. The effectiveness of another drink in overcoming the shakiness leads to a physical dependence on alcohol that becomes stronger as alcoholism progresses.

Long-term excessive consumption of alcohol can cause a condition known as the organic brain syndrome. Its manifestations include impaired judgment, poor powers of concentration, and memory lapses. The symptoms progress with continued drinking, but they may be reversed with abstinence.

Wernicke's encephalopathy is a brain disease often associated with chronic alcoholism, although it may have other causes such as thiamine deficiency. Wernicke's disease is a medical emergency in which the patient becomes mentally confused and disoriented and may suffer delirium tremens (DTs). Eye movements are abnormal and double vision may be experienced. **Nystagmus**—involuntary, rapid movement of the eyeball—is characteristic of the disease. The muscular coordination necessary for standing and walking is impaired. Treatment includes a highly nutritious diet and vitamin B supplements, particularly thiamine. If prompt treatment is administered, the symptoms can be reversed.

Thiamine, a B vitamin, is a coenzyme necessary for carbohydrate metabolism, and the lack of this vitamin particularly affects the cardiovascular and nervous systems. Nerve fibers become demyelinated, interfering with the transmission of nerve impulses. "Pins and needles" sensations are experienced, and the limbs become weak and numb. This can develop in chronic alcoholics who do not eat adequately. The effect on the nervous system causes mental confusion, an unsteady walk, and a paralysis of the muscles that move the eyes.

The effect of a niacin deficiency on the nervous system is variable, ranging from chronic depression to violent, irrational behavior. Degeneration of neurons in the brain results from the lack of this vitamin. Chronic alcoholics and drug addicts may develop the disease in the absence of adequate nutrition. The symptoms may be reversed through an improved diet and large doses of vitamin supplements.

Effects of Alcoholism on the Digestive System   Alcohol in excess is an irritant to the gastric mucosa, causing erosion and ulceration of the tissue. Gastritis is often a complication of alcoholism, as will be explained in Chapter 11. Ulceration that occurs because of the irritating effect of alcohol, particularly on an empty stomach, can lead to serious hemorrhaging. Some alcoholics experience nausea and vomiting in the morning after heavy drinking and are able to suppress the symptoms with another drink. This enables them to continue drinking during that day, and the cycle repeats itself.

Liver ailments caused by alcoholism are discussed in Chapter 12. Excessive alcohol has a toxic effect on the liver cells, causing tissue destruction and fibrosis. Alcoholic hepatitis and cirrhosis interfere with essential functions of the liver. Blood-clotting disturbances result from the inability of the liver to synthesize plasma proteins essential to coagulation, and hemorrhages in the gastrointestinal and urogenital tracts are common. Severe **ecchymoses**—hemorrhagic spots—develop in the skin and mucous membranes. **Epistaxis,** or bleeding from the nose, also results from the deficiency of proteins essential to clotting. **Esophageal varices,** described in Chapter 9, are a complication of cirrhosis and may lead to a fatal hemorrhage.

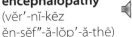
Wernicke's encephalopathy (vĕr'-nĭ-kēz ĕn-sĕf"-ă-lŏp'-ă-thē)

nystagmus (nĭs-tăg'-mŭs)

ecchymoses (ĕk-ĭ-mō'-sis)

epistaxis (ĕp"-ĭ-stăk'-sĭs)

esophageal varices (ē-sŏf"-ă-jē'-ăl văr'-ĭ-sēz)

gynecomastia
(jī″-nĕ-kō-măs′-tē-ă)

pancreatitis
(păn″-krē-ă-tī′-tĭs)

delirium tremens
(dē-lir′-ĭ-ŭm
trĕ′-mĭns)

Feminization of the male cirrhosis patient results from a hormonal imbalance. The nonfunctioning liver is unable to inactivate estrogen secreted by the adrenal cortex, and the hyperestrogenism that develops causes enlargement of the breasts (**gynecomastia**) and testicular atrophy. Pubic and axillary hair becomes sparse.

Pancreatitis, although it has other causes, is often related to chronic alcoholism (Chapter 12). The disease destroys the pancreas through enzymes that are abnormally released into the tissue. The patient generally experiences nausea, vomiting, and severe pain. As the pancreas becomes more and more necrotic, the likelihood of hemorrhaging increases. Treatment includes a nonirritating diet with no fat or alcohol.

Delirium tremens, DTs, is a medical emergency caused by heavy drinking over a long period of time and may occur after withdrawal from heavy alcohol intake. The symptoms include delirium with illusions and vivid hallucinations that are terrifying to the patient. The patient is extremely restless and shakes uncontrollably. The metabolic rate is increased, causing excessive sweating.

The patient with delirium tremens requires hospitalization in a quiet restful atmosphere. Attendants should show a calm, reassuring manner and observe the patient carefully to prevent self-injury. A comprehensive medical examination is essential to determine if there are any other complications, such as signs of heart failure or pneumonia. The patient is very susceptible to respiratory tract infections because of lowered resistance.

Fluid, electrolyte, and nutritional balance must be maintained, and this may require intravenous feeding. Sedation may be required, but it must be administered with caution to prevent overdosage. When the patient is able to take food, the diet should be high in protein and carbohydrates but low in fat and include vitamin B supplements. The complications of chronic alcoholism are summarized in Figure 6–7.

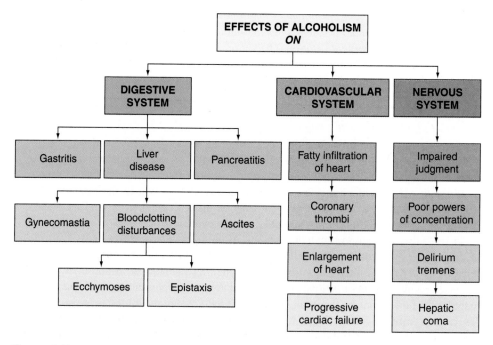

Figure 6–7
Complications of chronic alcoholism.

Hepatic coma develops in the final stages of advanced liver disease. This is caused by an accumulation of ammonia in the blood, which has a toxic effect on the brain. The ammonia accumulates when the liver is unable to detoxify it and form urea, the normal breakdown product of protein metabolism. The hepatic coma patient has periods of stupor or coma and manifests neurologic abnormalities. The flapping of outstretched arms is characteristic of the uncontrolled muscular contractions.

Oxygen or a combination of oxygen and carbon dioxide, the stimulus for the respiratory center of the brain, must be administered. Airways must be cleared using mechanical aids. If the patient is in shock, intravenous fluids or blood transfusions are required.

hepatic coma
(hĕ-păt′-ĭk kō′-mă)

Effects of Alcoholism on the Cardiovascular System Chronic alcoholism leads to progressive cardiac failure. Alcohol reduces the force of heart muscle contractions and an **arrhythmia,** (dysrhythmia) a deviation from the normal rhythm of the heart beat, develops. The heart enlarges, and **thrombi** (clots) frequently form in the coronary arteries. Fatty infiltration of the heart muscle generally occurs. If cirrhosis accompanies the alcoholism, circulation is impaired further as congestion develops in the veins. A severely damaged liver interferes with blood flow through the portal vein, causing a back pressure in the vessels emptying into it. This occurrence induces esophageal varices (mentioned previously).

arrhythmia
(ă-rĭth′-mē-ă)

thrombi
(thrŏm′-bī)

Alcohol and Pregnancy

There is an increasing awareness of how a mother's excessive consumption of alcohol during pregnancy affects the developing fetus. Alcohol readily diffuses into the bloodstream of the fetus through the placenta, just as nutrients and oxygen do. Because of its small size, the fetus is significantly affected by the alcohol and is likely to be born with physical and mental defects. The earliest weeks of pregnancy are the most critical for development and the most dangerous time for the mother to drink excessively.

Babies of alcoholic mothers are frequently born with fetal alcohol syndrome (FAS). Mental retardation is the most serious component of the syndrome, but physical growth before and after birth is also retarded. Heads tend to be smaller than those of normal babies, and limb and joint abnormalities are common. A characteristic facial appearance, particularly of the mouth and eyes, develops. The eye slits are small, the nose is short and pugged, and the jaws are underdeveloped. The babies are often born suffering withdrawal symptoms, manifested by stiffness and irritability. Fetal alcohol syndrome is most likely to occur if the mother has had a chronic drinking problem for many years.

Treatment of Alcoholism

Alcoholism is a treatable chronic disorder that is best controlled by early intervention and continuing attention. The treatment is directed toward enabling the alcohol-dependent patient to deal with problems and environment without using alcohol.

The best treatment for a particular alcoholic patient depends on the person. The patient may deny having a drinking problem and resist treatment for a time, but with the help of a physician, family member, employer, or friends, he or she may come to realize the need for assistance. Once the drinking problem has been recognized and the patient is willing to be treated, numerous facilities and resources are available.

Alcoholics Anonymous (AA) has been extremely effective for countless people and is very widespread geographically in its operation. Alcoholism Information Centers are listed locally and nationally. Many programs are offered for alcoholics by church organizations, the Veterans Administration, employers, and local community organizations.

The mental and physical health of the alcoholic patient determines the most appropriate type of treatment. A personal physician, a psychotherapist, group therapy, or behavior-modification programs are among the options. The emphasis is always directed toward rehabilitation.

Admission to a general or psychiatric hospital is often required for serious alcoholism problems. Comprehensive alcohol treatment centers are also available where the physical and mental problems of the alcoholic can be treated. Delirium tremens and hepatic coma are medical emergencies requiring hospitalization.

Other facilities include detoxification centers for the acutely intoxicated, who once would have been put in jail. Halfway houses or recovery houses are helpful for the alcoholic who is adjusting to coping with life without alcohol. Relapses occur, but as with any chronic illness, they should not indicate that the treatment has failed. The alcoholic who achieves control of the disease sees life in a new light and believes that the struggle was worth it.

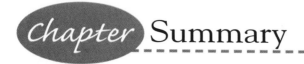

Chapter Summary

Malnutrition develops from a wide variety of causes: the unavailability of required nutrients, diseases that prevent use of ingested food, chronic alcoholism, eating unbalanced meals, and psychoneurotic disorders.

Vitamins are essential parts of cellular enzyme systems and must be obtained from fruits and vegetables because the body cannot synthesize them. Various diseases develop as a result of specific vitamin deficiencies.

A nutritional disease that has become increasingly recognized, especially among youths in this country, is anorexia nervosa, a condition resulting in starvation to the point of emaciation and even death. Psychoneurotic problems underlie the disease, and the individual has a misconception about proper body size and self-image, and envisions himself or herself as fat when, in fact, he or she is extremely thin.

Another problem related to food intake is obesity. Excessive eating and inadequate exercise are generally the causes of the problem. Obesity is a serious condition that adversely affects the cardiovascular and respiratory systems and may lead to adult-onset diabetes mellitus. Gallbladder disease and osteoarthritis are also aggravated by obesity.

The excessive consumption of alcohol over a prolonged period of time seriously impairs body functioning. Chronic alcoholism can lead to many diseases of the digestive system—gastritis, pancreatitis, cirrhosis of the liver—and is frequently accompanied by malnutrition. The cardiovascular system is affected together with the central nervous system. Manifestations of the effect of alcohol on the brain are impaired judgment, poor powers of concentration, and memory lapses. The medical emergencies, hepatic coma and delirium tremens, result from long-term alcohol abuse. Continued abuse of alcohol when pregnant may result in fetal alcohol syndrome (FAS), which produces an underweight child and sets the stage for future complications.

Treatment for the nutritional diseases discussed in this chapter is a balanced diet with adequate vitamin supplementation. Treatment for obesity includes diet, exercise, and, often, psychological counseling or group therapy. Alcoholism is treated medically and psychologically in a variety of ways, all of which are directed toward rehabilitation of the patient physically, mentally, and socially.

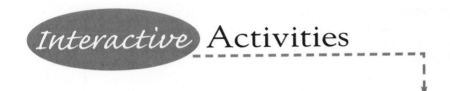

Interactive Activities

CASE FOR CRITICAL THINKING

An elderly, private man living alone was not able or interested in changing his simple diet of white bread, butter and cheap beer. After some years he notices that he tends to bruise easily, his gums bleed, his remaining teeth become loose, and he experiences overall weakness. What simple diet changes would improve his condition? Specifically what nutrient is required in this case? Would it have made any difference if wine were consumed instead of beer? Explain.

MULTIMEDIA EXTENSION ACTIVITIES

www.prenhall.com/mulvihill
Use the above address to access the free, interactive companion Website created for this textbook. Included in the features of this site are chapter specific activities, internet links, and an audio-glossary.

Audio Glossary
Use the CD-ROM disk enclosed with your textbook to hear the pronunciation of the key terms in this chapter.

Quick Self Study

MULTIPLE CHOICE

1. In women, anorexia nervosa is always accompanied by
   _____.
   a. Varicose veins   b. Goiter
   c. Amenorrhea   d. Tremors

2. An involuntary, rapid movement of the eyeball is called _____.
   a. Epistaxis   b. Nystagmus
   c. Conjunctiva   d. Osteomalacia

3. An accumulation of ammonia in the blood results in _____.
   a. Arrhythmia   b. Collagen
   c. Hypercalcemia   d. Hepatic coma

4. Blood clotting is facilitated by _____.
   a. Vitamin K   b. Glycogen
   c. Vitamin D   d. Potassium

TRUE OR FALSE

_____ 1. Vitamin A contributes to the integrity of mucous membranes.

_____ 2. An anorexia nervosa patient suffers from a severe vitamin deficiency.

_____ 3. High acidity causes tooth decay in bulimia.

_____ 4. Lack of calcium causes goiter.

_____ 5. Obesity in adults results from formation of new adipose cells.

FILL-INS

1. Night blindness is caused by a lack of vitamin _____.

2. A lack of vitamin D in adults results in a softening of the bones called
   _____.

3. Bleeding gums are caused by a lack of _____.

4. Weak muscles are a sign of a _____ deficiency.

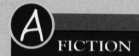

FICTION

It is true that beans are generally low in fat. Along with nuts and seeds, beans are a great source of fiber, protein, and vitamins. However, many types of nuts and seeds are high in fat and, therefore, high in calories. So, watch out for the choices at the salad bar, and your diet.

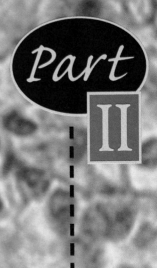

Diseases of the Systems

Part II

Each system can malfunction in its own unique way. Part II describes the normal structure and function of each system, and relates the diseases of the system to an organ or system failure.

chapters ←

Microscopic Image of a Kidney Carcinoma

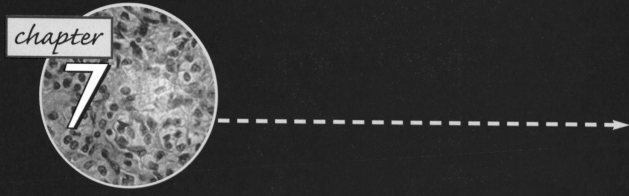

Diseases of the Blood

Our life depends on an adequate blood supply to all body tissues.
Blood distributes oxygen, nutrients, salts, and hormones to the cells
and carries away the waste products of cellular metabolism. Blood
also provides a line of defense against infection, toxic substances, and
foreign antigens.

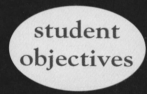

student
objectives

After studying this chapter, students should be able to

➤ Describe the cellular composition of blood
➤ Distinguish the causes and characteristics of the anemias
➤ List the detrimental effects of anemia
➤ Describe the detrimental effects and treatment of polycythemia
➤ Explain the causes, symptoms, and treatment of red blood cell abnormalities
➤ Define thrombocytopenia and idiopathic thrombocytopenia
➤ Define and distinguish among the different types of leukemias and
lymphomas
➤ Describe the general diagnostic procedures used to identify blood diseases

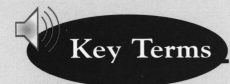

Key Terms

Allogenic

Anemia

Aplastic anemia

Autologous

Basophil

Bilirubin

Cobalamin

Crohn's disease

Dyspnea

Ecchymoses

Eosinophils

Erythrocytes

Erythropoiesis

Erythropoietin

Hematocrit

Hematoma

Hemoglobin

Hemolysis

Hemostasis

Hodgkin's disease

Hypochromic

Idiopathic
thrombocytopenia
purpura

Intrinsic factor

Jaundiced

Leukemia

Leukocytes

Lymphadenopathy

Lymphocytes

Lymphocytic

Lymphomas

Monocytes

Myelogenous

Neutrophil

Normoblasts

Partial thromboplastin
time

Pernicious anemia

Petechiae

Phlebotomy

Platelets

Proerythroblasts

Prothrombin time

Reticulocyte

Sickle cell anemia

Splenomegaly

Spheroidal

Thrombocytes

Thrombocytopenia

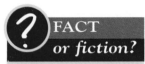

erythrocytes
(ĕ-rĭth′-rō-sīts)

leukocytes
(loo′-kō-sīts)

platelets
(plāt′-lets)

hematocrit
(hē″-măt′-ō-krĭt)

hemoglobin
(hē″-mō-glō′-bĭn)

neutrophil
(nū′-trō-fĭl)

lymphocytes
(lĭm′-fō-sīts)

monocytes
(mŏn′-ō-sīts)

eosinophils
(ē″-ŏ-sĭn′-ō-fĭls)

basophil
(bā′-sō-fĭl)

thrombocytes
(thrŏm′-bō-sīts)

hemostasis
(hē-măs′-tā-sĭs)

erythropoiesis
(ē-rĭth″-rō-poy-ē′-sĭs)

erythropoietin
(ĕ-rĭth″-rō-poy-ĕ-tĭn)

proerythroblasts
(prō″-ĕ-rĭth′-rō-blăsts)

normoblasts
(nor′-mō-blăsts)

reticulocyte
(rĕ-tĭk′-ū-lo-sīt)

➤ COMPOSITION OF BLOOD

The cellular components of blood are red blood cells or **erythrocytes,** white blood cells or **leukocytes,** and clotting elements or **platelets.** All are suspended in the plasma or the fluid portion of circulating blood. These formed elements comprise about 45% of the blood, and plasma comprises the remaining 55%. The ratio of red blood cell-volume to whole blood is called **hematocrit.**

Red bone marrow and lymph nodes are the blood-forming tissues of the body. Erythrocytes and platelets are formed in the red marrow. Leukocytes are formed in both red marrow and lymph tissue.

Red blood cells make up about half of the blood's volume. Erythrocytes are filled with **hemoglobin,** which enables them to carry oxygen from the lungs to all body tissues. Mature red blood cells are biconcave and possess no nucleus. Erythrocytes normally number about 5 million/mm^3 of blood in males, and about 4.5 million/mm^3 of blood in females.

White blood cells, the leukocytes, are fewer in number. There are five main types of white cells that provide the mechanisms for fighting infections. **Neutrophils** are the most prevalent white blood cells and help protect the body against bacterial and fungal infections. **Lymphocytes** consist of T-lymphocytes and B-lymphocytes. T-lymphocytes kill virus-infected cells, tumor cells, and foreign tissues; B-lymphocytes develop into cells that produce antibodies. **Monocytes** ingest dead cells and protect the body against many infective organisms. **Eosinophils** kill parasites and are involved in allergic responses. **Basophils** promote inflammation and participate in allergic responses (see Chapter 2).

Platelets or **thrombocytes** initiate blood clotting. As a part of the blood's protective mechanism for **hemostasis,** platelets gather at a bleeding site where they are activated to arrest bleeding.

➤ RED BLOOD CELL FORMATION

The process of red cell formation is called **erythropoiesis.** This takes place in the red marrow of flat bones such as the sternum, hip bones, ribs, and skull bones. A hormone, **erythropoietin,** synthesized principally by the kidney, stimulates this cell development. As erythrocytes mature, they go through several stages before entering the circulation. They begin as large, nucleated, primitive cells called **proerythroblasts** and, at this stage, possess no hemoglobin. The proerythroblasts multiply, but daughter cells, called erythroblasts, are small. The **normoblasts** contain a nucleus, but it begins to shrink as the cytoplasm fills with hemoglobin synthesized by the endoplasmic reticulum. The nucleus is eventually digested and absorbed, and the cell is then called a **reticulocyte.** When the reticulum is lost, the cells become mature erythrocytes ready to circulate. Figure 7–1 il-

Disease by the Numbers ✕ + ÷

EPIDEMIOLOGY

Anemia affects about 4 million Americans. In people younger than age 65, approximately six times as many women as men have anemia.

Reference: Mayo Clinic Health Information. August, 1999.

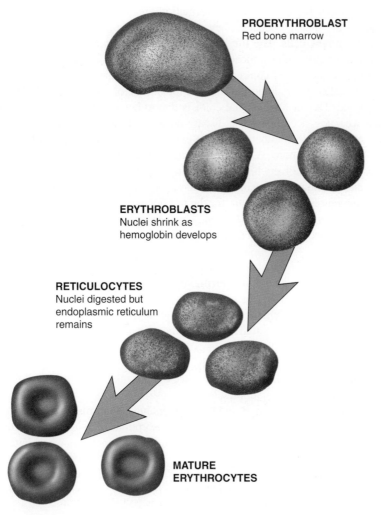

PROERYTHROBLAST
Red bone marrow

ERYTHROBLASTS
Nuclei shrink as
hemoglobin develops

RETICULOCYTES
Nuclei digested but
endoplasmic reticulum
remains

**MATURE
ERYTHROCYTES**

Figure 7–1
Red cell development—erythropoiesis.

lustrates red blood cell formation. Maturation of erythrocytes is more a degenerative process than one of differentiation, which makes these cells unique. Understanding this developmental pattern is important because certain serious blood conditions are evident when immature red cells, normoblasts, or reticulocytes, are found in the circulation. Examples of these conditions will be discussed.

➤ THE ANEMIAS

One of the most common blood diseases is anemia. Although there are many kinds of anemia and as many causes, there is one common denominator: a reduction in the amount of oxygen-carrying hemoglobin. **Anemia** can result from a loss of red blood cells due to prolonged bleeding (hemorrhage), or rupture of the cells, **hemolysis.** Anemia can also be caused by the improper formation of new red blood cells, which can be the result of poorly functioning bone marrow or an iron or vitamin deficiency. The most critical

anemia
(ăn-nē′-mĭ-ă)

hemolysis
(hē-mŏl′-ĭ-sĭs)

nutrients required for red blood cell formation are iron, vitamin B_{12}, and folic acid. Erythrocytes are unusual because they do not possess a nucleus and, therefore, cannot divide to form new cells. The life span of red blood cells is about 120 days, and new cells must constantly replace those that die.

Certain symptoms are common to all anemias. The anemic person is generally pale (a condition called *pallor*) and the mucous membrane of the mouth is light in color, as is the nail bed. This lack of normal color is due to hemoglobin deficiency. Fatigue and muscular weakness accompany the disease because of the inadequate oxygen supply to the cells and tissues. The anemic person experiences **dyspnea,** or shortness of breath. To meet the need for more oxygen, the respiration rate is quickened and the patient experiences palpitations of the heart as it attempts to pump more blood to the tissues.

dyspnea
(dĭsp-nē′-ă)

The anemias may be classified in several ways; they will be considered here on the basis of their causes. It is important for the physician to diagnose the cause of a patient's anemia, for this is what must be treated. The iron prescribed appropriately for one type of anemia is ineffective, even harmful, for another type.

Vitamin B_{12} Deficiency Anemia

pernicious anemia
(pĕr-nĭsh′-ŭs ă-nē-mē-ă)

cobalamin
(kō-bawl′-ă-mĭn)

intrinsic factor
(ĭn-trĭn′-sĭk făk′-tŭr)

Crohn's disease
(krōnzs dĭ-zēz)

Vitamin B_{12} deficiency anemia or **pernicious anemia** is caused by inadequate absorption or intake of vitamin B_{12} or **cobalamin.** Vitamin B_{12} is normally absorbed in the small intestine by the **intrinsic factor.** Intrinsic factor is produced in the stomach and carries vitamin B_{12} to the small intestine where it is absorbed into the bloodstream. Without intrinsic factor, vitamin B_{12} is excreted in the stool.

Vitamin B_{12} in the diet comes only from animal sources. Strict vegetarians who avoid all animal products including milk, cheese, eggs, and meat will develop pernicious anemia unless they take B_{12} supplements.

Other causes of vitamin B_{12} deficiency include abnormal bacterial growth that prevents absorption, diseases that result in malabsorption, such as **Crohn's disease** (see Chapter 11), and removal of part of the stomach or small intestine where vitamin B_{12} is absorbed.

The signs of pernicious anemia are a low red blood cell count, disturbances of the nervous system, a peculiar yellow and blue color blindness, a sore burning tongue, weight loss, and confusion.

Replacing vitamin B_{12} effectively treats pernicious anemia. Because vitamin B_{12} cannot be absorbed into the bloodstream, it must be replaced by injection. Vitamin B_{12} supplementation is required for life.

Iron Deficiency Anemia

Iron deficiency is one of the most common causes of anemia. Normally the body recycles iron. When red blood cells die, the iron in them is returned to the bone marrow to be used again in formation of new red blood cells. Iron deficiency anemia can result from excessive blood loss from an ulcer, malignant lesions, or monthly menstrual bleed. A diet deficient in iron may cause this anemia, especially in infants, children, and pregnant women.

hypochromic
(hī″-pō-krō′-mĭk)

Iron deficiency causes the red blood cells to appear lighter than normal or **hypochromic.** Hemoglobin is a protein containing iron and serves as the oxygen-carrier protein giving blood its characteristic color.

The first step in treating iron deficiency anemia is to identify and correct the cause of bleeding. Surgery may be required to repair a bleeding ulcer or to stop excessive menstrual bleeding. Oral and injectable iron supplements are effective in replacing the lost iron (see Figures 7–2 and 7–3).

side by side

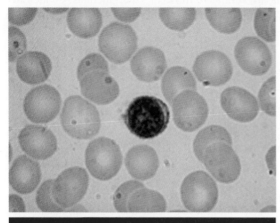

Figure 7–2

Normal red blood cells.

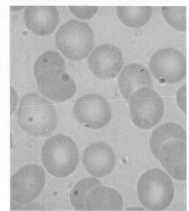

Figure 7–3

Iron deficiency anemia blood cells.

Folic Acid Deficiency Anemia

Folic acid is found in raw vegetables, fresh fruit, and meat. Folic acid deficiency is most common in the western world where consumption of raw vegetables is low. Other causes of folic acid deficiency include malabsorption due to chronic diseases, alcoholism, pregnancy, and use of certain medications.

Measurement of decreased folic acid levels in the blood is conclusive for folic acid deficiency anemia. Oral folic acid supplementation is effective in replacing folic acid. Supplementation for life is needed for those who have trouble absorbing folic acid.

PREVENTION *PLUS!*

The minimum daily adult requirement of folic acid is 50 μg, but because absorption from food is incomplete, a daily intake of 200 μg is recommended.

Hemolytic Anemia

Hemolytic anemia results from excessive destruction of red blood cells. With hemolysis or destruction of red cells, hemoglobin is released into the plasma. The hemoglobin breaks down, yielding a colored pigment, **bilirubin,** which is normally detoxified by the liver and converted into bile. This pigment is orange, and as it accumulates in the plasma, it causes a **jaundiced** or yellow-orange appearance in the tissues.

A number of factors can increase destruction of red blood cells. Normally, when red blood cells get old, scavenger cells in the bone marrow, spleen, and liver destroy them. The spleen can enlarge and increase destruction of red blood cells. Antibodies produced by the immune system may bind to red blood cells and destroy them in an autoimmune reaction (see Chapter 2). Red blood cells may be destroyed because of

bilirubin
(bĭl-ĭ-rōō′-bĭn)

jaundiced
(jon′-dĭsd)

abnormalities in the cells themselves either in shape, function, or hemoglobin content. Various drugs can cause hemolysis of red blood cells.

Symptoms of hemolytic anemia are similar to those of other anemias. Sudden hemolysis results in sudden fevers, chills, lightheadedness, and a significant drop in blood pressure.

➤ RED BLOOD CELL ABNORMALITIES

Sickle Cell Anemia

sickle cell anemia

(sĭk′-ŭl sĕl
ă-nē-mē-ă)

Sickle cell anemia is an inherited condition characterized by sickle-shaped red blood cells and chronic hemolytic anemia. Sickle cell disease is generally confined to African-Americans. Neither the hemoglobin molecule nor the red blood cell itself can form properly. Sickling only occurs when the cells release oxygen; they return to the normal biconcave shape after picking up oxygen. After many cycles of unloading and loading oxygen, an individual cell becomes permanently sickled and destroyed. The rapid destruction of erythrocytes stimulates production of new red cells but at a rate faster than they can mature (see Figure 7–4). As a result, many reticulocytes and nucleated red cells enter the circulation.

The symptoms of sickle cell anemia include jaundice of the sclera (the white of the eye); pain in the arms, legs, and abdomen; and recurrent fever. In a crisis period, headache, paralysis, and convulsions can develop from a cerebral blood clot that forms as a result of the abnormally viscous blood.

Most people with sickle cell disease initially develop an enlarged spleen. As the spleen becomes injured by trapped sickled cells, it shrinks and no longer functions. Because the spleen helps fight infection, bacterial and viral infections frequently occur.

Sickle cell anemia cannot be cured. Treatment is aimed at preventing sickle crises, controlling the anemia, and relieving symptoms.

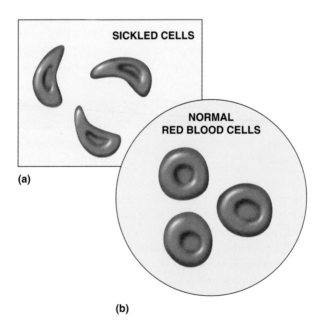

Figure 7–4
Sickled red blood cells (a) compared with normal red blood cells (b).

Hereditary Spherocytosis

Spheroidal or spherocytic anemia is an inherited disorder that results in spherical red blood cells rather than biconcave or disk-shaped. The abnormal shape of the cell makes it fragile and susceptible to rupture. A characteristic sign of this disease is jaundice caused by the release of hemoglobin, which is processed by the liver, forming excess bilirubin. The spleen becomes enlarged, **splenomegaly,** due to an accumulation of red cells, many of which are immature. The immature cells result from hyperactivity of the bone marrow as it attempts to compensate for the red cell destruction.

Treatment of spherocytic anemia is not needed for mild cases. Splenectomy, a removal of the spleen for severe cases reduces the number of cells that are destroyed, but it increases susceptibility to infection because defense provided by the spleen is lost.

Hemolytic anemias can be acquired. An allergic reaction to drugs such as the sulfonamides may cause this condition. The malarial parasite also causes hemolysis of red cells and severe anemia.

spheroidal
(sfir'-oi-dawl)

splenomegaly
(splē"-nō-mĕg'-ă-lē)

➤ APLASTIC ANEMIA

If the bone marrow fails to function, another type of anemia, **aplastic anemia,** results. The bone marrow stops producing erythrocytes, leukocytes, and platelets. The person then is not only anemic but cannot fight infection, a leukocytic function, and has a bleeding tendency due to platelet depletion. Exposure to excessive radiation, certain drugs, and industrial poisons can cause the bone marrow to stop functioning. This is a very serious condition that may or may not be reversed. Regular transfusion of red blood cells, white blood cells, and platelets are necessary. Regular injections of medications that stimulate the production of red blood cells and white blood cells are also beneficial.

aplastic anemia
(ă-plăs'-tĭc
ă-nē'-mē-ă)

➤ EXCESSIVE RED BLOOD CELLS

Polycythemia

Polycythemia is a disorder in which there is excessive production of red blood cells. This disorder is rare and is generally initiated by tumors that cause hyperactivity of the bone marrow. In polycythemia, the erythrocytes can number 7 to 11 million/mm^3 of blood. The hematocrit of a person with polycythemia may be as high as 70 to 80% compared with the normal of 45%. The elevated count increases blood volume; this raises the blood pressure, placing an increased workload on the heart. Blood flow is reduced because of increased viscosity and a tendency to clot. The excessive number of red cells gives the skin a purplish appearance. Mucous membranes are extremely red, and the eyes appear bloodshot. The spleen, a reservoir for erythrocytes, is always enlarged. Leukocytes and platelets, also produced in the bone marrow, show elevated counts. Treatment is aimed at correcting the underlying cause, reducing the red cell count and the blood volume. Periodic bloodletting **(phlebotomy)** is used to reduce the volume, and radiation therapy is used to decease red cell production.

phlebotomy
(flĕ-bŏt'-ŭ-mē)

➤ BLEEDING DISEASES

Hemophilia

Hemophilia is a bleeding disorder that results from a deficiency of clotting factors. In classic hemophilia, hemophilia A, there is a deficiency in clotting factor VIII. A deficiency of clotting factor IX is seen in hemophilia B. It is strictly a hereditary disease that generally affects males. A female may have the disease, inherited from a mother who is a carrier and a father who has hemophilia. This is rare but possible (see Chapter 5).

The hemophiliac can experience several episodes of prolonged and severe bleeding from minor cuts or injury. Injections into a muscle can result in a large bruise or **hematoma.** Excessive bleeding in the joints and muscles ultimately leads to joint abnormalities.

People with hemophilia should avoid situations that may provoke bleeding. Treatment involves transfusions of whole blood or plasma and injections of clotting factors.

hematoma
(hē″-mă-tō′-mă)

Thrombocytopenia

A deficiency in the number of platelets, which initiate the blood-clotting process, causes spontaneous hemorrhages in the skin (Figure 7–5), mucous membranes of the mouth, and internal organs. Small, flat, red spots called **petechiae,** appear, or larger hemorrhagic areas **(ecchymoses),** may develop. Gastrointestinal and urogenital hemorrhages, as well as severe nosebleeds, may also occur. The disease is known as **thrombocytopenia.** Thrombocyte is another name for platelet, and the suffix, *penia,* means a scarcity.

The disease may result from impaired platelet production, antibodies to platelets, or an allergic response to drugs. Thrombocytopenia may also be idiopathic, that is, of unknown origin. In the latter case, the patient may have a history of bleeding after injury or minor surgery, such as a tooth extraction. The condition is referred to as **ITP,** for **idiopathic thrombocytopenia purpura.**

Thrombocytopenia caused by allergic reactions to drugs can be corrected by stopping the drug. Bedrest is helpful to avoid accidental injury. Platelet transfusions are needed when the platelet count is critically low or if the thrombocytopenia results from impaired platelet production.

petechiae
(pĕ-tē′-kē-ī)

ecchymoses
(ĕk′-ĭ-mō″-sĕs)

thrombocytopenia
(thrŏm′-bō-sī-tŭ-pē″-nē-ŭ)

idiopathic
thrombocytopenia
purpura
(ĭd′-ē-ō-păth″-ĭk
thrŏm″-bō-sī″-pē′-nē-ă
pŭr-pū-ră)

➤ DISEASES OF WHITE BLOOD CELLS

Leukemia

Leukemia is a cancer of white blood cells or leukocytes. Leukemia means *white blood* in Greek. In this disease, the bone marrow produces a large number of abnormal white

leukemia
(loo-kē′-mē-ă)

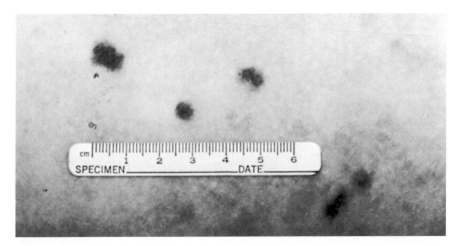

Figure 7–5
Photograph of ecchymotic hemorrhages in the skin. (*Courtesy of Dr. David R. Duffell.*)

blood cells. The leukocyte count is extremely elevated from the normal range of about 5000 to 10,000 mm^3 of blood to 200,000 to 1 million/mm^3 of blood. (Reference: *Laboratory Medicine,* Volume 30, Number 7, July, 1999.)

The signs and symptoms of leukemia include fever, swollen lymph nodes, **lymphadenopathy,** joint pain, and abnormal bleeding. Anemia, with its manifestation of weakness, shortness of breath, and heart palpitation, accompanies the leukemia. Red blood cell production is severely reduced by the overproduction of malignant white cells inasmuch as both types come from the same stem cells in the malignant bone marrow. Organs where blood is stored, the spleen and liver, become greatly enlarged with the infiltration of white cells. Figure 7–6 summarizes signs and symptoms of leukemia.

The cancerous tissues grow at a rapid rate, using up the body's nutrients, thus causing weight loss. White blood cells, the principal cells in fighting infection, are produced faster than they mature, so they are unable to fight infection normally. The person becomes

lymphadenopathy
(lĭmf-ăd′-ĭn-ŏp″-ŭ-thē)

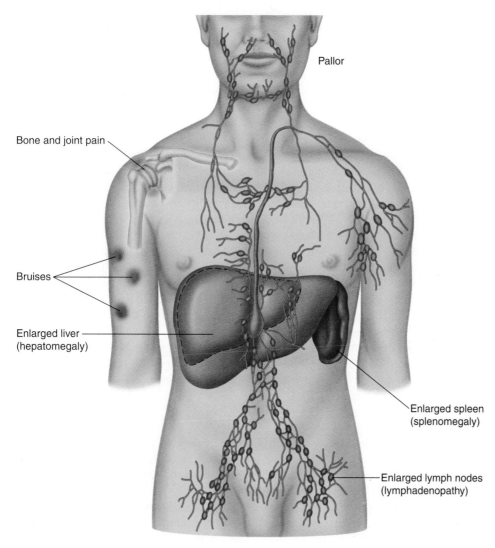

Figure 7–6
Signs and symptoms of leukemia.

highly susceptible to infection and must be protected against exposure to bacteria. As the number of leukocytes increases, the number of platelets decreases; this interferes with the blood-clotting mechanism, causing a tendency to hemorrhage and to bruise.

The two main types of leukemia are named on the basis of the site of the malignancy. If the cancer originates in the bone marrow, it is called **myelogenous** leukemia; the primitive white cells in this tissue are called *myelocytes*. In myelogenous leukemia, it is the granulocytes that are greatly increased, whereas both red blood cell and platelet production are decreased.

The other type of leukemia is **lymphocytic** leukemia and results from cancer of the lymphocytic stem cells, which are found both in the bone marrow and in the lymph nodes. The lymphocytes in this case are the only white cells that are increased, but they become disproportionately high in number and are immature and ineffective. Figure 7–7 gives a comparison of leukemia types.

The cause of leukemia is unknown, but it may be due to a virus, or exposure to radiation may be a factor. A high incidence of leukemia has been found in people exposed to fallout from nuclear weapons. Heredity may also play a part in its etiology.

Both kinds of leukemia can be chronic or acute. Acute lymphocytic leukemia is the more common form in children. Acute forms of leukemia produce immature cells that do not perform the normal white blood cell functions. Because the blood is filled with immature cell, the course of the disease is more swift (hence, acute). Acute lymphocytic leukemia has an abrupt onset and progresses rapidly. Acute myelogenous leukemia is more common in adults. Chronic forms of leukemia produce cells that undergo some maturation and are at least partially functional. Because the cells do function, the disease is slow to develop and is often discovered by accident, during routine blood tests. It also has a longer (hence, chronic) course.

Progress is being made in controlling leukemia and even curing it. Treatment goals include eliminating leukemic cells through chemotherapy and the use of antineoplastic agents to inhibit growth of cancerous tissue. The patient's ability to tolerate adverse affects of treatment is enhanced and psychosocial support is given. There are three stages of chemotherapy treatment—induction, consolidation, and maintenance. The induction stage utilizes intensive chemotherapy to induce complete remission. The largest number of leukemic cells are destroyed at this time. Intermittent cycles of chemotherapy are given during the consolidation stage to eliminate any remaining leukemic cells. If complete remission is achieved, the patient enters the maintenance stage, which is designed to continue the remission. Low doses of chemotherapeutic agents given in combination every 3 to 4 weeks prevent leukemic cells from returning to the bone marrow.

Depending on the type of leukemia, 50 to 90% complete remission is possible, which means that there is no evidence of the leukemia in serum studies and the bone marrow returns to normal.

Malignant Lymphomas

Lymphomas include several types of malignancies of the lymphatic system. The lymphatic system carries infection-fighting lymphocytes through lymph vessels to all parts of the body. Cancerous lymphocytes or **lymphoma cells** can be confined to a single lymph node or can spread to any organ of the body.

The two major types of lymphoma are **Hodgkin's disease** and non-Hodgkin's lymphoma. Hodgkin's disease is distinguished by the presence of characteristic *Reed-Sternberg* cells in affected lymph nodes. These cells are large, cancerous lymphocytes that have more than one nucleus. Non-Hodgkin's lymphoma originates in the lymphatic system and usually spreads throughout the body. These lymphomas may progress slowly over many years or rapidly in a few months.

myelogenous
(mī-ĕ-lō-jĕn′-ŭs)

lymphocytic
(lĭm′-fō-sĭt-ĭk)

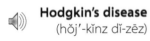

lymphomas
(lĭm-fō′-măs)

Hodgkin's disease
(hŏj′-kĭnz dĭ-zēz)

TYPE	INCIDENCE	SIGNS AND SYMPTOMS	PROGNOSIS	MALIGNANT CELLS
Acute myelogenous leukemia (AML)	Most common nonlymphocytic leukemia Usually develops in persons between ages 30 and 60 Slightly more common in men	Usual: anemia, pallor, fatigue, weakness, fever Possible: bleeding, bruising, bone and joint pain, headache, enlarged lymph nodes, liver and spleen, recurrent infections	Generally poor Death usually results from infection or hemorrhage	Granulocytes (neutrophils, eosinophils, and basophils)
Acute lymphocytic leukemia (ALL)	Most common cancer in children Usually diagnosed before age 14 (peak incidence between ages 2 and 9) Males slightly more affected than females	Usual: anemia, pallor, fatigue, weakness, swollen lymph nodes, recurrent infections Possible: bleeding, bruising, and headache	Generally good (initial treatment usually induces remission in 95% of patients) Overall cure rate is 50%	Lymphocytes
Chronic myelogenous leukemia (CML)	About 20% of blood cancers Usually affects adults between ages 40 and 60	Usual: loss of appetite, weight loss, fatigue, weakness, enlarged spleen and liver Possible: bleeding, bruising, bone and joint pain, fever, enlarged lymph nodes	Generally poor Average survival time of 3 years No treatment produces satisfactory results	Granulocytes
Chronic lymphocytic leukemia (CLL)	Most common form of blood cancer in industrial countries Affects primarily older adults, males more frequently than women	Usual: loss of weight, enlarged lymph nodes and spleen Possible: fever	Depends on patient's age, signs, and symptoms Median survival time is 4 to 6 years	B lymphocytes

Figure 7–7
Comparison of leukemia types.

The causes of lymphomas are unknown, although viral infections are suspect. Non-Hodgkin's lymphoma is a complication of AIDS.

Signs and symptoms of lymphomas are painless, swollen lymph nodes, fever, and weight loss. The likelihood of cure depends on the type of lymphoma. Chemotherapy, radiation, and bone marrow transplants are helpful in bringing these diseases into remission. The cure rate increases if the disease is detected and treated early.

on the Practical Side

Bone Marrow Transplantation

Bone marrow transplantation is now being used effectively to treat leukemia, non-Hodgkin's lymphoma, Hodgkin's disease, and other diseases of blood-forming tissues. The type of bone marrow transplant depends on who donates the bone marrow. **Autologous** transplants allow the patient to donate his/her own bone marrow. Only 30% of patients who need **allogenic** or donor transplants have suitable, genetically matched donors. Recent advances in technology reduce the need for a match between the donor and the recipient. Certain cells of the immune system, T lymphocytes, which would cause rejection, are removed from the donor's bone marrow. The remaining suspension of normal bone marrow cells is given like a blood transfusion. The cells enter the general circulation of the recipient and grow in the bone marrow cavities.

autologous
(ăw-tŏl'-ō-gŭs)

allogenic
(al'-ō-jĕn'-ĭk)

➤ DIAGNOSTIC PROCEDURES FOR BLOOD DISEASES

Blood tests are extremely significant diagnostically for systemic diseases as well as specific blood conditions. Blood tests reveal cholesterol levels, important enzyme levels, electrolyte (salt) balances as well as blood components.

A bone marrow smear may be done when certain blood disorders are suspected. The smear is obtained by introducing a sharp needle into the bone marrow cavity (usually of the iliac crest) and withdrawing a sample of the marrow. The test shows if the bone marrow is adequately manufacturing normal red and white blood cells and platelets. The smear is particularly helpful in diagnosing aplastic and pernicious anemias, leukemia, and purpura when used in conjunction with other tests.

A total white blood cell count (WBC) can suggest infection or inflammation as well as a serious blood disease. Additional testing is required if warranted by the clinical condition of the patient.

A differential white blood cell count can reveal abnormalities in the ratio of leukocyte types. Figure 7–8 lists conditions indicated by an increased number of specific leukocyte types.

Important tests in the determination of anemia and polycythemia are the red blood cell count (RBC) and hematocrit or packed red cell volume (PCV). The word *hematocrit* means to separate blood, which is done when a blood sample is centrifuged to separate cells from plasma. The ratio of red blood cells to the total sample roughly meas-

TYPE OF LEUKOCYTE INCREASED	CAUSE
Neutrophils	Acute bacterial infections, inflammatory disorders, certain drugs, stress
Eosinophils	Allergies, parasitic infestations
Lymphocytes	Viral infections
Monocytes	Chronic severe infections when controlled

Figure 7–8
Conditions indicated by an increased number of specific leukocyte types.

ures the concentration of erythrocytes. Hemoglobin content of a venous blood sample can be determined in several ways and is expressed in grams of Hb/100 ml blood. A variety of laboratory tests are used to determine the nature and extent of coagulation disorders. Platelet counts on a blood smear are often checked in those who have thrombocytopenia. Testing the activity of factors VIII and IX is used to determine the type and severity of hemophilia. Bleeding time or **prothrombin time** or **partial thromboplastin time** measures defects in coagulation. Bleeding time is prolonged in thrombocytopenia, severe liver disease, leukemia, and aplastic anemia.

prothrombin time
(prō-thrŏm′-bĭn tīm)

partial thromboplastin time
(pǎr′-shāl thrŏm″-bō-plăs′-tĭn tīm)

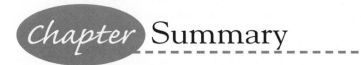

Chapter Summary

The principal diseases of the blood considered have been those involving erythrocytes, leukocytes, and platelets. Each of these formed elements of the blood has a specific function. If any is insufficient in number, improperly formed, or immature, that function cannot be adequately performed. In distinguishing the various anemias, the symptoms were related to their cause, and the best treatment for each was explained. The inability to clot blood and prevent hemorrhaging was seen in hemophilia. In one, a protein factor in plasma was lacking, and in the other, platelets were too few in number. A malignancy of blood-forming tissues and blood cells causes leukemia. Its complications of anemia, susceptibility to infection, and a tendency to hemorrhage were considered. The incidence, signs and symptoms, and the prognosis of the various leukemias were compared. Malignant lymphomas were classified, the most common of which is Hodgkin's disease. Finally, the significance of the various blood tests was explained.

Diseases at a Glance: Diseases of the Blood

Categories	Disease	Signs and Symptoms
Malignancies	Myelogenous leukemia	Fever, swollen lymph nodes, lymphadenopathy, joint pain, abnormal bleeding, anemia, pallor
	Lymphocytic leukemia	Fever, swollen lymph nodes, lymphadenopathy, joint pain, abnormal bleeding, anemia, pallor
	Lymphoma	Enlarged, painless lymph nodes
	Hodgkin's disease	Enlarged, painless lumps, usually in neck, intermittent fever, anemia, weakness
Other abnormal structure/function	Polycythemia	Purplish skin, red mucous membranes, eyes bloodshot, splenomegaly, increased blood pressure
	Hemophilia	Bleeding in joints, with swelling and intense pain, excessive bleeding
	Purpura thrombocytopenia	Spontaneous hemorrhages, petechiae, ecchymosis, nosebleed, internal hemorrhages
Anemias * Hemolytic type	Anemia	Low red cell count, pallor, fatigue, muscle weakness, dyspnea, palpations of heart (common to all types, usual)
	* Sickle cell	Usual and jaundice in sclera, pain in arms, legs, abdomen, recurrent fever; in crisis, headache, paralysis, and convulsions
	* Spheroidal	Usual and jaundice, splenomegaly
	Pernicious anemia	Usual and stomach acid absent, digestive disturbances, tongue sore and smooth; numbness and tingling due to lack of B_{12}, remission and exacerbation
	Iron deficient anemia	Usual, but normal number of pale cells, iron deficiency
	Aplastic anemia	Usual, with unusual hemorrhage, increased number of infections

Affected Organ/Body Region	Diagnostic Procedure	Treatment
Bone marrow	Differential blood count, marrow biopsy	Chemotherapy
Lymph nodes	Differential blood count, marrow biopsy	Chemotherapy
Lymph nodes, lymphoid tissue	Biopsy	Radiation, chemotherapy
Lymph nodes, lymphoid tissue	Biopsy, typical cell type	Radiation, chemotherapy
Red and white cells and platelets	Excess number cells, blood volume	Phlebotomy, radiation therapy
Clotting proteins	Lack of clotting proteins	Transfusions of clotting proteins, whole blood
Platelets	Low number of thrombocytes	Corticosteroids, splenectomy
Red blood cells	Red cell count and hematocrit for all types	Blood transfusions may be used in all types
Red blood cells	Sickled red cells	Preventive to avoid crisis; bone marrow transplant
Red blood cells	Spheroidal red cells	Splenectomy
Red blood cells	Absence of intrinsic factor, B_{12} levels low	Vitamin B_{12} injections
Red blood cells	Pale cells, count normal, iron deficiency	Reduce blood loss, iron supplements
Red and white blood cells and platelets	Low count of all cells, prolonged bleeding time	Blood transfusion Drug therapy

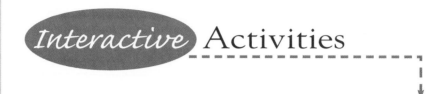

Interactive Activities

CASE FOR CRITICAL THINKING

1. A 25-year-old male presents to the emergency room with complaints of fever, severe abdominal pain, shortness of breath, jaundice, and swelling of his hands and feet. This patient has been severely incapacitated by his disease. What disease does this patient most likely have? How should this patient manage his disease?
2. A 35-year-old female is seen in the doctor's office with complaints of dizziness, weakness, and severe stomach pain. She has a history of peptic ulcer disease and is a mother of 5 children who are 1, 3, 5, and 7 years of age. What factors predispose this woman to iron deficiency anemia?
3. A 60-year-old male is seen by his physician with a one-year history of emotional instability, and weakness. This patient also complains of a sore tongue, and a tingling sensation in his feet. What type of anemia based on these symptoms does this patient most likely have?

MULTIMEDIA EXTENSION ACTIVITIES

www.prenhall.com/mulvihill
Use the above address to access the free, interactive companion Website created for this textbook. Included in the features of this site are chapter specific activities, internet links, and an audio-glossary.

Audio Glossary
Use the CD-ROM disk enclosed with your textbook to hear the pronunciation of the key terms in this chapter.

Diseases at a Glance: Diseases of the Blood

Use the chart on page(s) 116–117 to answer the following:

1. List 5 types of diseases or conditions of the blood.

2. What are the major signs and symptoms of the diseases or conditions you named?

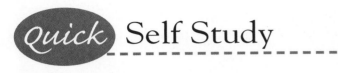 **Self Study**

TRUE OR FALSE

_____ 1. Hemolytic anemia can be caused by drugs.

_____ 2. A differential white blood cell count shows increased lymphocytes in bacterial infections.

_____ 3. The main function of red blood cells is to fight infection.

_____ 4. Aplastic anemia is best treated by administration of iron.

_____ 5. Pernicious anemia is due to a deficiency of intrinsic factor.

FILL-INS

1. _____ anemia results if the bone marrow fails to function.

2. _____ anemia is caused by inadequate absorption or intake of cobalamin.

3. _____ _____ anemia can result from excessive blood loss from an ulcer, malignant lesion, or monthly menstrual bleed.

4. _____ anemia is an inherited condition characterized by sharply curved red blood cells.

MULTIPLE CHOICE

1. Jaundice would occur in _____.
      a. aplastic   b. sickle cell
      c. pernicious anemia

2. Which of the following anemias are associated with hemolysis?
      (1) aplastic   (2) congenital spheroidal
      (3) sickle cell   (4) pernicious
      (5) hypochromic
      a. (2) and (4)   b. (1) and (3)
      c. (2) and (3)   d. (3) and (5)

3. Cells contain normal amounts of hemoglobin but are few in number in
   _____.
      a. hypochromic anemia   b. sickle cell anemia
      c. pernicious anemia

4. Acute myelogenous leukemia affects _____.
      a. lymphocytes   b. granulocytes
      c. monocytes

 FACT

A 14-year health study from the Harvard School of Public Health analyzed data from more than 88,000 women enrolled in the Nurses Health Study. The research team found that women who had a main meal of beef, pork, or lamb daily were more than twice as likely to develop non-Hodgkin's lymphoma as those who had such meals less than once a week. Reference: Journal of the National Cancer Institute 1999; *91: 1751–1758.*

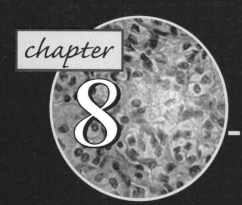

Diseases of the Heart

No one questions the importance of a well-functioning heart. It is the pump that keeps blood flowing to all the cells and tissues of the body.

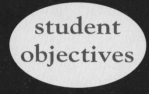

student objectives

After studying this chapter, students should be able to

➤ Describe normal heart function

➤ Depict pulmonary and systemic circulation

➤ Describe regulatory mechanisms of the heart's conduction system

➤ Summarize notable characteristics of heart disease

➤ Compare and contrast the features of hypertensive heart disease with cor pulmonale

➤ Describe the abnormalities associated with congenital heart disease

➤ Distinguish between valvular insufficiency and valvular stenosis and their consequences on the chambers of the heart

➤ Distinguish between rheumatic heart disease and infectious endocarditis

➤ Define abnormal heart rhythms

➤ Summarize procedures used to diagnose heart disease

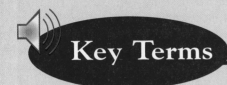

Key Terms

Angina pectoris

Angiocardiography

Angioplasty

Aortic stenosis

Atherosclerosis

Auscultation

Autoimmune disease

Bradycardia

Bundle of His

Cardiac catheterization

Cardiac cycle

Coarctation

Congenital

Cor pulmonale

Coronary arteriography

Coronary thrombosis

Cyanosis

Defibrillator

Diastole

Dyspnea

Echocardiography

Electrocardiogram

Endocarditis

Endocardium

Foramen ovale

Friable

Heart block

Heart murmurs

Hemolytic streptococci

Hypertrophy

Infarct

Ischemia

Mitral stenosis

Mitral valve

Myocardial infarction

Myocardium

Nitroglycerin

Patent ductus arteriosis

Pericardium

Petechiae

Pulmonary edema

Pulmonary stenosis

Purkinje's fibers

Resuscitation

Sclerotic

Sinoatrial node

Stasis

Syncope

Systole

Tachycardia

Tetralogy of Fallot

Thrombolytic

Tricuspid valve

Valvular insufficiency

Vegetations

Venae cavae

Ventricular fibrillation

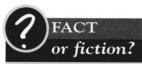
Read this chapter to find the answer.

 myocardium
(mī-ō-kăr′-dē-ŭm)

 endocardium
(ĕn″-dō-kăr′-dē-ŭm)

 pericardium
(per″-ĭ-kar′-dē-ŭm)

 mitral valve
(mī′-trăl vălv)

 tricuspid valve
(trī-kŭs′-pĭd vălv)

➤ STRUCTURE AND FUNCTION OF THE HEART

The heart is a hollow muscular organ that is located in the center of the chest. The heart consists of four chambers: a right and left atrium and a right and left ventricle. The walls of these chambers are cardiac muscle, or **myocardium.** Lining these chambers is a smooth delicate membrane, the **endocardium,** that is continuous with the lining of the blood vessels. The heart is enclosed in a double membranous sac, the **pericardium.** Figure 8–1 shows these tissues of the heart, any of which can become diseased.

A partition, or septum, separates the right and left sides of the heart. The right and left sides of the heart each have an upper chamber or atrium that collects blood, and a lower chamber or ventricle that ejects blood. Between the atria and the ventricles are valves that assure a one-way blood flow, the atrioventricular or AV valves. The valves are delicate but very strong and are continuous with the endocardium. The valve between the left atrium and left ventricle has two flaps, or cusps, that meet when the valve is closed and is called the bicuspid or **mitral valve.** The valve between the right atrium and right ventricle has three cusps and is called the **tricuspid valve.** Figure 8–2 shows these valves in the closed position. Valves are frequently damaged by rheumatic fever and endocarditis, diseases that will be explained.

At the entrance to the great vessels leaving the heart, the aorta and pulmonary artery, is another set of valves, the semilunar valves. The function of all the valves is to prevent the backflow of blood. The atria are the receiving chambers for blood returning from the body and the lungs; the ventricles serve as pumps sending blood throughout the body and to the lungs.

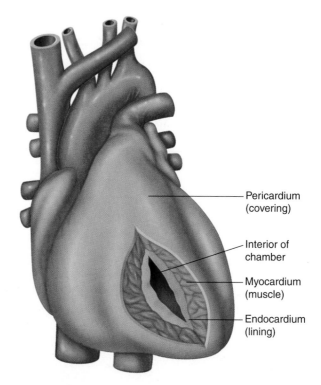

Pericardium (covering)

Interior of chamber

Myocardium (muscle)

Endocardium (lining)

Figure 8–1
Tissues of the heart.

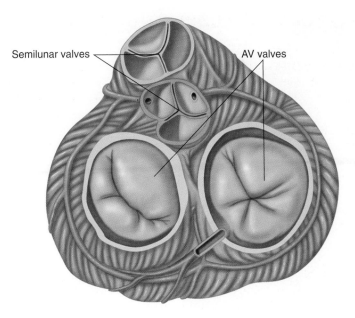

Figure 8–2
Heart valves in closed position viewed from the top.

During each heartbeat, each heart chamber relaxes as it fills, and then contracts as it pumps blood. This filling period is the **diastole,** or the diastolic phase, of the atria. The atria then contract and the relaxed ventricles fill in their diastolic phase. The contracting phase of each is the **systole,** or systolic phase. The alternate contraction and relaxation of atria and ventricles comprises the **cardiac cycle.**

The heart muscle itself needs a good blood supply, which is provided by the coronary arteries that cross over the surface of the heart (Figure 8–3). These are the small vessels that frequently become blocked, causing a heart attack.

An understanding of the blood flow pattern through the heart and lungs will make the various diseases of the heart more meaningful. Valve defects, septal defects, heart attacks, and other diseases will be considered in the light of their interference with heart action.

diastole
(dī-ăs′-tō-lē)

systole
(sĭs′-tō-lē)

cardiac cycle
(kăr′-dĭ-ăk sī′-kŭl)

➤ MOVEMENT OF BLOOD BETWEEN THE HEART AND LUNGS

Blood that has circulated throughout the body has given up most of its oxygen and has picked up waste products and carbon dioxide from cellular metabolism. This oxygen-poor blood flows from the body through the two largest veins or **venae cavae** into the right atrium. When the atrium fills, it propels the blood into the right ventricle. The right ventricle propels blood through the pulmonary valve into the pulmonary artery that further branches to the right and left lung. The blood in the lungs flows through capillaries and absorbs oxygen and gives up carbon dioxide, which is then exhaled. Figure 8–4 shows this path of blood flow.

Oxygenated blood from the lungs flows through the pulmonary veins into the left atrium. The left atrium fills and propels blood through the mitral valve into the left

venae cavae
(vē′-nē kā′-vē)

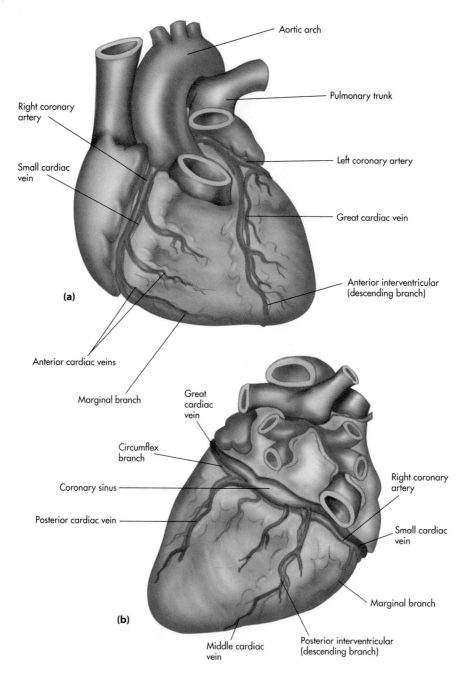

Figure 8–3
Coronary arteries and major blood vessels.

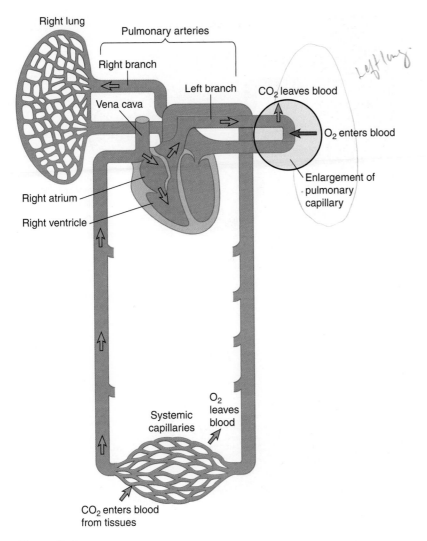

Figure 8-4
Venous return to heart and blood flow to lungs.

ventricle. After the left ventricle fills, it pumps blood through the aortic valve into the aorta. The aorta carries blood that is distributed to all parts of the body except the lungs. Figure 8–5 shows the return of blood to the left side of the heart. Figure 8–6 shows the flow of blood through the heart.

➤ CONTROL OF THE HEART AND THE INFLUENCE OF THE AUTONOMIC NERVOUS SYSTEM

Unlike other muscles, the cardiac muscle can contract continuously and rhythmically without nerve stimulation. A small patch of tissue, the **sinoatrial node** or the pacemaker of the heart, initiates the heartbeat. The impulse for contraction spreads over the atria and the ventricles via the **bundle of His,** and terminates in the **Purkinje fibers,** which further branch through the ventricles. This conduction system is illustrated in Figure 8–7.

sinoatrial node
(sĭn″-ō-ā′-trĭ-ăl nōd)

bundle of His
(bŭn′-dŭl of Hĭs)

Purkinje fibers
(per-kĭn-jŭ fī′-bŭrs)

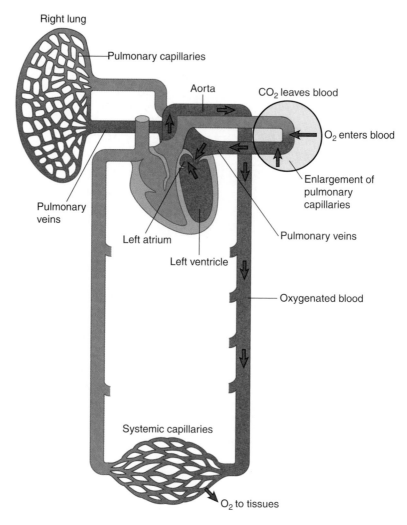

Figure 8–5
Return of oxygenated blood to heart and entry into aorta (red = oxygenated blood, blue = deoxygenated blood).

Although the heart muscle is not dependent on nerve stimulation for contraction, it is influenced by nerves of the autonomic nervous system for its rate of beating, the pulse rate. Two sets of nerves work antagonistically, one slowing the heart, the other accelerating it. The vagus nerve slows heart action by means of a chemical it secretes, acetylcholine. This vagus nerve action is important because it prevents the heart from overworking by slowing it down during rest and sleep. The cardiac accelerator nerve of the sympathetic portion of the autonomic nervous system speeds up the action of the heart during periods of stress, strenuous physical activity, and excitement, when the body needs a greater blood flow. The sympathetic system triggers (or stimulates) the release of epinephrine into the bloodstream. As this reaches the pacemaker of the heart, the speed of contraction is increased.

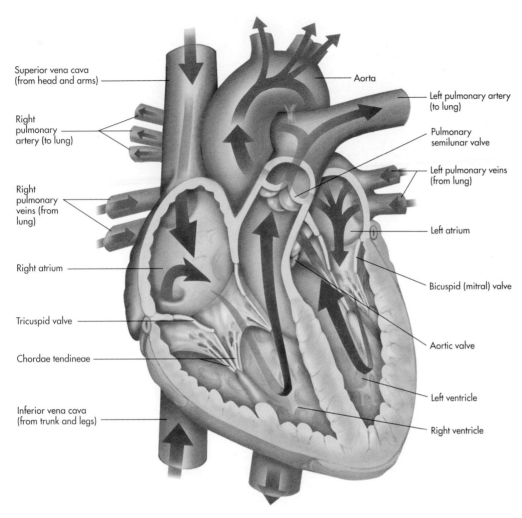

Figure 8–6
The flow of blood through the heart.

 PREVENTION *PLUS!*

Women can reduce their risk of coronary heart disease by 30 to 40 percent by walking briskly for 3 or more hours each week.

➤ DISEASES OF THE HEART

Coronary Artery Disease

The heart muscle itself receives a fraction of the large volume of blood flowing through the atria and the ventricles. A system of arteries and veins or coronary circulation supplies the heart with oxygen-rich blood and returns oxygen-depleted blood to the right atrium. Unfortunately, these small vessels can become blocked (occluded). This results

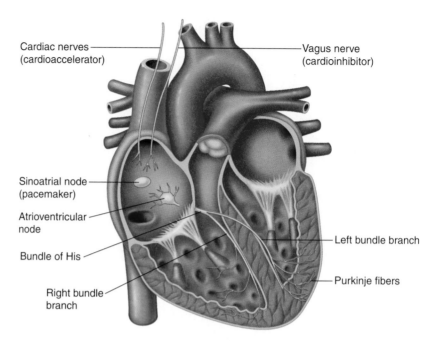

Cardiac nerves (cardioaccelerator)

Vagus nerve (cardioinhibitor)

Sinoatrial node (pacemaker)

Atrioventricular node

Bundle of His

Right bundle branch

Left bundle branch

Purkinje fibers

Figure 8–7
Conducting system of the heart.

coronary
thrombosis
(kŏr′-ō-nă-rē
thrŏm-bō′-sĭs)

atherosclerosis
(ăth″-ĕr-ō-sklĕ-rō′-sĭs)

ischemia
(ĭs-kē′-mē-ă)

infarct
(ĭn-fărkt′)

myocardial
infarction
(mī″-ō-kăr′-dĭ-ăl
ĭn-fărk′-shŭn)

resuscitation
(rĭ-sŭs″-ĭ-tā-shŭn)

when a blood clot forms on the inner wall of a coronary artery, causing a **coronary thrombosis,** or from a narrowing of the lumen, the opening within the vessel.

The narrowing of the lumen is due to accumulation of fatty material under the inner lining of the arterial wall, a condition termed **atherosclerosis** (see Chapter 9). Figure 8–8 illustrates possible means of occlusion or blockage. An atherosclerotic vessel eventually becomes occluded or blocked. **Ischemia,** a deficiency of blood supply to the heart muscle, results in a heart attack. Cardiovascular diseases are the leading cause of death in the United States.

If the lumen of the coronary artery narrows slowly, some heart muscle cells die and are replaced by scar tissue. When an area of the myocardium is suddenly deprived of blood due to occlusion of the coronary artery, that tissue dies and the dead muscle is called an **infarct.** This is a true heart attack or **myocardial infarction.** Severe chest pains generally accompany the attack, but the pain may be referred to the neck or left arm, and the person may feel nauseous, restless, cold, and clammy.

The prognosis for the person with a myocardial infarction depends on many factors. The speed with which medical attention is given is very important. Thus, cardiopulmonary **resuscitation** (CPR) can be of great assistance while waiting for an emergency care unit to arrive.

on the Practical Side

Diet
A low-salt diet can decrease blood volume and fluid accumulation in congestive heart failure. Dietary sodium can easily be reduced to 2 to 4 g per day by eliminating cooking salt.

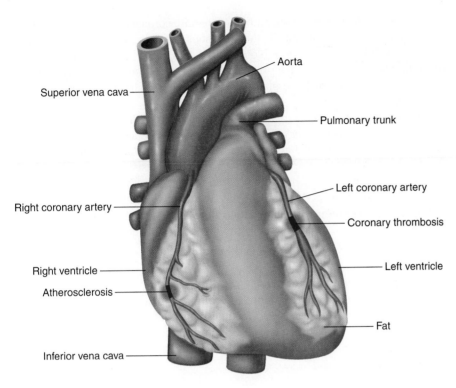

Aorta

Superior vena cava

Pulmonary trunk

Left coronary artery

Right coronary artery

Coronary thrombosis

Left ventricle

Right ventricle

Atherosclerosis

Fat

Inferior vena cava

Figure 8–8
Blockage of coronary arteries.

The size of the coronary artery that is occluded and the extent of heart muscle damage, which is indicated by the level of certain blood enzymes, are also factors in the prognosis. If a collateral circulation is established—that is, if blood from a surrounding area channels into the damaged tissue—recovery will be better.

The damaged area can repair itself with scar tissue, but it will never serve as heart muscle again. There will be a tendency for blood clots to form or for a weakened area to rupture. Rest is needed for the repair period, but after this time, controlled exercise is advised to maintain circulation. In today's society, the predisposing causes of coronary artery disease are generally well known: obesity, hypertension, smoking, a sedentary lifestyle, and a high-cholesterol diet.

Remarkable advances have been made in recent years in the treatment of heart disease. Severe damage to heart muscle after a heart attack has been greatly reduced by early administration of **thrombolytic** (blood clot-dissolving) drugs. Such drugs commonly used are TPA (tissue plasminogen activator) and streptokinase. Other anticoagulants—aspirin and heparin—are used in conjunction with the thrombolytic drugs.

thrombolytic
(thrŏm″-bō-lĭt′-ĭk)

Disease by the Numbers X + ÷

Approximately 250,000 sudden cardiac deaths occur each year in the United States

Reference: American Heart Association, 1996.

angioplasty
(ăn'-jĭ-ō-plăs"-tē)

angina pectoris
(ăn-jī'-nah
pĕk'-tor-ĭs)

nitroglycerin
(nī-trō-glĭs'-ĕr-ĭn)

Treatment of a myocardial infarction may require coronary bypass surgery in which a portion of the patient's vein, usually the saphenous vein, is used to reroute blood around the occlusion. When obstruction to blood flow is less severe, **angioplasty** may be performed. In this procedure, a balloon-tip catheter is inserted into the coronary arteries and expanded to break and crush the plaques. Laser techniques have also been used to reduce the plaques.

Angina pectoris is temporary chest pain or sensation of chest pressure that is caused by transient oxygen insufficiency. The person feels pressure and pain below the breastbone, which may radiate to the neck, jaw, and arms. There is also a feeling of tightness and suffocation. Angina is triggered by physical activity, lasts no more than a few minutes, and subsides with rest. Angina attacks may be triggered by heavy meals, exposure to cold, or emotional stress. Medication such as **nitroglycerin** is administered to dilate coronary arteries, permitting adequate blood flow. A person who experiences recurring attacks of angina is said to have chronic unstable angina. Control of exercise and physical activity is necessary for all cases of angina.

Hypertensive Heart Disease

This condition is caused by long-standing high blood pressure or hypertension. The heart pumps against resistance of narrowed blood vessels. The hypertensive heart enlarges as it tries to meet the demands of the body. The ventricle that does most of the work finally enlarges or dilates, becomes exhausted, and eventually fails to pump blood adequately.

Cor Pulmonale

cor pulmonale
(kŏr pŭl-mō-nă'-lē)

hypertrophy
(hī-pĕr'-trō-fē)

Cor pulmonale is a serious heart condition in which the right side of the heart fails as a result of long-standing chronic lung disease. As respiratory failure develops, pressure in the blood vessels to the lung increases a condition termed pulmonary hypertension. This hypertension overworks the right ventricle, which pumps blood into the pulmonary artery, causing dilation and **hypertrophy** of the right ventricle. Treatment is aimed at relieving the causative lung disease by administration of bronchodilator medication and the use of a ventilator.

Congestive Heart Failure

Congestive heart failure is a progressive heart condition in which the quantity of blood pumped by the heart is insufficient to meet the needs of the body. Any disease that affects the heart and interferes with circulation can lead to heart failure. Coronary heart disease impairs blood flow to the heart and can cause a heart attack that permanently damages the heart. An infection of the heart caused by viruses, bacteria, and other microorganisms may damage the heart muscle and heart valves. Heart valve disorders and hypertension increase the size of the heart muscle and cause it to work harder initially. Over time, the enlarged heart weakens and fails to pump adequately. The heart's conduction system may fail, resulting in slow, fast, or irregular heartbeats that cannot pump blood effectively.

**pulmonary
edema**
(pŭl'-mō-nĕr-ē
ĕ-dē'-mă)

Congestive heart failure may involve either the right or left side of the heart. Right-sided disease tends to result in a build-up of blood flowing into the right side of the heart. This build-up results in edema of the ankles, distention of the neck veins, and enlargement of the spleen because of congestion in the veins that cannot empty properly into the heart. Left-sided failure leads to a build-up of fluid in the lungs or **pulmonary edema,** which causes shortness of breath. Figure 8–9 shows the effect of each type of congestive heart failure.

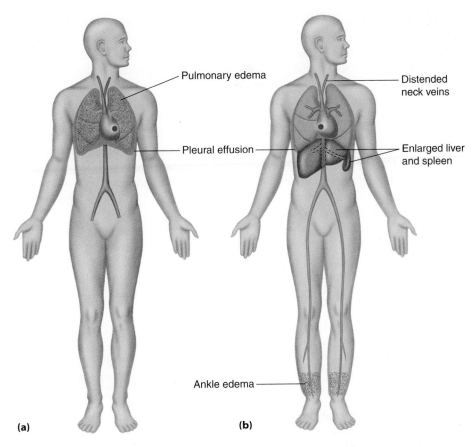

Figure 8–9
(a) Left-sided congestive heart failure. (b) Right-sided congestive heart failure. (*From Kent, Hart. Introduction to Human Disease, Appleton & Lange, 1987.*)

Disease by the Numbers X + ÷

Approximately 32,000 babies are born each year with cardiovascular defects.

Reference: American Heart Association, 1996.

Congenital Heart Disease

The tremendous accomplishments in open heart surgery have drastically reduced the mortality rate of children born with heart defects. Most of the **congenital** abnormalities are in the septum that separates the right and left side of the heart. An opening in this septum allows a mixing of deoxygenated and oxygenated blood, which causes the heart to overwork.

Septal defects may be large or small, with the smaller defects causing no problem. An example of a small septal defect is failure of the foramen ovale to close after birth. The **foramen ovale** is a small opening that allows blood from the right side of the heart to enter the left directly, bypassing the nonfunctional fetal lungs. Failure of this opening to close is the most common but least serious septal defect.

congenital
(kŏn-gĕn'-ĭ-tăl)

foramen ovale
(fō-rā'-mĕn ō-văle)

The septal defect may be in the wall between the two atria, atrial septal defect (ASD), or between the ventricles, ventricular septal defect (VSD), and it may be large. Because blood pressure is higher on the left side than on the right side of the heart, blood is generally shunted through the opening in a left-to-right direction. This factor alone would not be significant for oxygenation of the blood. Blood from the left side is already oxygenated, and blood from the right side is on its way to the lungs, but the right side of the heart is overworked. It receives blood as usual from the vena cava but also from the left side of the heart. To accommodate this blood volume, the right side dilates. Because it is required to pump more blood to the lungs, the right ventricle enlarges (hypertrophies). The left ventricle is overworked if a ventricular septal defect is large. Blood is shunted to the right ventricle, yet the left ventricle must pump enough blood into the aorta. This ventricle can become exhausted and fail. Figure 8–10 shows a normal ventricular wall and Figure 8–11 shows a hypertrophied ventricular wall.

cyanosis
(sī-ăn-ō-sĭs)

Cyanosis, a blue color in the tissues, does not occur if the shunt of blood through the septal defect remains left to right. If the pressure becomes greater in the right ventricle than in the left, the shunt reverses and cyanosis occurs. The deoxygenated blood from the right side of the heart then enters the general circulation; the blue color is because of deoxygenated hemoglobin. Figure 8–12 illustrates the routine shunt and that which causes cyanosis.

tetralogy of fallot
(tĕ-trăl′-ō-jē of
fă-lō′)

Tetralogy of Fallot is one of the most serious of the congenital defects and consists of four *(tetra)* abnormalities. The baby with this condition is the true "blue baby"; it is born cyanotic, with all the tissues a definite blue; cyanosis is because of poorly oxy-

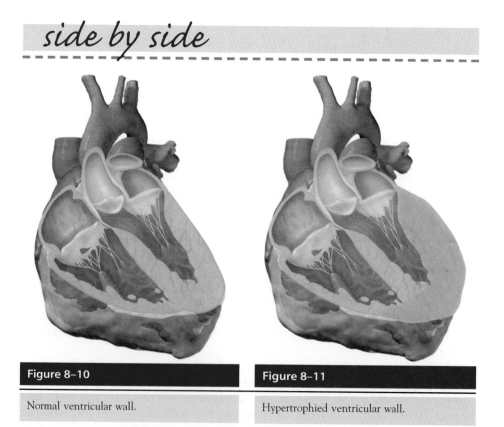

side by side

Figure 8–10	Figure 8–11
Normal ventricular wall.	Hypertrophied ventricular wall.

SMALL SEPTAL DEFECT

Aorta

Left atrium

Oxygenated blood
Higher Pressure

Normal shunt
Left to right
No cyanosis

Left ventricle

Deoxygenated blood
Lower pressure

(a)

Right atrium

Right ventricle

Oxygenated blood
Pressure decreases

Deoxygenated blood
Pressure increases

(b)

Pulmonary artery

Deoxygenated blood

Right ventricle

(c)

LARGE SEPTAL DEFECT
Pressure increases in
deoxygenated side

SHUNT REVERSES RIGHT TO LEFT
Deoxygenated blood enters
aorta—cyanosis develops

Figure 8–12
Effect of septal defects (a) Normal shunt—no cyanosis. (b) Increased pressure in right ventricle.
(c) Shunt reverses—cyanosis develops.

genated blood. The union of oxygen with hemoglobin gives normal arterial blood its bright red color.

The first cause of the cyanosis is **pulmonary stenosis.** Remember, a valve leads into the pulmonary artery. Stenosis of a valve means that the opening is too small. Because of the narrow opening, an inadequate amount of blood reaches the lungs to be oxygenated, and all body tissues suffer from this lack of oxygen.

Second, accompanying the pulmonary stenosis is a large ventricular septal defect, the seriousness of which has already been discussed. Third, a misplaced aorta overrides the ventricular septum. Normally, only oxygenated blood from the left ventricle enters the aorta, but in this case, the right ventricle also feeds into the aorta, permitting the mixing of oxygenated and deoxygenated blood. Last, because of the increased strain on the right ventricle attempting to pump through a stenotic valve, the ventricle hypertrophies.

In addition to cyanosis, other signs accompany the disease. There is secondary polycythemia, a disease described in Chapter 7 as a compensatory mechanism. The inadequate oxygen supply stimulates erythropoiesis, and an excessive number of red blood cells are formed.

The fingers are clubbed and fingernails curled caused by poor oxygenation of tissues at the fingertips. The child experiences **dyspnea** after any exertion, even crying. The child may assume a squatting position after exercise, which provides some relief from the breathlessness. Surgical repair of the problem consists of patching the ventricular septal defect, opening the narrowed passageway from the right ventricle and the narrowed

pulmonary stenosis
(pŭl′-mō-něr-ē stě-nō′-sĭs)

dyspnea
(dĭsp′-nē-ă)

**patent ductus
arteriosis**
(pā′-těnt dŭk-tŭs
ăr-těr-ē-ō′-sĭs)

coarctation
(kō-ărk-tā′-shŭn)

pulmonary valve, and closing any abnormal connection made between the aorta and the pulmonary artery. Figure 8–13 shows the four abnormalities in the Tetralogy of Fallot.

Patent ductus arteriosis (PDA) is a common congenital disease. The ductus arteriosis is a fetal blood vessel that connects the pulmonary artery and the aorta, shunting blood from the nonfunctional fetal lungs. Figure 8–14 shows this vessel diagrammatically. Soon after birth, it normally closes, but if it remains open or patent, blood intended for the body flows from the aorta to the lungs overloading the pulmonary artery. This blood is oxygenated so there is no cyanosis. There is long-term danger of heart failure and infection at the site of the lesion. The ductus may be closed surgically by dividing the connection between the pulmonary artery and the aorta.

Coarctation of the aorta is a narrowing, or stricture, of the artery that provides blood to the entire body. The stricture occurs beyond the branching of blood vessels to the head and arms, so the blood supply to the upper part of the body is adequate. Little blood, however, flows through the constricted area to the abdomen and legs. Blood pressure is very low in the legs, but is high in the arms. Many collateral blood vessels develop to compensate for this poor blood supply. This is comparable to the collateral circulation that develops after a myocardial infarction. The coarctation can be corrected

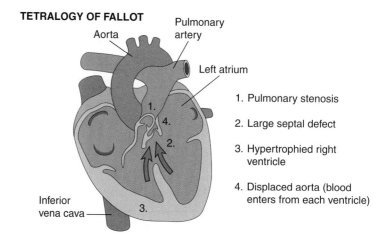

TETRALOGY OF FALLOT

Aorta
Pulmonary artery
Left atrium

1. Pulmonary stenosis

2. Large septal defect

3. Hypertrophied right ventricle

4. Displaced aorta (blood enters from each ventricle)

Inferior vena cava

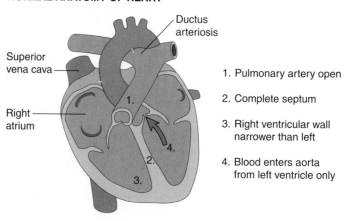

NORMAL ANATOMY OF HEART

Ductus arteriosis

Superior vena cava

Right atrium

1. Pulmonary artery open

2. Complete septum

3. Right ventricular wall narrower than left

4. Blood enters aorta from left ventricle only

Figure 8–13
Tetralogy of Fallot (**top**) compared to normal anatomy (**bottom**).

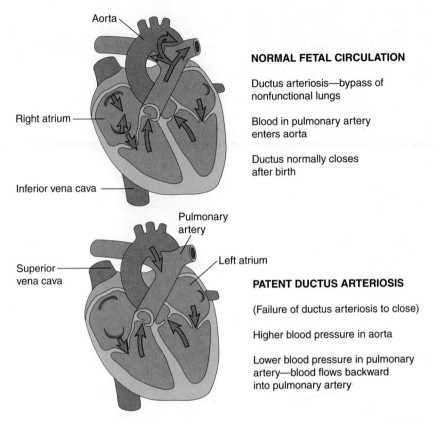

NORMAL FETAL CIRCULATION

Ductus arteriosis—bypass of nonfunctional lungs

Blood in pulmonary artery enters aorta

Ductus normally closes after birth

PATENT DUCTUS ARTERIOSIS

(Failure of ductus arteriosis to close)

Higher blood pressure in aorta

Lower blood pressure in pulmonary artery—blood flows backward into pulmonary artery

Figure 8–14
Patent ductus arteriosis.

surgically by cutting out (excising) the narrow segment and sewing the good ends of the aorta together. Coarctation of the aorta is pictured in Figure 8–15**a** as compared with the normal branching of the aorta (Figure 8–15**b**).

Disease by the Numbers x + ÷

In 1996, 71,000 valve replacements were performed in the United States.

Valvular Disorders
The valves assure a unidirectional flow of blood through the heart. Closed, they allow a heart chamber to fill with blood; open, they let blood flow forward.

Valves can malfunction in one of two ways. The opening may be too small (stenotic) for sufficient blood flow, or it may be too large to prevent backflow, valvular insufficiency. Valve defects cause **heart murmurs** with characteristic sounds that indicate the nature of the defect. If a valve problem is particularly serious, it can be corrected surgically by reconstruction or replacement. Some of the various valve defects and the effect they have on the heart are considered below.

In **mitral stenosis,** the mitral valve opening is too small and the cusps that form the valve, normally flexible flaps, become rigid and fuse together. A deep funnel-shaped

heart murmurs
(hart mŭr′-mŭrs)

mitral stenosis
(mī′-trăl stĕ-nō′-sĭs)

side by side

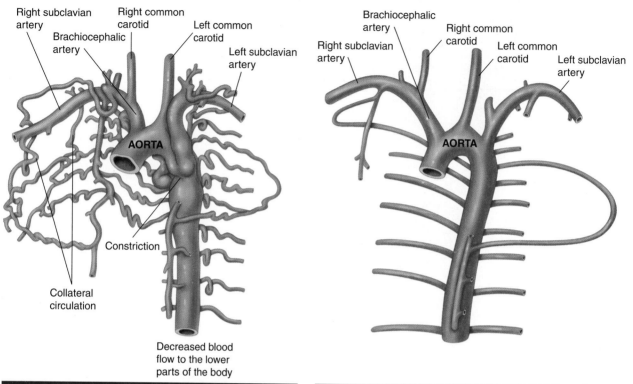

Figure 8–15a

Coarctation of the aorta.

Figure 8–15b

Normal branching of the aorta.

valve is formed, and much pressure is required to force enough blood through the narrow opening. The narrow mitral valve increases resistance of blood flow from the left atrium to the left ventricle. Mitral stenosis often follows rheumatic fever and is more common in women than in men. Rheumatic heart disease will be described in the next section.

The chambers that contain blood that must pass through this valve become greatly dilated. Blood pressure builds in the left atrium and in the veins of the lungs. The right side of the heart would also be affected. This is illustrated in Figure 8–16. The left atrium also becomes hypertrophied because of overwork in pumping blood through the stenotic valve.

One of the complications of any valve defect is the tendency for a thrombus, or clot, to form on the affected area. As blood flows over the malfunctioning valve, clotting elements of the blood are deposited. If the thrombus becomes detached, it will travel as an embolism and possibly occlude a blood vessel to the brain, kidney, or other vital organ.

The damming up of blood behind the stenotic mitral valve causes a congestion in the veins. The veins, attempting to empty into the right atrium, do so with difficulty. The veins in the neck stand out prominently. As the congestion builds in the veins, fluid from the blood leaks out into the tissue spaces, causing edema.

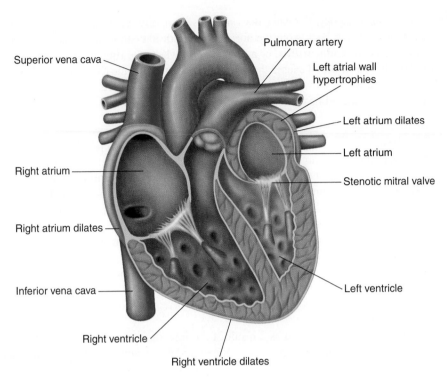

Superior vena cava

Pulmonary artery

Left atrial wall hypertrophies

Left atrium dilates

Left atrium

Right atrium

Stenotic mitral valve

Right atrium dilates

Inferior vena cava

Left ventricle

Right ventricle

Right ventricle dilates

Figure 8–16
Effect of mitral stenosis on the heart.

Poor circulation causes cyanosis because an inadequate amount of oxygen is reaching the tissues. The backup of blood and congestion cause the heart to become exhausted, and congestive heart failure can result.

Mitral insufficiency, or incompetence, means that the opening in the mitral valve is too large and cannot close completely. Blood leaks back through the mitral valve each time the ventricle contracts. As the left ventricle pumps blood out of the heart and into the aorta, some blood leaks back into the atrium, increasing the pressure and volume there. This, in turn, increases blood pressure in the vessels leading from the lungs to the heart, resulting in lung congestion. This can occur if the cusps become hardened, **sclerotic,** and retract. Another cause is the failure of specialized muscles, called *papillary muscles,* in the ventricle. These are attached to the underside of the cusps by means of little cords and normally prevent the cusps from swinging up into the atria when the ventricles contract. If the papillary muscles fail to contract, the cusps open toward the atria under the force of ventricular blood.

Aortic stenosis, the narrowing of the valve leading into the aorta, occurs more often in men than in women and most frequently in men over 50 years old. It may result from rheumatic fever but not as frequently as does mitral stenosis. Sometimes it is a congenital defect or it may occur with hardening of the arteries; the cusps become rigid and adhere together. Masses of hard, calcified material are deposited, giving a warty appearance to the valve. Because the left ventricle of the heart must pump through this valve into the aorta, this chamber hypertrophies greatly through overwork. An inadequate amount of blood may be pumped into the aorta to meet the requirements of the body. An insufficient blood supply to the brain can cause **syncope** (fainting). This valve defect, like others, can be corrected surgically.

sclerotic
(sklĕ-rŏt'-ĭk)

aortic stenosis
(ā-ŏr'-tĭk stĕ-nō'-sĭs)

syncope
(sĭn'-kō-pē)

endocarditis
(ĕn″-dō-kăr′-dī-tĭs)

In aortic insufficiency, the valve does not close properly. Each time the left ventricle relaxes, blood flows back from the aorta. This condition can result from inflammation within the heart, **endocarditis,** or a dilated aorta where the ring around the valve is too large. Back flow of blood causes the ventricle to dilate, become exhausted, and eventually fail. Figure 8–17 shows a normal bicuspid valve, and Figure 8–18 shows valve vegetation from endocarditis.

Rheumatic Heart Disease

hemolytic streptococci
(hē-mō-lĭ′-tĭk strep′-tō-kok′-sī)

Rheumatic heart disease is a peculiar disease that results from a streptococcal infection, although the organisms are no longer present when the disease presents itself. Rheumatic fever develops from a throat or ear infection caused by Group A **hemolytic streptococci.** The symptoms are fever, inflamed and painful joints, and sometimes a rash. There is a latent period of a few weeks between the infection and the development of rheumatic fever. The disease usually strikes children or very young adults.

autoimmune disease
(ău-tō-ĭ-mūn′ dĭ-zēz′)

Rheumatic fever is an **autoimmune disease.** It results from a reaction between streptococcal antigens and the patient's own antibodies against them. All parts of the heart may be affected, but most frequently it is the mitral valve that is damaged. The exact mechanism that causes the valve lesion is not known. There seems to be an attraction of the antigen-antibody complex for the mitral valve. The aortic semilunar valve is also affected at times.

vegetations
(vĕj-ĕ-tā′-shŭnz)

The valves become inflamed as a result of the infection, and clotting elements are deposited by blood flowing over the valves. Small nodular structures called **vegetations** form along the edge of the cusps. The normally delicate cusps thicken and adhere to each other. Later, fibrous tissue develops, which has a tendency to contract.

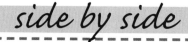

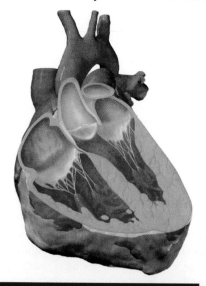

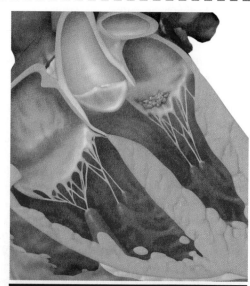

Figure 8–17

Normal bicuspid valve.

Figure 8–18

Valve vegetations from endocarditis.

If the adhesions of the cusps seriously narrow the valve opening, the mitral valve becomes stenotic. The effects of mitral stenosis are described in this chapter (see Valvular Diseases). An inadequate amount of blood flows from the left atrium to the left ventricle. **Stasis,** or slowed blood flow, frequently causes thrombus formation.

It is possible for the cusps to retract to the extent that they fail to meet, and the valve cannot close. The mitral valve is then insufficient, or incompetent, and there is a backflow of blood, regurgitation, from the left ventricle to the left atrium. Fortunately, rheumatic fever is not as common today as it once was. This is because of the widespread use of antibiotics in treating streptococcal infections.

Infectious Endocarditis

Infectious endocarditis is a disease that was once considered fatal but that now responds well to antibiotics if treated early. The endocardium is the inner lining of the chambers of the heart and covers the valves. Endocarditis is an inflammation of this lining caused by a strain of *Streptococcus* bacteria. These organisms can enter the bloodstream from an infected tooth, a skin infection, urinary tract infection, or other infections. Frequently, this inflammation occurs on a rheumatic fever lesion, an already damaged valve, or on a congenital heart defect. Various routes of bacterial invasion are illustrated in Figure 8–19.

The nodules or vegetations that form in endocarditis are larger than those of rheumatic fever. They are also **friable,** tending to break apart easily and enter the bloodstream. The vegetations are filled with bacteria, unlike rheumatic fever vegetations. Typical lesions of endocarditis are shown in Figure 8–20. As fragments of the vegetations break apart, they enter the bloodstream to form emboli, which can travel to the brain, kidney, lung, or other vital organs, causing a variety of symptoms. The emboli can lodge in small blood vessels of the skin or other organs and cause the blood vessels to rupture. These small hemorrhages produce tiny red spots called **petechiae.**

stasis
(stā′-sĭs)

friable
(frī′-ă-bl)

petechiae
(pĕ-tē′-kē-ē)

➤ ABNORMALITIES OF HEART CONDUCTION

In reviewing the anatomy and physiology of the heart, a specialized patch of tissue, the pacemaker, was mentioned as establishing heart rate. Normally, the impulse for contraction then spreads over the atria and is conducted to the ventricles through a conduction bundle. This conduction system can fail and, if the impulse does not spread from the atria to the ventricles, the pulse is drastically reduced; this failure in passage of the impulse is known as **heart block.** Heart block can result from scar tissue interfering with the conduction bundle, and it may be necessary to implant an electric pacemaker if the block is complete.

Heart block is graded as first, second, or third degree. When conduction to the ventricle is slightly delayed, first degree heart block occurs and usually produces no symptoms. In second degree heart block, not every impulse from the atria reaches the ventricles. Some forms of second degree heart block progress to third degree heart block in which impulses from the atria are completely blocked. The ventricle beats slowly and less efficiently. Eventually heart failure ensues.

At times, the impulse for contraction spreads over the atria and the ventricle in an uncoordinated fashion. Atrial fibrillation and atrial flutter are very fast impulses. These fast impulses produce rapid and incompetent contraction of the ventricles. Medications can be administered to slow the conduction through the bundle of His to the ventricles. This allows the ventricles to fill properly before contraction.

heart block
(hart blŏk)

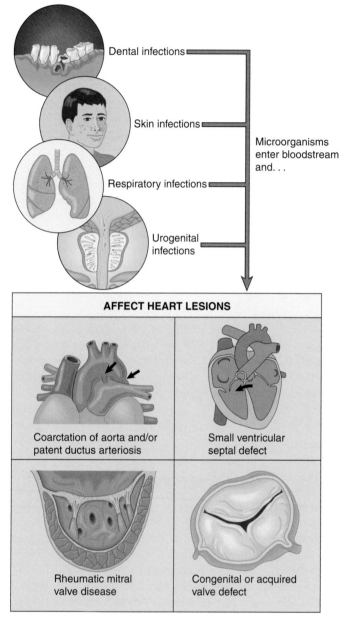

Figure 8–19
Infections resulting in bacterial endocarditis.

ventricular fibrillation
(vĕn-trĭk-ū-lăr fĭ″-brĭl-ā-shŭn)

defibrillator
(dĭ-fĭ″-brĭ-lā′-tŭr)

Ventricular fibrillation is far more serious than atrial fibrillation, and it is potentially fatal. A series of uncoordinated impulses spread over the ventricles causing them to twitch or quiver rather than contract. The ventricle does not carry out effective coordinated contractions. Because no blood is pumped from the heart, ventricular fibrillation is a form of cardiac arrest. Immediate attempts at resuscitation must be made or death will result. Permanent damage to other organs, particularly the brain, results when blood supply to them is compromised. A machine called a **defibrillator** delivers electrical shocks, and is used to re-establish normal heart rhythm.

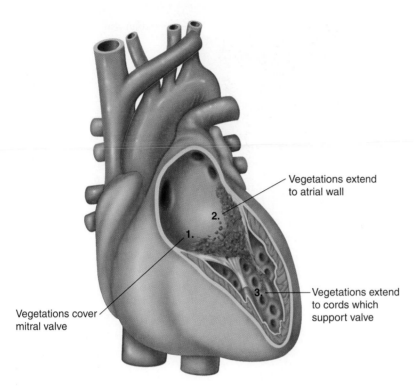

Vegetations extend
to atrial wall

Vegetations cover
mitral valve

Vegetations extend
to cords which
support valve

Figure 8–20
Bacterial endocarditis.

Heart beat rhythm may become irregular and is known as cardiac arrhythmia. Beats may be skipped or come in prematurely; these beats are called premature ventricular contractions (PVCs). The heart rate may increase significantly, **tachycardia,** or be abnormally slow, **bradycardia.**

tachycardia
(tăk″-ĭ-kăr′-dĭ-ă)
bradycardia
(brăd″-i-kăr′-dĭ-ă)

➤ DIAGNOSTIC PROCEDURES FOR HEART DISEASES

Modern medicine provides many techniques for diagnosing and treating heart problems. **Auscultation**—listening through a stethoscope for abnormal sounds—and the electrocardiogram provide valuable information regarding heart condition. The **electrocardiogram** (ECG) is an electrical recording of heart action and aids in the diagnosis of coronary artery disease, myocardial infarction, valvular heart disease, and some congenital heart diseases. It is also useful in diagnosing arrhythmias and heart block. **Echocardiography** (ultrasound cardiography) is also a noninvasive procedure that utilizes high-frequency sound waves to examine the size, shape, and motion of heart structures. It gives a time-motion study of the heart, which permits direct recordings of heart valve movement, measurements of the heart chambers, and changes that occur in the heart chambers during the cardiac cycle. Color Doppler echocardiography explores blood flow patterns and changes in velocity of blood flow within the heart and great vessels. It enables the cardiologist to evaluate valvular stenosis or insufficiency.

Another valuable procedure is **cardiac catheterization** in which a catheter is passed into the heart through appropriate blood vessels to sample the blood in each chamber

auscultation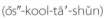
(ŏs″-kool-tā′-shŭn)
electrocardiogram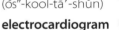
(ē-lĕk″-trō-kăr′-dĭ-ō-grăm)
echocardiography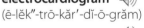
(ĕk″-ō-kăr″-dē-ŏg′-rah-fē)

**cardiac
catheterization**
(kăr′-dĭ-ăk
kăth″-ĕ-tĕr-ĭ-zā′-shŭn)

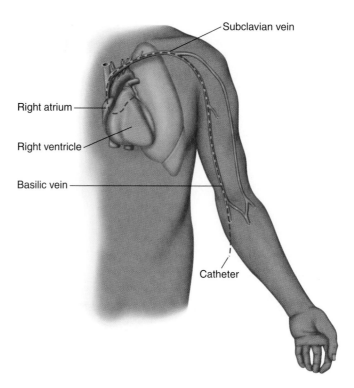

Figure 8–21
Cardiac catheterization.

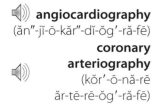

(()) **angiocardiography**
(ăn″-jĭ-ō-kăr″-dĭ-ŏg′-ră-fē)
coronary
arteriography
(kŏr′-ō-nă-rē
ăr-tē-rē-ŏg′-ră-fē)

for oxygen content and pressure. The findings can indicate valvular disorders or abnormal shunting of blood and aids in determining cardiac output (Figure 8–21).

X-rays of the heart and great vessels, the aorta and pulmonary artery, can be taken by means of **angiocardiography** in which a contrast indicator (dye) is injected into the cardiovascular system. A blockage is indicated by an area in which the dye fails to penetrate; coronary bypass surgery may be indicated by this procedure. **Coronary arteriography** employs selective injection of contrast material into coronary arteries for a film recording of blood vessel action, and it too is valuable for possible indication of coronary bypass surgery.

An exercise tolerance test is diagnostic for the existence of coronary artery disease and other heart disorders. This test monitors the ECG and blood pressure during exercise. Problems that normally do not occur at rest are revealed.

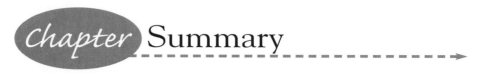

Chapter Summary

After reviewing the normal structure and function of the heart, heart diseases such as coronary artery disease, myocardial infarction, and angina pectoris were discussed. Myocardial infarction and angina pectoris cause severe chest pain or referred pain in the arm or neck. Dyspnea is a common symptom of many heart diseases; the lack of oxygen in the tissues stimulates the respiratory center, causing the person to experience difficulty in breathing or shortness of breath. Fainting or loss of consciousness occurs when the brain is deprived of an adequate blood supply. All of the tissues and organs are affected by poor circulation. Cyanosis occurs when blood is not properly oxygenated and fluid accumulates in the tissues, causing edema when veins become congested.

Hypertensive heart disease develops from long-standing hypertension, and cor pulmonale results from chronic lung disease. Congestive heart failure means that the heart is pumping inadequately to meet the needs of the body.

Congenital heart diseases, tetralogy of Fallot, patent ductus arteriosis, and coarctation of the aorta were explained. It was noted that a congenital defect is frequently the site of a bacterial infection.

Valvular diseases, valves that are stenotic or insufficient, cause heart murmurs. The abnormal sounds result from blood being forced through a stenotic valve or being regurgitated through an insufficient valve. Rheumatic heart disease is a common cause of valvular disease.

Abnormalities of heart action, heart block, fibrillation, and arrhythmia were described. Diagnostic procedures include auscultation, electrocardiography, ultrasound cardiography (echocardiography), cardiac catheterization, and exercise tolerance testing. The condition of coronary arteries and the great vessels can be evaluated through angiocardiography and coronary arteriography.

Advances in open heart surgery have made possible the correction of congenital heart defects, valve replacement, and electric pacemaker implantation. Antibiotics have reduced the danger of endocarditis and the frequency of rheumatic heart disease. Coronary bypass surgery and angioplasty reduce heart damage by increasing coronary circulation.

Diseases at a Glance: Heart

Categories	Disease	Signs and Symptoms
Infections	Endocarditis	Fever, anorexia, weight loss, back pain, night sweats, petechiae, heart murmur
Inflammation	Rheumatic disease	Follows infection by Group A hemolytic streptococci; latent period followed by fever, inflamed and painful joints, rash, heart murmur
Cardiac muscle injury and malfunction	Coronary artery disease	Angina pectoris following exercise, stress, heavy meal
	Myocardial infarct (MI)	Chest pain, radiating to jaw, neck, left arm, back, feeling of tightness, suffocation, nausea and vomiting may occur; may be "silent" (no symptoms)
	Hypertensive heart disease	Long-standing high blood pressure, enlargement of heart, later pulmonary edema with dyspnea, dilation and weakness of ventricles
	Congestive heart failure	Fatigue, difficulty breathing; left side failure leads to pulmonary edema, right side failure leads to systemic edema; both may occur
	Cor pulmonale	Chronic lung disease, right heart failure with systemic edema, fatigue, rapid heart rate

Abnormal Valves and Functions

Categories	Abnormality	Signs and Symptoms
Valvular abnormality and malfunction	Mitral stenosis	Heart murmur, dyspnea, fatigue, lower oxygen in arteries, pulmonary edema may develop
	Mitral insufficiency (mitral prolapse)	Heart murmur, may be asymptomatic, palpitations, fatigue, dyspnea may develop
	Aortic stenosis	Lower output of blood with syncope, heart murmur
	Aortic insufficiency	Heart murmur, back-flow into ventricle, ventricle enlarges

Affected Organ/Body Region	Diagnostic Procedure	Treatment
Valves of heart	Echocardiography	Antibiotics
Valves of heart	Patient history of strep infection; physical exam, strep antibody tests	Anti-inflammatory, steroids, diuretics, bed rest
Coronary arteries, ischemia in heart muscle	Angiocardiography, coronary arteriography	Drug therapy, nitroglycerin, angioplasty, bypass surgery
Heart muscle, any part of organ	ECG, blood test (serum enzymes), physical exam	Thrombolytic drugs (TPA, streptokinase) angioplasty, bypass surgery
Ventricles	BP, scans show enlarged heart, x-ray, physical exam	Drug therapy, oxygen
Ventricles	Physical exam, x-ray, scans show enlarged heart	Drug therapy, diuretics, oxygen
Right ventricle	Patient history, physical exam	Bronchodilators, ventilator

Affected Structure	Diagnostic Procedures	Treatment
Mitral (left atrioventricular) valve	Echocardiography, auscultation	Valve replacement surgery
Mitral valve	Echocardiography, auscultation	Valve replacement surgery only if severe
Aortic semilunar valve	Echocardiography, auscultation	Valve replacement surgery
Aortic semilunar valve	Echocardiography, auscultation	Valve replacement surgery

Abnormal Valves and Functions (continued)

Categories	Abnormality	Signs and Symptoms
Abnormal activities	Heart block	Pulse reduced, palpitations or irregular beat
	Atrial fibrillation	Palpitations as ventricle contraction is affected
	Ventricular fibrillation	Collapse, since blood flow stops; cardiac arrest may follow
	Cardiac arrthymia	Palpitations as beat is uncoordinated
	Tachycardia	Rapid heart rate, not due to exercise
	Bradycardia	Slow heart rate, not increasing in exercise

Congenital Deformities of the Heart

Categories	Defect	Signs and Symptoms
Congenital defects	Atrial septal defect (ASD)	Small ones without symptoms; large ones may lead to pulmonary hypertension
	Ventricular septal defect (VSD)	Loud murmur during contraction of ventricles; right heart failure may occur with large defect; cyanosis if blood shunts right to left
	Tetralogy of Fallot	Cyanotic "blue baby," murmurs, excess number of red cells, dyspnea, fingers and nails clubbed
	Patent ductus arteriosus (PDA)	Murmur develops
	Coarctation of aorta	BP low in legs, high in arms; congestive heart failure can result

Affected Structure	Diagnostic Procedures	Treatment
Pacemaker, conduction system	ECG	Artificial pacemaker
Atria	ECG	Medication, such as lanoxin
Ventricles	ECG	Cardiopulmonary resuscitation, defibrillator
Ventricles	ECG	Medication
Ventricles	ECG	Medication
Ventricles	ECG	Pacemaker may be needed

Affected Structures	Diagnostic Procedures	Treatments
Wall between left and right atria	Chest x-ray, ECG	Large defects surgically repaired
Wall between left and right ventricles	Chest x-ray, ECG, cardiac catheterization, angiography, or echocardiography	Large defects surgically repaired; small ones may spontaneously close
Pulmonary stenosis, VSD, displaced aorta, right ventricular hypertrophy	Chest x-ray, ECG, cardiac catheterization, angiography	Surgical repair
Connects aorta to pulmonary artery	Chest x-ray, cardiac catheterization, angiography	Medication, ligation (tying shut) of defect
Aorta (lumen narrow)	Chest x-ray, cardiac catheterization	Surgery

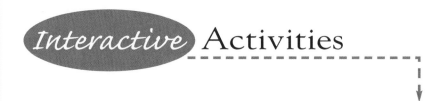

CASES FOR CRITICAL THINKING

1. A 59-year-old male calls paramedics after experiencing an episode of chest pain while shoveling snow. He describes his pain as a crushing, tight feeling that radiates to his left arm and jaw. What type(s) of heart disease is this patient experiencing?
2. A 60-year-old male has been experiencing an increase in shortness of breath, a productive cough, and tiredness over the past few months. On examination, the doctor hears congestion in the lungs. What type of heart failure is this patient currently experiencing?
3. A 12-year-old child experiences high fever and chills. He also says that his heart feels like it's pounding. Two weeks before these symptoms, the child fell of his bike and "skinned" his knee. This child also has a history of a "heart murmur." What disease should we consider?

MULTIMEDIA EXTENSION ACTIVITIES

www.prenhall.com/mulvihill
Use the above address to access the free, interactive companion Website created for this textbook. Included in the features of this site are chapter specific activities, internet links, and an audio-glossary.

Audio Glossary
Use the CD-ROM disk enclosed with your textbook to hear the pronunciation of the key terms in this chapter.

Diseases at a Glance: Heart

Use the chart on page(s) 144–147 to answer the following:

1. List 5 types of diseases or conditions that affect the heart.

2. What are the major signs and symptoms of the diseases or conditions you named?

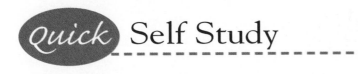 Self Study

TRUE OR FALSE

_____ 1. The left atrium hypertrophies and dilates when the mitral valve is stenotic.

_____ 2. Pain of a myocardial infarction is relieved by nitroglycerin.

_____ 3. Tachycardia refers to a decreased heart rate.

_____ 4. Aortic insufficiency causes back flow of blood from aorta to ventricle.

MULTIPLE CHOICE

_____ 1. Congestive heart failure involving the _____ of the heart causes shortness of breath due to pulmonary edema.
   a. right side   b. left side

_____ 2. Which defects are part of the tetralogy of Fallot?
   (1) mitral insufficiency   (2) hypertrophy of right ventricle
   (3) atrial septal defect   (4) pulmonary stenosis
   (5) aortic stenosis   (6) ventricular septal defect
   (7) misplaced aorta   (8) hypertrophy of left ventricle
   a. (1), (2), (4), (8)   b. (3), (5), (7), (8)
   c. (2), (3), (5), (7)   d. (2), (4), (6), (7)
   e. (1), (3), (5), (8)

_____ 3. _____ causes cyanosis.
   a. Failure of the foramen ovale to close
   b. Failure of the ductus arteriosis to close
   c. Pulmonary stenosis

_____ 4. _____ requires immediate attempts at resuscitation to prevent cardiac arrest.
   a. Atrial fibrillation   b. Ventricular fibrillation

_____ 5. Hypertension in a patient's arms but no femoral pulse indicates
   _____.
   a. Tetralogy of Fallot   b. coarctation of the aorta
   c. patent ductus arteriosis   d. failure of the foramen ovale to close

FILL-INS

1. _____ uses high frequency sound waves to examine the heart.

2. Enlargement of the walls of the heart is _____.

3. Oxygen poor blood flows from the body through the _____ and into the _____.

4. The left ventricle pumps blood to the body via the _____.

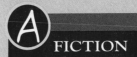 FICTION

Aspirin therapy should be given to all patients that have experienced an acute myocardial infarction (AMI). As the initial clot from an AMI dissolves there is a paradoxical increase in local thrombin, and platelet aggregation, which may lead to re-thrombosis and another AMI. Aspirin therapy minimizes re-thrombosis, platelet aggregation, and the reoccurrence of an AMI.

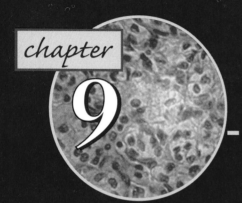

chapter

9

Diseases of the Blood Vessels

The heart is an effective pump only if the blood vessels through which it distributes blood are unobstructed.

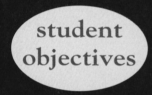

student objectives

After studying this chapter, students should be able to

➤ Describe the distribution of blood from the heart to the body and back to the heart

➤ Recite the structure and function of arteries, arterioles, capillaries, and veins

➤ Outline the common problems associated with diseases of the arteries and veins

➤ Distinguish between the terms atherosclerosis and arteriosclerosis

➤ Outline the formation of atherosclerosis

➤ Outline thrombus formation

➤ Describe the development of an embolism and the problems and complications that result from an embolism

➤ Outline the basis of aneurysm formation

➤ Describe the complications that arise from an aneurysm

➤ Recount the treatment of aneurysms

➤ Describe the symptoms and treatment for Raynaud's phenomena

➤ Distinguish the difference between phlebitis and thrombophlebitis

➤ Outline the causes, treatment, and complications of varicose veins

➤ Outline the effects of hemorrhoids and esophageal varicies

➤ Distinguish between primary, secondary, and malignant hypertension

➤ Describe the blood pressure reading and relate blood pressure to the phases of heart activity

➤ Distinguish and describe the various control mechanism for blood pressure

➤ Describe the relationship between hypertension and kidney disease

➤ Describe the effects of uncontrolled hypertension

➤ Outline the various treatments for hypertension

➤ Define shock and describe the different causes of shock

➤ Describe the diagnostic procedures used to diagnose vascular disease

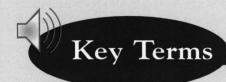
Key Terms

Anaphylactic shock

Aneurysm

Anticoagulant

Aorta

Atherosclerosis

Cardiogenic shock

Carotid audiofrequency analysis

Cerebral vascular accident

Compression sclerotherapy

Computed tomography

Diuretic

Doppler imaging

Ecchymosis

Embolism

Endoscopic sclerotherapy

Esophageal varices

Gangrene

Hemorrhage

Hemorrhoids

Hypovolemic shock

Intima

Ischemia

Ligated

Necrotic

Neurogenic shock

Petechiae

Phlebitis

Plaques

Purpura

Raynaud's disease

Sclerosis

Septic embolism

Spider veins

Stasis

Thrombophlebitis

Thrombosis

Thrombus

Ultrasound arteriography

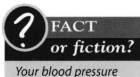

FACT
or fiction?

*Your blood pressure
may be high and you
might not even know it.*

*Read this chapter to find the
answer.*

aorta
(ā-ŏr′-tă)

➤ BLOOD VESSELS AND CIRCULATION

The importance of a well-functioning heart acting as a pump to provide blood to all parts of the body has been discussed. Another factor essential to this distribution of blood, is a good vascular system, that is, healthy blood vessels.

The cardiovascular system is also called the *circulatory system* because of the distribution of blood from the heart, through the body, and back to the heart. This is accomplished by the arrangement of blood vessels in a circular fashion.

Two circulatory systems function concurrently: the systemic circulation and the pulmonary circulation. The systemic circulation distributes oxygenated blood from the heart to all parts of the body, and it returns unoxygenated blood to the heart. The pulmonary system carries unoxygenated blood to the lungs to be oxygenated and returns the blood to the heart for systemic distribution (Figure 9–1). A partition in the heart maintains the separation of oxygenated from deoxygenated blood (see Chapter 8).

Blood vessels that carry blood away from the heart are the arteries, the largest of which is the **aorta.** The aorta branches, sending blood to the head through the carotid arteries, to the upper extremities and throughout the body. These arteries continue to divide into smaller and smaller vessels called *arterioles*. Arterioles lead into capillaries, the connecting links between arteries and veins. Blood then flows into the smallest veins, venules, and then into larger veins. Veins return blood to the heart.

PULMONARY CIRCULATION

Arteries — Veins

Veins — Arteries

SYSTEMIC CIRCULATION

Figure 9–1
Pulmonary and systemic circulation.

➤ STRUCTURE AND FUNCTION OF THE BLOOD VESSELS

The structure of different blood vessel types varies. The walls of arteries are thick and strong with considerable elastic tissue and are lined with endothelium, which comprises the intima. Arterioles are not only smaller in diameter but their walls are thinner, consisting mostly of smooth muscle fibers arranged circularly; arterioles are also lined with endothelium. Capillaries are minute vessels about 1/2 to 1 mm long with a lumen as wide as a red blood cell. Their wall consists of a layer of endothelium. Veins have walls that are much thinner than their companion arteries, but the lumen is considerably larger. Veins tend to collapse when empty.

Arterioles can change their diameter, that is, they constrict and dilate, which alters blood flow to the tissues as needed. This is controlled by the autonomic nervous system.

Capillaries, the thinnest-walled vessels, allow for the exchange of oxygen and carbon dioxide between the blood and tissues. Nutrients and waste products of cellular metabolism are also exchanged through capillary walls by diffusion.

Veins, particularly those of the legs, contain valves that help return blood upward to the heart against gravity. The largest veins are the inferior vena cava, from the lower part of the body, and the superior vena cava, from the upper part, both of which empty into the heart.

➤ DISEASES OF THE ARTERIES

Arteriosclerosis

Arteriosclerosis is caused by several conditions in which the wall of an artery becomes thicker and less elastic. The most common of these diseases is atherosclerosis in which fatty material accumulates under the inner lining or **intima** of the arterial wall (Figure 9–2).

intima
(ĭn'-tĭ-mă)

Atherosclerosis

Atherosclerosis begins with inflammatory processes such as a tear in the artery wall. Monocytes or white blood cells then accumulate at that site. These white blood cells, in turn, transform into cells that accumulate fat. Fatty deposits, called **plaques,** narrow the lumen of the blood vessels and, in some instances, completely occlude it. This fatty material consists mostly of cholesterol. Plaque may also consist of complex carbohydrates, blood and blood products, fibrous tissue, and calcium deposits. The aorta and its branches can be affected as well as smaller coronary and cerebral arteries (Figure 9–3). Occlusion of these vessels interferes with blood flow to the heart muscle, causing a myocardial infarction, and to the brain, causing a stroke or **cerebral vascular accident** (CVA). Lack of blood to any organ is called **ischemia** and promotes tissue damage.

atherosclerosis
(ăth-ĕr-ō-sklĕ-rō'-sĭs)

plaques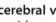
(plăkz)

cerebral vascular accident
(sĕ-rē'-brăl văs'-kū-lar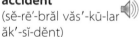
ăk'-sĭ-dĕnt)

ischemia
(ĭs-kē'-mē-ă)

Disease by the Numbers **x + ÷**

Fifty percent of all deaths due to atherosclerosis of the coronary arteries are sudden.

Reference: American Heart Association, 1999 Heart and Stroke Statistical Update, Dallas, Texas.

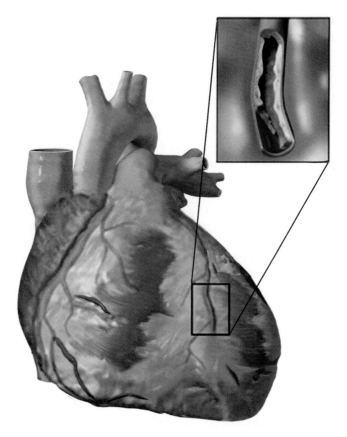

Figure 9–2
An atherosclerotic artery.

The cause of atherosclerosis is not completely known, but it does have a hereditary basis. Atherosclerosis is a common complication of diabetes, also a disease with a hereditary tendency. A low-cholesterol diet and regular exercise should reduce the risk of developing atherosclerosis. Figure 9–4 summarizes the possible effects of artery disease on the heart and brain.

Thrombosis and Embolism

One of the body's protective devices is the blood-clotting mechanism. When there is injury to tissues and blood vessels, excessive bleeding is prevented as the blood starts to clot. This same mechanism can function within the intact blood vessels, and this intravascular clotting produces a **thrombus.**

 thrombus
(thrŏm′-bŭs)

 thrombosis
(thrŏm-bō′-sĭs)

Several factors lead to **thrombosis,** the forming of blood clots on blood vessel walls. Clots tend to form where blood flow is slower. Because blood flows more slowly in veins than in arteries, veins are the more common site of thrombus formation. Clots are also likely to form where there is turbulence in the bloodstream, as there is over the heart valves. A diseased valve is a likely site for a clot formation.

Platelets, which normally initiate the blood-clotting mechanism, are deposited on the inner wall of a blood vessel or on a heart valve. Normally, these surfaces are very smooth, and platelets do not adhere. But when they are injured or diseased, the platelets

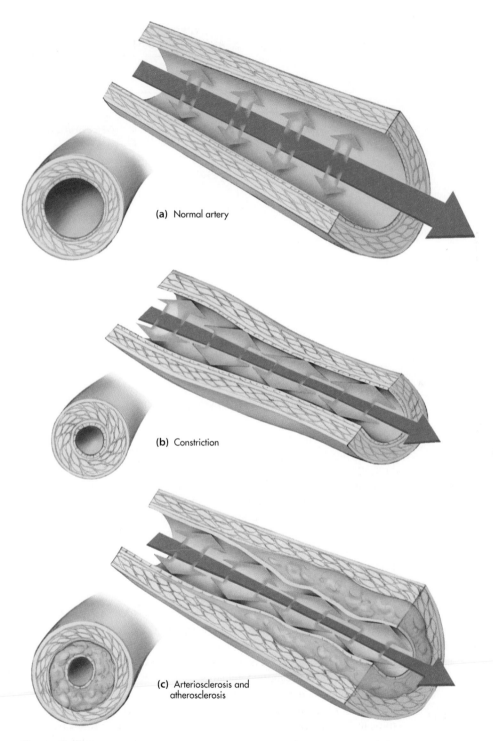

Figure 9-3
Blood vessels: (**a**) Normal artery. (**b**) Constriction. (**c**) Arteriosclerosis and atherosclerosis.

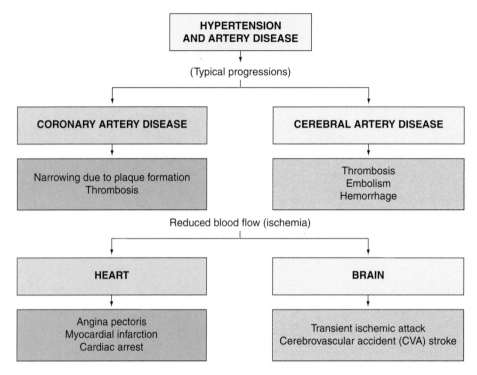

Figure 9–4
Possible effects of artery disease on the heart and brain.

stick and the clot begins to form. Atherosclerosis and rheumatic heart disease are predisposing causes of thrombus formation. Clots frequently form in coronary and cerebral arteries and in the legs when circulation is poor. Figure 9–5 illustrates thrombus formation. Changes in the blood itself can cause thrombosis. The blood may become too viscous or the platelet count may be excessively high.

anticoagulant
(ăn″-tĭ-kō-ăg′-ū-lănt)

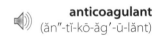

Anticoagulant medication may be administered to prevent intravascular clotting or to promote resolution of and prevent recurrence of a thrombus. These medications must be monitored closely for adverse effects because they interfere with platelet function. (For additional information, refer to Chapter 7.)

The thrombus may retract and allow blood to flow, or it may permanently occlude the vessel. The thrombus can become detached and travel in the bloodstream as an embolus. Infected tissue around the thrombus can cause this detachment as can sudden movement.

embolism
(em′-bō-lĭzm)

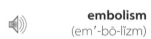

Let us imagine a thrombus in a leg vein and follow its course as it travels as an **embolism.** Veins become larger as they approach the heart, so the clot travels easily to the heart. Vessels become smaller as they leave the right side of the heart toward the lungs. The embolus can then get stuck in a pulmonary artery and even occlude it. A pulmonary embolus is illustrated in Figure 9–6.

A damaged mitral valve often results from rheumatic heart disease and is a potential site for thrombus formation. A clot formed on this valve can break loose and enter the aorta. It then may travel to the brain, kidney, or some other organ. Figure 9–7 shows an embolus traveling to the brain through the carotid artery.

septic embolism
(sĕp′-tĭc ĕm′-bō-lĭzm)

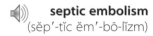

An embolism may contain infected material from pyogenic bacteria and is then called a **septic embolism.** This sometimes results from a lack of sterile technique during labor and delivery or an abortion. Substances other than blood can comprise an em-

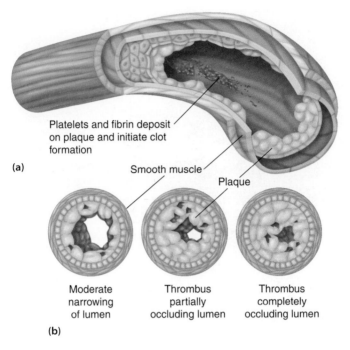

(a)

Platelets and fibrin deposit
on plaque and initiate clot
formation

Smooth muscle

Plaque

Moderate
narrowing
of lumen

Thrombus
partially
occluding lumen

Thrombus
completely
occluding lumen

(b)

Figure 9–5
Thrombus formation in an atherosclerotic vessel. Depicted are the
initial clot formation (a) and the varying degrees of occlusion (b).

bolism. Air introduced into a vein during surgery produces air bubbles; these air bubbles, fat globules, and groups of cancer cells can all travel in the blood as emboli with the potential of closing a blood vessel.

Lack of blood due to a closed blood vessel causes tissue death, an infarct. Bacteria can enter the **necrotic,** or dead, tissue and cause **gangrene** or gangrenous necrosis. The localized tissue death distal to the clot is called *coagulation necrosis.*

If this occurs in the foot, a greenish color develops that turns to black, and the condition spreads up the leg.

Aneurysms
A weakening in the wall of a blood vessel can cause localized dilation known as an **aneurysm.** Aneurysms most commonly occur in the aorta and result primarily from arteriosclerosis. Aneurysms can also develop in arteries other than the aorta. The danger of an aneurysm is the tendency to increase in size and rupture, resulting in hemorrhage, possibly in a vital organ such as the heart, brain, or abdomen. Figure 9–8 shows a normal aorta and Figure 9–9 shows an aortic aneurysm.

Aneurysms usually produce no symptoms and are detected by an x-ray or routine physical exam. Ultrasound techniques can diagnose and measure aneurysms. A **computed tomography** or CT scan is accurate in determining the shape and size of an aneurysm. Early detection prevents rupture.

Surgical procedures have been very successful in repairing blood vessels affected by aneurysm formation. The diseased area of the vessel is removed and replaced with a plastic graft or segment of another blood vessel. This procedure reduces the risk of hemorrhage and thrombus formation.

necrotic
(nĕ-krō-tĭk)

gangrene
(găng-grēn′)

aneurysm
(ăn′-ū-rĭzm)

computed tomography
(kŏm-pū′-tĕd tō-mŏg′-ră-fē)

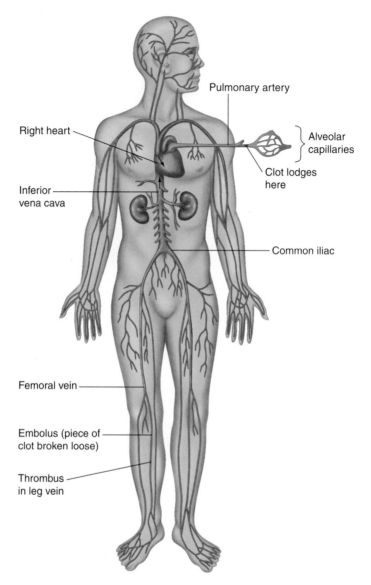

Figure 9–6
Pulmonary embolism.

Hemorrhages

The rupture of blood vessels with subsequent bleeding is discussed in several contexts throughout the text. A large loss of blood in a short period of time, either internally or externally, is termed a **hemorrhage.** Aneurysms, just described, head injuries (Chapter 6), and bleeding diseases (Chapter 7) are often causes of hemorrhage. The size and location of the ruptured blood vessels determine the result. Minute blood vessels that rupture in the skin cause tiny red or purple spots called **petechiae** (Chapter 7). Small hemorrhages into the tissue beneath the skin or mucous membranes are termed **purpura.** Trauma to underlying blood vessels, which causes discoloration of an area is an **ecchymosis** or bruise. The colors of a bruise or "black and blue" spot are the result of the breakdown of hemoglobin when blood vessels are damaged.

hemorrhage
(hĕm′-ĕ-rĭj)

petechiae
(pĕ-tē′-kē-ē)

purpura
(pŭr′-pū-ră)

ecchymosis
(ĕk-u-mō′-sĭs)

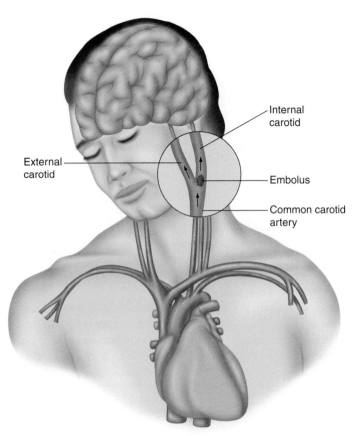

Internal carotid

External carotid

Embolus

Common carotid artery

Figure 9–7
Embolus traveling to the brain.

side by side

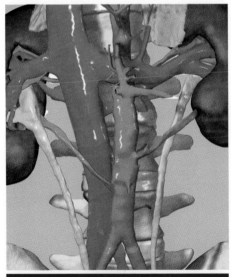

Figure 9–8

A normal aorta.

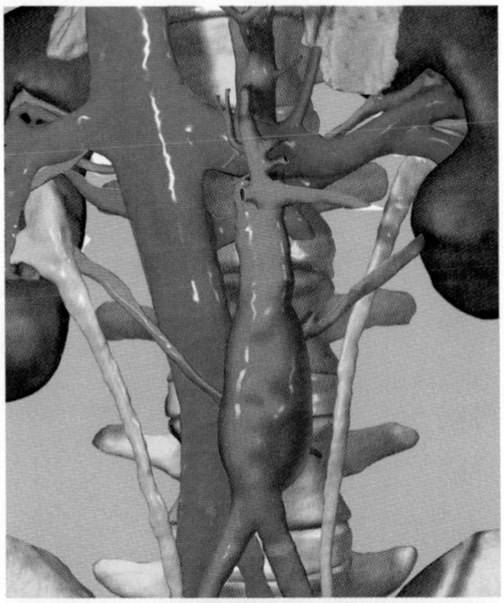

Figure 9–9

An aortic aneurysm.

**Raynaud's
disease**
(rā-nōz' dĭ-zēz')

Raynaud's Disease

Raynaud's disease is a condition in which small arteries or arterioles in the fingers and toes constrict. Symptoms of spasms including numbness, discoloration of the local skin of the fingers and toes, and pain result (see Figure 9–10).

Spasms come and go and are most commonly triggered by cold. As vessels constrict, blood flow temporarily decreases causing the fingers and toes to turn white. As the episode resolves, the affected areas may turn pink or bluish in color.

Raynaud's disease can usually be controlled by protection from cold. Smoking should be avoided as it constricts blood vessels. Relaxation techniques can help reduce stress, which may bring about an attack.

on the Practical Side

Colors in a "Black and Blue" Mark
Trauma may injure soft tissue without breaking the skin. Tiny blood vessels are ruptured, and blood flows into the tissue spaces. The bruise is red at first, then becomes purple, blue, green, and yellow before fading. The changes in color are due to the rupture of red blood cells with the release of hemoglobin. The breakdown of hemoglobin produces the colored molecules of the bruise.

➤ DISEASES OF THE VEINS

Phlebitis

phlebitis
(flē-bī'-tĭs)

Phlebitis is an inflammation of a vein, usually in the leg. Veins are both superficial and deep. It is only when the deep veins are affected that the condition is considered potentially serious. Several factors may cause phlebitis: injury, general infection, poor circulation, and obesity, to name a few.

thrombophlebitis
(thrŏm"-bō-flē-bī'-tĭs)

The greatest danger in the deep veins is thrombus formation, and the condition is then called **thrombophlebitis** (Figure 9–11). If a vein becomes occluded by a clot, edema develops. The blood cannot return properly to the heart, the veins become congested

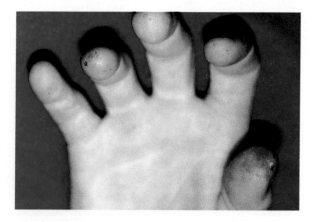

Figure 9–10
Raynaud's disease (*Courtesy of Jason L. Smith, MD*).

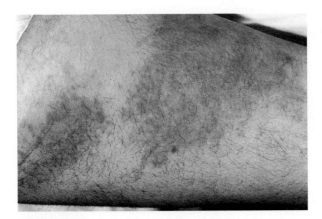

Figure 9–11
Thrombophlebitis (*Courtesy of Jason L. Smith, MD*).

with blood, and fluid seeps out into the tissues. It is important that the clot does not become dislodged and travel as an embolism. Anticoagulants may be administered to prevent further clot formation, and antibiotics are administered to prevent infection. Surgery is sometimes required to remove the thrombus.

Varicose Veins

Varicose veins generally develop in the superficial veins of the leg, most commonly the greater saphenous, near the medial side of the leg. The veins become swollen, painful, and appear knotty under the skin. The condition is caused by stagnation of blood in the veins that can result from several factors.

Development of varicose veins can be an occupational hazard for someone who stands or sits still for long periods of time. Normally the action of the leg muscles helps move the blood upward from one valve to the next. In the absence of this "milking action" of the muscles, the blood exerts a pressure on the closed valves and thin walls of the veins. The veins then dilate to the extent that the valves are no longer competent. The blood then collects, becomes stagnant, and the veins become more swollen.

Pregnancy or a tumor in the uterus can also cause varicose veins. The return flow of blood from the legs encounters resistance and a back pressure of blood results, breaking down more and more valves. Heredity often plays a part in the development of varicose veins as does obesity. Figure 9–12 illustrates normal veins and the flow of blood upward through the valves and varicose veins where the valves have become incompetent. Ulcers tend to develop because of poor circulation. The slowing blood flow (**stasis**) often causes infection. The distended veins can rupture, causing hemorrhage into the surrounding tissues.

Treatment varies with the severity of the symptoms. At times, an elastic bandage or wearing support hose is adequate. Walking, elevating the legs when seated, and weight control can lessen the severity. A surgical procedure called "stripping the veins" is very successful. The superficial veins are tied off, **ligated,** and removed. A collateral circulation to the deep veins takes over. Small, dense, red networks of veins, called **spider veins,** can be effectively treated with laser. The light overheats and scars the tiny superficial veins, which closes them off to blood flow (Figure 9–13).

stasis
(stā′-sĭs)

ligated
(lī′-gāt-ĕd)

spider veins
(spī′-dĕr vāns)

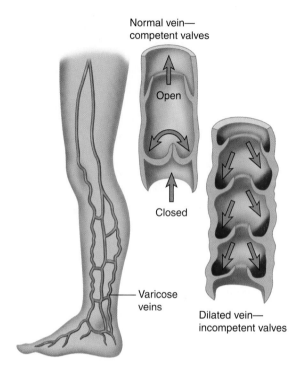

Figure 9–12
Development of varicose veins.

**compression
sclerotherapy**
(kŏm′-prĕ-ssĭon
sklĕr-ō-thar′-ă-pē)

hemorrhoids
(hĕm′-ō-roydz)

Another treatment is **compression sclerotherapy** in which a strong saline solution is injected into specific sites of the varicose veins. The irritation causes scarring of the inner lining and fuses the veins shut. The procedure is followed by uninterrupted compression for several weeks to prevent reentry of blood. A daily walking program during the recovery period is required to activate leg muscle venous pumps.

Hemorrhoids are varicose veins of the rectum and cause pain, itching, and bleeding. Like varicose veins in the leg, hemorrhoids can develop from pressure on the veins.

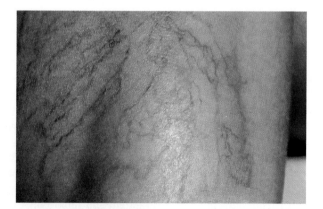

Figure 9–13
Spider veins (*Courtesy of Jason L. Smith, MD*).

Straining due to constipation, pressure on the veins from a pregnant uterus, or a tumor may promote their development (Chapter 11).

Esophageal varices, or varicose veins of the esophagus, frequently accompany cirrhosis of the liver. They result from pressure that develops within the veins as they try to empty. Because of blocked blood vessels within the damaged liver, there is a backup of blood and general congestion. A fatal hemorrhage from these varices can occur.

A relatively new procedure for treating esophageal varices is called **endoscopic sclerotherapy.** In this procedure, a retractable needle is guided into the esophagus by means of a fiberoptic endoscope. The gastroenterologist punctures the varicosities and injects a caustic **sclerosis** (hardening) solution to occlude the swollen veins. This prevents engorgement, rupture, and hemorrhage, or stops a hemorrhage that has already begun.

esophageal varices
(ĭ-sŏf″-u-jē′-ul var′-u-sēz″)

endoscopic sclerotherapy
(ĕn′-du-skŏp″-ĭk skli-rō-thar′-ă-pē)

sclerosis
(sklĕ-rō′-sĭs)

➤ HYPERTENSION

Hypertension or "high blood pressure" is a condition of abnormally high blood pressure in the arteries. Called the "silent killer," hypertension is usually not diagnosed until complications arise. The causes of primary hypertension are not known, though there tends to be a hereditary basis. Secondary hypertension results from other diseases, such as brain tumors, kidney disease, and endocrine disorders. Primary hypertension is aggravated by obesity, lack of exercise, and excessive alcohol and salt intake. Hypertension may have a gradual onset and continue for a long time, or it may be malignant, with sudden onset and rapid progression resulting in death if not treated immediately.

A blood pressure reading has two parts corresponding to the two phases of heart activity: the systolic and diastolic pressure. The systolic pressure is the highest pressure in the arteries caused by the force of contraction of the ventricles. Diastolic pressure corresponds to the pressure in the arteries when the ventricles are relaxing and refilling. A normal adult has an average blood pressure of 120 mm Hg (systolic) over 80 mm Hg (diastolic) or 120/80 mm Hg.

Blood pressure normally varies throughout the day increasing with activity and decreasing with rest. Because of these fluctuations, high blood pressure is not considered abnormal unless there are three elevated readings in a row, each taken at different times under similar conditions. Generally, pressures that are consistently greater than 140/90 mm Hg are considered high.

Control Mechanisms
In the normal person, several mechanisms function to control blood pressure. Adjustments of blood pressure are governed by changes in kidney function and nervous system. The autonomic nervous system regulates many body functions automatically and includes the sympathetic and parasympathetic nervous systems (Chapter 16).

Blood pressure is increased in various ways. The heart can pump with greater force through less space or vasoconstricted arteries. As more fluid is added to the system, the blood pressure increases until arteries dilate or expand, and the kidneys are able to excrete the excess fluid. During the "fight or flight" response, the sympathetic nervous system temporarily increases blood pressure.

The kidney compensates for a decrease in blood volume by secreting a substance called renin. Renin activates angiotensin, a hormone that causes the walls of the arteries to constrict, and increases blood pressure. Angiotensin also triggers the release of another hormone, aldosterone, which causes the kidneys to retain salt (sodium) and water, thus expanding blood volume and further increasing blood pressure. Frequently, vaso-constriction of blood vessels due to high blood pressure causes increased renin, angiotensin, and aldosterone secretion. If this cycle is not broken, blood pressure continues to increase.

The parasympathetic nervous system works antagonistically to the sympathetic nervous system and decreases blood pressure. Another means of reducing blood pressure is by reducing blood volume via a capillary shift mechanism. When blood volume is high, the pressure in the arteries is higher than that of the tissue outside. The high pressure forces the fluid through the walls of the capillaries into the tissue spaces, thus reducing blood volume and pressure.

Hypertension and Kidney Disease

A close relationship exists between hypertension and kidney disease. Hypertension can contribute to kidney disease, and kidney disease can contribute to hypertension. Decreased function of the kidneys leads to water and salt retention, causing increased blood volume and elevated blood pressure levels. Long-standing hypertension causes arteriosclerosis of the renal artery, which reduces blood flow to the kidneys and damages them.

Effects of Hypertension

Untreated high blood pressure increases the risk of heart disease, kidney disease, and stroke. Increased blood pressure damages all arteries of the body, including the coronary arteries. Damaged arteries become sclerotic (hardened) and weak. Thrombi form in weakened vessels leading to ischemia and necrosis with loss of function in vital organs.

Hypertension overworks the heart, causing the left ventricle to hypertrophy. The left ventricle eventually fails and is unable to pump enough blood to meet the demands

---

PREVENTION *PLUS!*

Save Your Life by Changing It

Lose weight	■ The single most effective nondrug method to decrease blood pressure
Exercise	■ 30 to 35 minutes of exercise three times per week can decrease blood pressure, especially when combined with weight loss
Limit alcohol	■ Alcohol raises your blood pressure even if you don't have hypertension
Eat a low-fat and high-fruit and vegetable diet	■ A diet higher in vitamins and low in fat is associated with lower blood pressure.
	■ 40% of patients who reduced weight through diet management were able to stop their high blood pressure medication
Hold the salt	■ African-Americans and women over the age of 65 years seem to benefit when daily salt intake is reduced to no more than 2400 mg of salt per day, which is about 1 tsp

Reference: Mayo Clinic Women's Health Source, September, 1997.

of the body. As coronary vessels constrict and become occluded, attacks of angina pectoris (see Chapter 8) and myocardial infarction, or true heart attacks, result.

Weakened blood vessels can rupture and bleed because of high pressure within. Ruptured vessels cause local tissue damage in the brain (stroke), kidney, or other organs.

Treatment of Hypertension

Primary hypertension cannot be cured, but it can be treated to prevent complications. A combination of medication, diet changes, and exercise is the ideal method for controlling high blood pressure. Because there are usually no symptoms of high blood pressure, treatments that make people feel bad or interfere with lifestyle are avoided.

Overweight individuals are advised to reduce their weight. Changes in diet for those who have diabetes and high cholesterol levels are important for overall cardiovascular health. Cutting down on salt and alcohol intake may make drug therapy for high blood pressure unnecessary. Moderate exercise can help control weight and improve circulation.

Drug therapy can help reduce blood pressure by several different mechanisms. In choosing a drug, consider the person's age, sex, and race; severity of high blood pressure; the presence of other conditions (such as diabetes, or high cholesterol); potential side effects and drug interactions; cost; frequency of administration and safety. Drug therapy is started when lifestyle modification is not effective or produces an inadequate response. One or more drugs with different actions may be used to control blood pressure. For example, a **diuretic** that controls blood volume in combination with a drug that blocks sympathetic stimulation may be prescribed; a drug that blocks the renin-angiotensin-aldosterone cascade in combination with a sympathetic nervous system blocker is another alternative. In general, the best combination of drug therapy is one that fits the patient's lifestyle with minimal side effects.

diuretic
(dī-ū-rĕt-ĭk)

Treatment of secondary hypertension depends on the underlying cause. Treatment of kidney disease can normalize or lower blood pressure. Inserting a balloon-tipped catheter and inflating the balloon may dilate a narrowed artery. A narrowed or blocked artery may be bypassed. Tumors that produce high blood pressure can usually be removed surgically.

➤ SHOCK

Shock is a life-threatening condition in which blood pressure is too low to sustain life. Any condition that reduces the heart's ability to pump effectively or decreases venous return can cause shock. This low blood pressure causes an inadequate blood supply to the cells of the body. The cells can be quickly and irreversibly damaged and die. **Hypovolemic shock** (hemorrhagic) results from fluid volume loss after severe hemorrhage or loss of plasma in burn patients. Treatment includes administration of plasma or whole blood. **Neurogenic shock** is due to generalized vasodilation, resulting from decreased vasomotor tone. The reduced blood pressure causes poor venous return to the heart and, hence, poor cardiac output. The decreased vasomotor tone may be due to spinal anesthesia, spinal cord injury, or certain drugs. **Anaphylactic shock** accompanies a severe antigen-antibody reaction, such as occurs in an incompatible blood transfusion. **Cardiogenic shock** is the result of extensive myocardial infarction. It is often fatal, but drugs to combat it are sometimes effective. The types of shock are summarized in Figure 9–14.

hypovolemic shock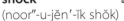
(hī″-pō-vŏl-ē-mĭk shŏk)

neurogenic shock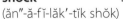
(noor″-u-jĕn′-ĭk shŏk)

anaphylactic shock
(ăn″-ă-fĭ-lăk′-tĭk shŏk)

cardiogenic shock
(kar″-dē-u-jĕn′-ĭk shŏk)

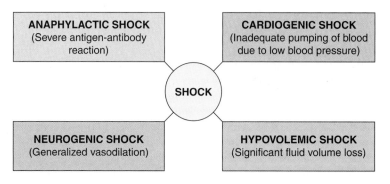

Figure 9–14
Various types of shock.

➤ DIAGNOSTIC PROCEDURES FOR VASCULAR DISEASE

carotid audiofrequency analysis
(ka-rŏt'-ĭd ăw'-dē-ō-frē'-kwĕn-sē ăn'-a-līs-sĭs)

ultrasound arteriography
(ŭl'-tră-sownd ăr-tē-rē-ŏg'-ră-fē)

Doppler imaging
(Dŏp'-lĕr ĭm-ĭj-ĭg)

Great advances have been made in noninvasive diagnostic techniques for peripheral vascular disease. This reduces the need for invasive angiography for many people. Carotid phonoangiography (CPA), also called **carotid audiofrequency analysis,** is an extension of auscultation. Special microphones are placed over areas of abnormal sounds that are heard with a stethoscope. The sound is pictured on an oscilloscope and photographed. Sound-frequency patterns can then be analyzed by computers, and the degree and location of carotid stenosis can be documented.

Ultrasound arteriography can show the anatomy of arteries, particularly the carotid bifurcation and the internal carotid artery. The **Doppler imaging** instrument uses echoes of moving blood columns to produce images of the vessel wall outline. The velocity of the blood is measured, and the degree of carotid stenosis can be determined. The noninvasive test is very useful for patients who have had strokes or transient ischemic attacks.

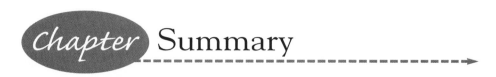

Chapter Summary

Healthy blood vessels are essential to adequate distribution of blood to all the tissues of the body. The condition of arteriosclerosis makes vessels susceptible to rupture and the roughened inner lining a site for clot formation. In atherosclerosis, the fatty deposits that build up in the intima of the arteries narrow the lumen, greatly reducing blood flow. These lipid plaques can actually occlude the opening.

Although clotting within blood vessels does not normally occur, certain factors can promote it. Rough or diseased surfaces provide a site for thrombus formation. The clot may become detached and travel as an embolism, possibly lodging and blocking a critical artery. Veins may become congested with blood and distended to the extent that the valves cannot function. The stagnation of blood causes the infection and ulceration associated with varicose veins.

Hypertension is the leading cause of strokes and congestive heart failure. Its causes, effects, and treatment were described. Noninvasive procedures for diagnosing vascular disease were explained.

Diseases at a Glance: Blood Vessels

Categories	Disease	Signs and Symptoms
Functional	Hypertension	None obvious, "silent killer"
	Hypovolemic (hemorrhagic) shock	Severe hemorrhage, severe and extensive burns
	Neurogenic shock	Falling blood pressure, slow heart rate
	Anaphylactic shock	Hives, itching, wheezing, increased heart rate, increased respiratory rate
	Cardiogenic shock	Myocardial infarction, fast heart rate, cool, clammy skin
	Raynaud's disease	Numbness, discoloration, pain, cold digits
Arterial disease	Arteriosclerosis, Atherosclerosis	Varies with arteries affected and severity, thrombus (clot) may block artery, embolus (traveling clot) may be released & block artery elsewhere
	Aneurysm	No symptoms until rupture
Vein disease	Thrombophlebitis	Pain, edema, inflammation, thrombus (clot) formation
	Varicose veins	Swelling of veins, stasis, rupture may occur Spider veins, hemorrhoids, esophageal varices

Affected Organ/Body Region	Diagnostic Procedure	Treatment
Systolic and diastolic pressures	BP measures consistently high	Weight loss, reduced salt and fat in diet, exercise, stop smoking, medication
Cardiovascular system	Physical exam	Fluid replacement, transfusion
Parasympathetic activation causes systemic vasodilation	Physical exam, cardiovascular monitoring	Elevation of legs, compressive stockings, drugs, fluids
Mast cells—massive histamine release	Physical exam	Epinephrine, steroids, fluids
Cardiovascular system	Physical exam, cardiovascular monitoring	Treatment of heart failure, drugs
Arteries	Physical exam	Protection from cold, no smoking
Artery walls	Ultrasound arteriography, Doppler imaging	Low cholesterol diet, exercise, weight loss, stop smoking; balloon angiography, bypass surgery
Artery walls	X-ray, MRI, ultrasound	Surgical repair
Deep veins, legs	Physical exam	Anticoagulants, antibiotics, surgery
Legs, rectal veins, esophageal veins	Physical exam	Endoscopic sclerotherapy, surgery

Interactive Activities

CASES FOR CRITICAL THINKING

1. A 40-year-old man is admitted to the emergency room with sudden, sharp pain in his leg. His left lower leg is bluish. This man has a history of smoking and is a recovering alcoholic. What diseases should we suspect or rule out?
2. A 28-year-old man confronts his druggist after checking his blood pressure and noting that it is in the "high range." What type of advice should this druggist give to this man?
3. A 37-year-old pregnant female has been complaining of leg cramps. She gained more weight than normal. Her mother had surgery on her legs to "repair her veins." At what vascular condition is this woman at risk? How should this condition be managed?

MULTIMEDIA EXTENSION ACTIVITIES

www.prenhall.com/mulvihill
Use the above address to access the free, interactive companion Website created for this textbook. Included in the features of this site are chapter specific activities, internet links, and an audio-glossary.

Audio Glossary
Use the CD-ROM disk enclosed with your textbook to hear the pronunciation of the key terms in this chapter.

Diseases at a Glance: Blood Vessels

Use the chart on page(s) 168–169 to answer the following:

1. List 5 types of diseases or conditions that affect the blood vessels.

2. What are the major signs and symptoms of the diseases or conditions you named?

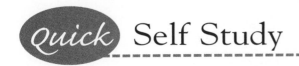

Quick Self Study

MULTIPLE CHOICE

1. The depositing of fatty patches within the arteries is called _____.
   a. arteriosclerosis   b. atherosclerosis

2. Phlebitis is an inflammation of the _____.
   a. veins   b. arteries

3. A bubble-like protrusion of an arterial wall is a/an _____.
   a. hematoma   b. petechia
   c. aneurysm

4. An embolus traveling from the leg to the heart would be more likely to block the
   _____.
   a. aorta   b. pulmonary artery

5. Raynaud's disease causes _____ of the arterioles.
   a. constriction   b. dilation

TRUE OR FALSE

1. Long-standing hypertension causes the left ventricle to hypertrophy.

2. An embolism in the brain may result from a thrombus on the mitral valve.

3. Neurogenic shock results from severe fluid volume loss.

4. After a severe hemorrhage, blood pressure increases.

FILL-INS

1. Raynaud's disease results in _____ of the arterioles.

2. The highest pressure in a blood pressure reading indicates _____.

3. Anticoagulant medication is administered to promote _____ of a
   thrombus and prevent _____.

4. In primary hypertension the causes are _____. Whereas in secondary hypertension the causes are _____.

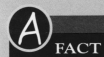

FACT

It is estimated that one-third of 50 million Americans who have high blood pressure don't even know that they have high blood pressure. Regular check-ups are important.

Reference: Mayo Clinic Women's Health Source, September, 1997.

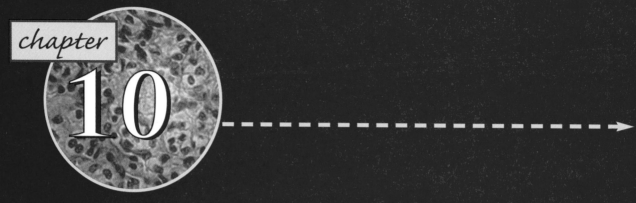

Diseases of the Urinary System

The kidneys are very interesting and complex organs. Not only do the kidneys remove waste products from the body, but they also help maintain blood pH, blood pressure, and perform other major tasks as homeostatic organs.

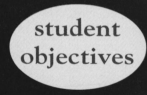

student objectives

After studying this chapter, students should be able to
➤ Identify the major diseases of the kidney
➤ Relate how infectious agents or their products may travel to the kidney
➤ Name the most common diagnostic procedures used to determine kidney and kidney-related diseases
➤ Recognize complications of kidney-related diseases
➤ Relate infectious precursors to kidney-related diseases
➤ Distinguish between pyelonephritis and glomerulonephritis
➤ Recognize specific signs and symptoms associated with urinary tract disorders
➤ Identify potential causes and treatments for renal calculi or kidney stones
➤ Describe complications of renal calculi
➤ Distinguish between the two types of kidney dialysis
➤ Define lithotripsy
➤ Define incontinence and give related symptoms and treatment
➤ Describe procedures and treatments for bladder cancer

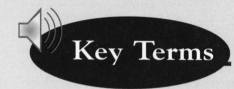

Key Terms

Acidosis

Albuminuria

Alkalosis

Anuria

Azotemia

Bowman's capsule

Casts

Creatinine

Cystitis

Cystoscope

Diabetic nephropathy

Dialysis

Dysuria

Edema

Electrolyte balance

Glomerulonephritis

Glomerulus

Hematuria

Hydrolithotripsy

Hydronephrosis

Hydroureters

Hyperkalemia

Hypernephroma

Intravenous pyelogram

Juxtaglomerular apparatus

Lithotripsy

Nephron

Nephrotripsy

Oliguria

Polycystic kidney

Prolapses

Pyelitis

Pyelonephritis

Pyuria

Renal pelvis

Renin

Staghorn calculus

Urea

Uremia

Ureterocele

Ureters

Urethra

Urethritis

Urinalysis

Urinary calculi

Wilms' tumor

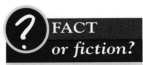

electrolyte balance
(ē-lĕk′-trō-līt băl′-ăns)

acidosis
(ăs″-ĭ-dō′-sĭs)

alkalosis
(ăl″-kă-lō′-sĭs)

juxtaglomerular apparatus
(jŭks″-tă-glō-mĕr′-ū-lăr ăp″-ă-rā′-tŭs)

renin
(rĕn′-ĭn)

nephron
(nĕf′-rŏn)

Bowman's capsule
(bō′-măns kăp′-sūl)

glomerulus
(glō-mĕr′-ū-lŭs)

renal pelvis
(rē′-năl pĕl′-vĭs)

ureters
(ū′-rĕ-tĕrs)

➤ FUNCTIONS OF THE KIDNEYS

The kidneys play an essential role in maintaining **electrolyte balance,** a factor essential to normal nerve and muscle physiology. The proper balance of salts like sodium, potassium, and calcium is required for normal heart activity.

Another kidney function is to help maintain the correct pH, or acid-base balance, of blood and body fluids. The body tolerates a very limited pH range of 7.35 to 7.45. If the pH of blood is lower than this, the blood is too acidic, and a condition called **acidosis** develops. The effect of acidosis will be discussed with diabetes mellitus because it is a complication of this disease. If the pH of blood is higher than 7.45, the blood is too alkaline, and the condition is called **alkalosis.** Death can result from either of these extremes. The kidneys help regulate blood pH by excreting an acidic urine when blood and body fluids are too acidic, and an alkaline urine when the pH is abnormally high. The kidneys also produce a hormone, erythropoietin, that stimulates red blood cell production. When kidneys become diseased, the hormone is not secreted and severe anemia develops. Specialized cells within the arterioles leading to the functional kidney area comprise the **juxtaglomerular apparatus.** These cells secrete **renin** that converts angiotensinogen to angiotensin, an active enzyme to help elevate blood pressure.

The Nephron

The functional unit of the kidney is the **nephron.** There are about a million nephrons in each kidney. It is the work of these minute structures to filter waste products from the blood, to reabsorb water and nutrients such as glucose and amino acids from the tubular fluid, and to secrete excess substances from the body fluids.

Each nephron consists of a **Bowman's capsule,** a proximal convoluted tubule, loop of Henle, and a distal convoluted tubule that leads to a collecting tubule. Urine is formed in the nephron. Figure 10–1 illustrates the parts of the nephron. As the various kidney diseases are considered, the effect of the malfunction of these parts will become clear.

Formation of Urine

Blood (plasma) to be filtered is carried to a tuft of capillaries called the **glomerulus,** which is situated inside Bowman's capsule. These capillary walls are very thin. Their surface area is large, and the blood pressure within them is higher than the pressure in Bowman's capsule. These factors cause the filtration of fluid into Bowman's capsule. This fluid is initial urine or filtrate and is equivalent to protein-free plasma. In a healthy nephron, neither protein nor red blood cells pass through the filter into Bowman's capsule.

In the proximal convoluted tubule, most of the nutrients and a large amount of water are reabsorbed and taken back into blood capillaries surrounding the tubules. Salts, particularly sodium and chloride, are selectively reabsorbed according to the body's needs. Water is also reabsorbed with the salts.

The nitrogen-containing waste products of protein metabolism, urea and creatinine, pass on through the tubules to be excreted in the urine. Substances that are in excess in the body fluids, such as hydrogen ions if the fluid is too acidic, are secreted into the distal tubules to be excreted.

Two hormones play a very important role in the regulation of salt and water reabsorption. They are aldosterone, secreted by the adrenal glands, and antidiuretic hormone, secreted by the posterior pituitary gland. More will be said of these hormones when the diseases of the endocrine glands are discussed (Chapter 14).

Final urine from all the collecting ducts empties into the **renal pelvis,** the juncture between the kidneys and the **ureters.** It then moves down the ureters to be stored in the

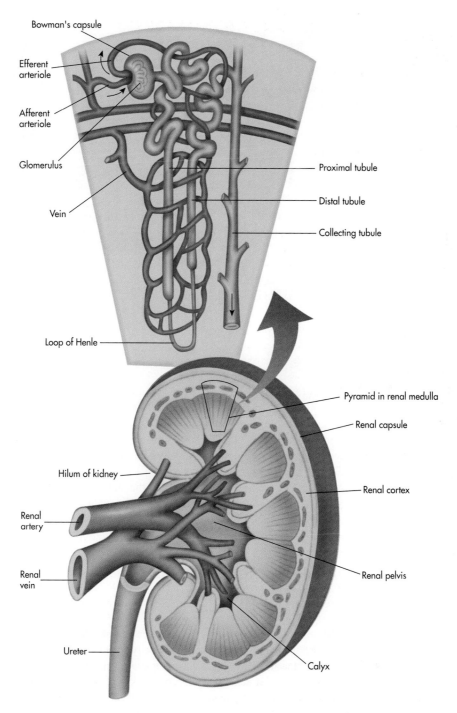

Figure 10-1
The kidney with an expanded view of a nephron.

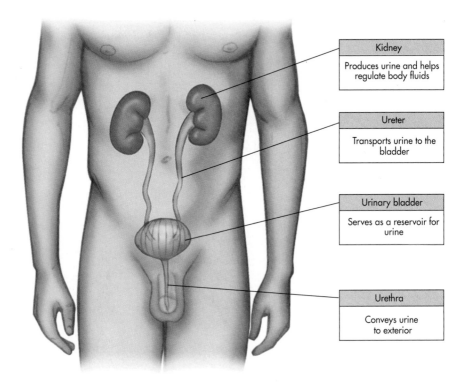

Figure 10–2
The urinary system.

urethra
(ū-rē′-thră)

urinary bladder, which empties to the outside through a single tube called the **urethra.** Figure 10–2 illustrates the urinary system.

An obstruction along this path can set the stage for infection. The obstruction may be a kidney stone; an enlarged prostate gland, the male gland that surrounds the urethra, or a tumor. Any blockage causes stasis and a diminished flow of urine, and bacteria thrive in the stagnant fluid.

➤ DISEASES OF THE KIDNEY

Glomerulonephritis

glomerulonephritis
(glō-mĕr″-ū-lō-nĕ-frī′-tĭs)

edema
(ĕ-dē′-mă)

albuminuria
(ăl-bū-mĭ-nū′-rē-ă)

hematuria
(hē″-mă-tū′-rĭ-ă)

casts
(kăsts)

Acute Glomerulonephritis   Acute **glomerulonephritis** is a common disease primarily affecting children and young adults. It usually results from a previous streptococcal infection: strep throat, scarlet fever, or rheumatic fever. The symptoms are chills and fever, loss of appetite, and a general feeling of weakness. There may be **edema,** or puffiness, particularly in the face and ankles. A urinalysis shows **albuminuria,** the presence of the plasma protein albumin in the urine. **Hematuria,** blood in the urine, is also commonly found. **Casts,** which are molds of kidney tubules consisting of coagulated protein and blood, are present. The signs and symptoms of acute glomerulonephritis are presented in Figure 10–3.

The presence of blood, albumin, and casts in the urine indicates that the glomeruli are diseased. Glomerulonephritis is a degenerative inflammation of the glomeruli. It is nonsuppurative, that is, no pus formation is associated with it, nor are any bacteria found.

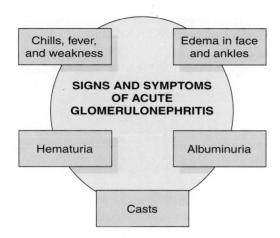

Figure 10–3
Signs and symptoms of acute glomerulonephritis.

Glomerulonephritis is a type of allergic disease caused by an antigen–antibody reaction. Approximately 1 to 4 weeks before the onset of the kidney inflammation, the strep infection triggers antibody production against the strep antigen. The antigen–antibody complexes become trapped in the glomeruli, blocking them and causing the inflammatory response. Numerous neutrophils crowd into the inflamed loops of the glomeruli, and blood flow to the nephrons is reduced. Less filtration into Bowman's capsule occurs, and less urine is formed.

Many glomeruli degenerate along with the nephrons they serve. This effect causes a shrinking of the kidney tissue. The remaining glomeruli become extremely permeable, allowing albumin and red blood cells to enter the nephrons and appear in the urine, Figure 10–4.

The prognosis for acute glomerulonephritis is generally good. Normal kidney function is restored after a period of time. Repeated attacks of acute glomerulonephritis, however, can lead to the chronic condition.

Chronic Glomerulonephritis Chronic glomerulonephritis may persist for many years with periods of remission and exacerbation. Hypertension generally accompanies this disease. The relationship between high blood pressure and kidney disease was discussed in Chapter 9. As more and more glomeruli are destroyed, the work of filtering the blood is accomplished by the remaining ones. Elevated blood pressure makes this possible.

A significant test to determine the extent of kidney function is to measure the specific gravity of a urine specimen. Specific gravity indicates the amount of dissolved substances in a sample compared with distilled water. Distilled water has a specific gravity of 1.000. The normal range for specific gravity of urine is 1.015 to 1.025, with variations throughout the day.

In advanced chronic glomerulonephritis, the specific gravity is low and fixed. This measurement indicates that the kidney tubules are unable to concentrate the urine.

After a long period of this disease, the kidneys shrink severely and are referred to as granular contracted kidneys. They gradually atrophy, dry up, and cease functioning.

Uremia, a toxic condition of the blood, is the end result of kidney failure. Waste products not excreted by the kidney accumulate to a poisonous level in the blood.

uremia
(ū-rē′-mĭ-ă)

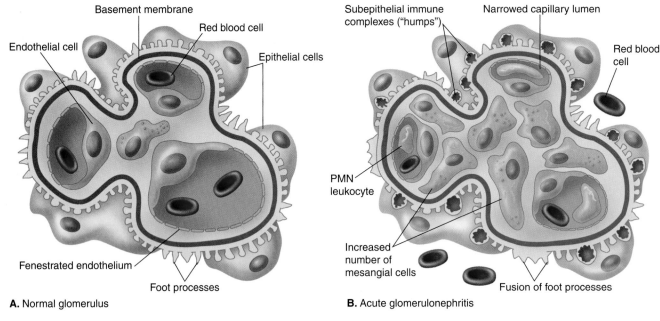

A. Normal glomerulus

B. Acute glomerulonephritis

Figure 10–4
Normal glomerulus and acute glomerulonephritis are shown.

Individuals suffering uremic toxicity feel nausea, headache, dizziness, and have faint vision. If unchecked, this condition may result in convulsions and coma. Dialysis treatment is quickly needed to restore blood nitrogen and electrolyte balance.

➤ RENAL FAILURE

urea
(ū-rē′-ă)

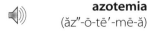

creatinine
(krē-ăt′-ĭn-ĭn)

azotemia
(ăz″-ō-tē′-mē-ă)

Several factors can cause the renal system, or kidneys, to stop functioning. Lack of blood flow to the kidneys due to severe hemorrhage, various poisons, and severe kidney diseases are some causes of renal failure. The kidneys are unable to clear the blood of **urea** and **creatinine,** which are nitrogen-containing waste products of protein metabolism. Urea is formed in the liver and is the primary method of nitrogen excretion from the body. If the kidneys are unable to excrete urea normally, it accumulates in the blood and a toxicity develops. The urea nitrogen can be analyzed as blood urea nitrogen, or BUN. An increase in the BUN is referred to as **azotemia** and the condition is known as uremia.

Measurement of the glomerular filtration rate (GFR) is used to assess the severity of renal disease or to follow its progress. Glomerular filtration rate is evaluated through clearance tests, most commonly, clearance of the waste product, creatinine. Serum creatinine level rises and creatinine clearance rate falls when the GFR is impaired.

$$\text{Creatinine clearance} = \frac{\text{Urine creatinine concentration (mg\%)} \times \text{Urine volume (ml/min)}}{\text{Plasma creatinine concentration (mg\%)}}$$

Normal levels for creatinine clearance are 88 to 128 ml/min in women and 97 to 137 ml/min in men. As may be expected, creatinine clearance levels decline in renal insufficiency and with aging.

Acute Renal Failure

Acute renal failure is a condition that develops suddenly and that can usually be treated successfully. The cause is often decreased blood flow to the kidneys resulting from surgical shock, shock after an incompatible blood transfusion, or severe dehydration. Kidney disease or trauma can also cause renal failure.

There is a sudden drop in urine volume, or **oliguria,** or even a total stoppage of urine production known as **anuria.** The person experiences headache and gastrointestinal distress. The breath has the odor of ammonia because of accumulation in the blood of nitrogen-containing compounds. Another concern is excess of potassium, **hyperkalemia,** which causes muscle weakness and can slow the heart to the point of cardiac arrest.

If proper treatment is administered, the prognosis is good. The condition causing the kidney failure must be corrected, and restoration of the patient's blood volume to normal is very important. Oral fluid intake should be restricted, allowing the kidneys to rest and the nephrons to regenerate. A dialysis machine may be used temporarily to clear the patient's blood of toxic substances in the interim.

oliguria
(ŏl-ĭg-ū′-rĭ-ă)

anuria
(ăn-ū′-rĕ-ă)

hyperkalemia
(hī″-pĕr-kă-lē′-mē-ă)

Chronic Renal Failure

Chronic renal failure is a very serious disease, generally ending in death. The condition develops slowly; there is no sudden drop in urinary output as there is in acute renal failure. Chronic renal failure can be the result of long-standing kidney disease such as chronic glomerulonephritis, hypertension, or **diabetic nephropathy,** a kidney disease resulting from diabetes mellitus.

Poisonous substances accumulate in the blood with adverse effects on all the systems. Urea is converted to ammonia, which acts as an irritant in the gastrointestinal tract to produce nausea, vomiting, and diarrhea. The nervous system is affected; vision becomes dim, mental ability is decreased, and convulsions or coma may ensue. Manifestations of chronic renal failure are summarized in Figure 10–5.

diabetic nephropathy
(dī-ă-bĕt′-ĭk nē-frŏp′-ă-thē)

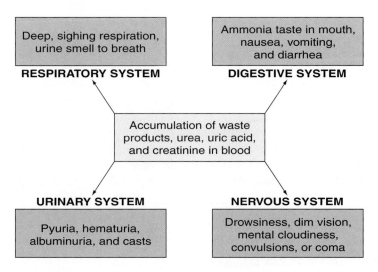

Figure 10–5
Manifestations of chronic renal failure.

🔊

dialysis
(dī-ăl′-ĭ-sĭs)

Dialysis—the artificial cleansing of the blood—may be done by tapping into blood vessels directly and is called *hemodialysis* (Figure 10–6). Another more indirect procedure is *peritoneal dialysis* (PD). The PD approach allows dialyzing fluid to be introduced into the abdominal cavity and uses the patient's peritoneum as the exchange medium. When a collapsible bag is attached externally it provides more freedom and flexibility during treatment. Dialysis may not be successful in advanced chronic renal failure, however. At the same time, kidney transplants pose many problems. However, improved antirejection medications, with fewer side effects, have reduced complications and allowed kidney transplants to prolong and save thousands of lives in the past 45 years (Figure 10–7).

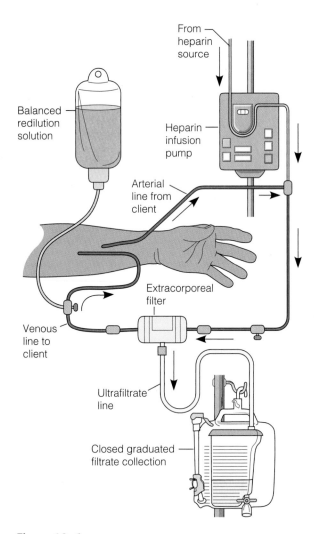

Figure 10–6
Continuous arteriovenous hemofiltration (CAVH).

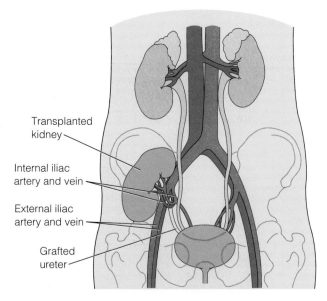

Figure 10–7
Placement of a transplanted kidney.

➤ PYELONEPHRITIS

Pyelonephritis is a suppurative inflammation of the kidney and renal pelvis. The renal pelvis is the cavity in the center of the kidney formed by the expanded, upper portion of the ureter that fits into it. Pyelonephritis is caused by pyogenic (pus-forming) bacteria. *Escherichia coli,* streptococci, and staphylococci are examples of such bacteria. Interstitial tissue, the kidney tissue between the tubules, is the site of the inflammation.

  The infection may be an ascending one that originates in the lower urinary tract, possibly the bladder, and spreads up into the kidneys, or it may be a descending infection carried by the bloodstream or lymph. Figure 10–8 shows the possible routes of infection. Any obstruction of the urinary tract—a congenital defect, a kidney stone, or an enlarged prostate gland—paves the way for an infection because of stagnation of the urine.

  Abscesses frequently form and rupture. Pus can then enter the renal pelvis and appear in the urine. This condition is called **pyuria.** The abscesses can fuse until the whole kidney is filled with pus. Renal failure occurs and uremia develops.

  If the infection is less severe, healing can occur, but scar tissue will form. Fibrous scar tissue tends to contract, and as it does, the kidney shrinks and becomes a granular contracted kidney.

  The symptoms of pyelonephritis are chills, high fever, and sudden back pain that spreads over the abdomen. Painful urination, **dysuria,** is experienced. Microscopic examination of the urine reveals numerous pus cells and bacteria. Hematuria is also common. Antibiotics are prescribed to counteract the infection.

pyelonephritis
(pī″-ĕ-lō-nĕ-frī′-tĭs)

pyuria
(pī-ū′-rĭ-ă)

dysuria
(dĭs-ū′-rĭ-ă)

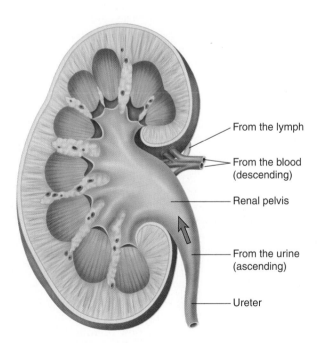

— From the lymph

— From the blood (descending)

— Renal pelvis

— From the urine (ascending)

— Ureter

Figure 10–8
Routes of infection for pyelonephritis.

➤ PYELITIS

pyelitis
(pī″-ĕ-lī′-tĭs)

Pyelitis is an inflammation of the renal pelvis, the juncture between the ureter and the kidney. Pyelitis, like pyelonephritis, is caused by *E. coli* or other pyogenic bacteria. It can result from a bladder infection, or the organism can be carried by the blood.

Pyelitis occurs commonly in young children, particularly girls, because the urethra in females is shorter than that of males. Microorganisms from fecal material can enter from the outside and travel easily to the bladder. The infection can then spread up the ureter to the renal pelvis. Painful urination as well as increased frequency and urgency are common symptoms of pyelitis. A urinalysis will reveal numerous pus cells.

This disease responds well to treatment with antibiotics. Early diagnosis and treatment are important in preventing the spread of the infection into the kidney tissue, thus becoming pyelonephritis.

➤ RENAL CARCINOMA

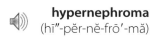

hypernephroma
(hī″-pĕr-nĕ-frō′-mă)

Carcinoma of the kidney, also called **hypernephroma,** causes enlargement of the kidney and destroys the organ. The tumor may not manifest itself for a long time. Painless hematuria will eventually become the chief symptom. When the tumor becomes large, an abdominal mass may be felt. This mass can then be detected on an x-ray as a tumor of the kidney.

Metastasis to other organs often occurs before the presence of the kidney tumor is known. The malignancy frequently spreads to the lungs, the liver, bones, and the brain.

Besides pain, signs include, loss of appetite, weight loss, anemia, and an elevated white blood cell count. Surgical removal is the best treatment.

Wilms' tumor
(vĭlmz tū′-mor)

A malignant tumor of the kidney that develops in very young children is **Wilms' tumor.** The tumor grows very fast and metastasizes through the blood and lymph vessels. The symptoms are the same as those described in renal carcinoma of an adult. Prognosis for this fast-growing cancer has improved in recent years.

➤ KIDNEY STONES

urinary calculi
(ū′-rĭ-nār″-ē
kăl′-kū-lī)

Urinary calculi predominantly form in the kidney; therefore, these structures are called renal calculi or kidney stones. Urinary calculi may be present and cause no symptoms until they become lodged in the ureter. The stones then cause intense pain that radiates from the kidney area to the groin.

Calculi are formed when certain salts in the urine form a precipitate, that is, come out of solution and grow in size. Small stones are often passed spontaneously in the urine, but larger stones may require surgery or other treatment. A stone may become so large that it fills the renal pelvis completely, blocking the flow of urine. A stone of this type, named for its shape, is the **staghorn calculus** illustrated in Figure 10–9. A kidney containing numerous small calculi is also shown. Calcium excess often leads to stone formation. Hyperactive parathyroid glands can cause the excess of circulating calcium, thus promoting formation of urinary calculi.

staghorn calculus
(stăg′-hŏrn
kăl′-kū-lŭs)

Stones can also form in the urinary bladder. The presence of stones causes urinary tract infections as they frequently obstruct the flow of urine. The converse is also true; urinary tract infections can lead to stone formation.

lithotripsy
(lĭth′-ō-trĭp″-sē)

Urinary calculi are sometimes partially dissolved by medication and then passed in the urine. **Lithotripsy,** the crushing of kidney stones, is now the preferable procedure

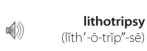

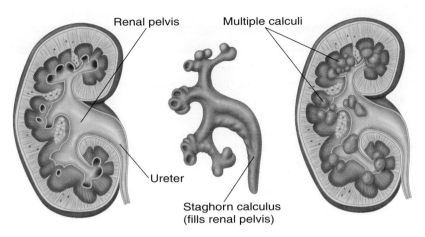

Figure 10-9
Urinary calculi.

to remove them, replacing the need for surgery. Sonic vibrations have been effectively used in crushing stones, either with the patient immersed in a tank of water, a procedure called **hydrolithotripsy** or performed out of water, **nephrotripsy** (Figure 10–10). In the newest technique, the patient is immersed in a tank of water to which acoustic shock waves from a lithotripter are emitted. These shock waves shatter the hard stones into sand-sized particles that are eliminated through the urine. Recovery from the procedure

hydrolithotripsy
(hī″-drō-lĭth′-ō-
trĭp″-sē)

nephrotripsy
(nĕf′-rō-trĭp″-sē)

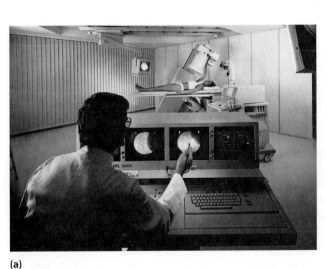

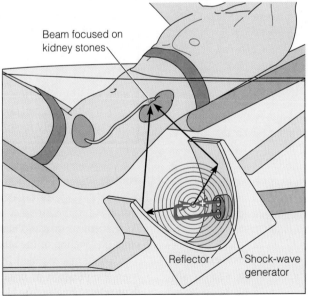

(a)   (b)

Figure 10-10
Extracorporeal shock-wave lithotripsy. Acoustic shock waves generated by the shock-wave generator travel through soft tissue to shatter the renal stone into fragments, which are then eliminated in the urine. (a) A shock-wave generator that does not require water immersion. (b) An illustration of water immersion lithotripsy procedure.

PREVENTION *PLUS!*

To prevent cases of kidney stones or recurring formation, which is common, it is recommended that urine output be increased. Therefore, drinking greater quantities of fluids, especially water, will dilute the urine and continually flush the kidney. The quantity of drinking fluids may need to more than double.

So have the water bottle on the tennis court or in your backpack to drink as you need it, instead of waiting until the end of the exercise for a cool beverage. Also, decrease any suspected factors in the diet that may help in the formation of kidney stones. These factors include an excess of dietary calcium or vitamin D, which also reduces the possibility of urinary tract infections (UTI).

is very rapid, and the patient usually requires only 2 to 3 days of hospitalization. Drugs that prevent certain types of new stones i.e., uric acid stones from recurring are a significant advance in treating urinary calculi, because some patients tend to develop stones repeatedly. With recurring kidney stones, the parathyroid becomes a suspect source of the problem (see Chapter 13).

Disease by the Numbers   x + ÷

The pH of urine may range from a strongly acidic 4.6 to a very alkaline 7.9. Normally, the urine pH fluctuates from about 5.5 to just over 7 in a 24-hour period. Consistently high alkaline numbers like 7.2 to 7.7 tend to cause calcium phosphate or magnesium ammonium phosphate stones. When persistently highly acidic urine is produced with a pH of 4.6 to 5.4, for example, the stone composition is cystine or uric acid.

Renal calculi occur in 1 of 1000 individuals in the U.S., especially between the ages of 30 to 50. However, autopsies show an incidence of kidney stones at 1 per 100, a much higher rate than reported cases in the public at large. Men are three times more likely to suffer kidney stones than are women.

➤ HYDRONEPHROSIS

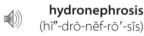

hydronephrosis
(hī″-drō-nĕf-rō′-sĭs)

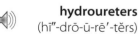

hydroureters
(hī″-drō-ū-rē′-tĕrs)

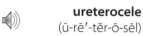

ureterocele
(ū-rē′-tĕr-ō-sēl)

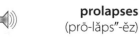

prolapses
(prō-lăps″-ĕz)

As a result of urinary calculi, a tumor, an enlarged prostate gland, congenital defect, or other obstruction of the renal pelvis, the kidney can become extremely dilated with urine. This condition is called **hydronephrosis.** The ureters above the obstruction are dilated from the pressure of urine that is unable to bypass the obstruction and are called **hydroureters.** Figure 10–11 shows this dilated condition. A **ureterocele** can cause hydronephrosis. In this instance the terminal portion of the ureter **prolapses** or slips into the bladder. When detected by tests (see "Diagnostic Tests"), it can be corrected surgically.

The degree of pain accompanying hydronephrosis depends on the nature of the blockage. Hematuria is generally present. If an infection develops because of the stagnation of urine, pyuria may be detected. Fever would then be a symptom too. Figure 10–12 depicts hydronephrosis of the kidney.

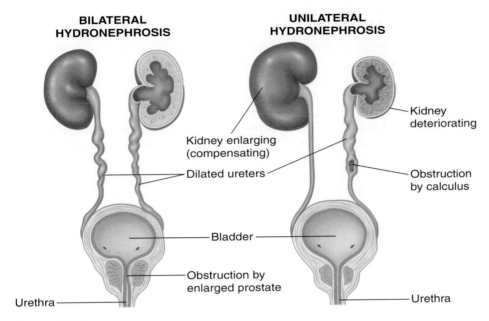

Figure 10–11
Hydronephrosis.

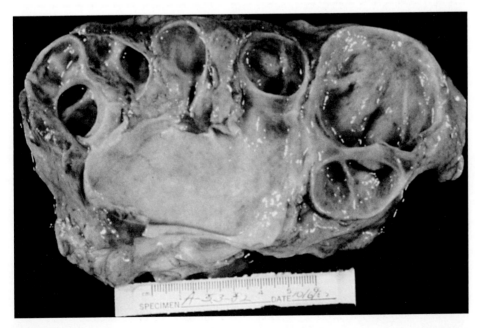

Figure 10–12
Hydronephrosis (*Courtesy of Dr. David. R. Duffell*).

➤ POLYCYSTIC KIDNEY

polycystic kidney
(pŏl″-ē-sĭs′-tĭk kĭd′-nē)

Polycystic kidney is a congenital anomaly, an error in development (Figures 10–13 and 10–14). Both kidneys are usually involved in this hereditary disease. In children this condition is caused by autosomal recessive genes whereas in adults, it is the autosomal dominant gene. Adult polycystic kidney disease affects 1 of 500 to 1000 individuals. The multiple cysts are dilated kidney tubules that do not open into the renal pelvis as they should. The cysts enlarge, fuse, and usually become infected. As the cysts enlarge, they compress the surrounding kidney tissue. Figure 10–15 illustrates the polycystic kidney of an adult. The patient demonstrates flank pain, hematuria, polyuria, and often renal calculi. Hypertension develops as a result of this long-standing kidney disease. Without a transplant, the kidneys eventually fail, and death is caused by uremia.

➤ DISEASES OF THE URINARY BLADDER AND URETHRA

Cystitis

cystitis
(sĭs-tī′-tĭs)

Cystitis is an inflammation of the urinary bladder. Commonly called a "bladder infection," it is more common in women than in men because of their shorter urethra. The chief causative agent is one present in fecal material, *Escherichia coli,* which can reach the urinary opening and travel upward to the bladder. Cystitis can also develop from sexual intercourse when infecting organisms around the vaginal opening spread to the urinary opening.

The symptoms of cystitis are increased urinary frequency and urgency, plus a burning sensation during urination. Microscopic examination of the urine reveals bacteria, pus, and casts. Leukocytes are typically present too.

side by side

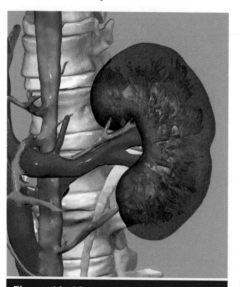

Figure 10–13

Normal kidney.

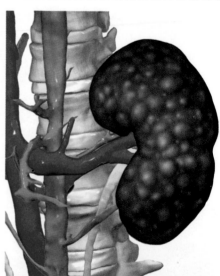

Figure 10–14

Polycystic kidney.

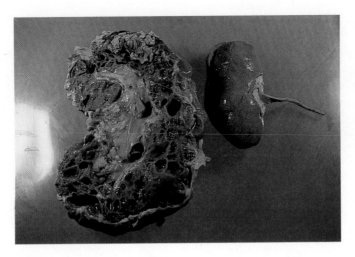

Figure 10–15
A cut view of polycystic kidney.

Carcinoma of the Bladder

Certain chemicals used in industry have been linked to carcinoma of the urinary bladder. (Figures 10–16 and 10–17). The tumor may grow, sending fingerlike projections into the lumen of the bladder. These tumors can be seen with a **cystoscope** and removed, but they tend to recur. A more invasive pattern of growth develops where the tumor

cystoscope
(sĭst′-ō-skōp)

side by side

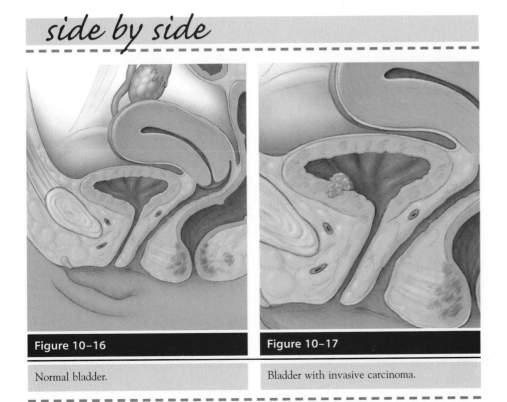

Figure 10–16

Normal bladder.

Figure 10–17

Bladder with invasive carcinoma.

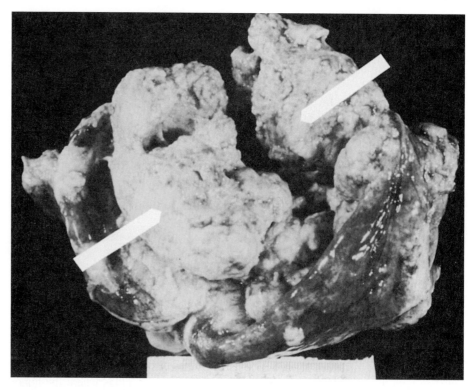

Figure 10–18
Advanced carcinoma of the bladder **(white arrow)** (*Courtesy of Dr. David R. Duffell*).

infiltrates the bladder wall. Surgery is then required to remove the malignant section (Figure 10–18).

If the whole urinary bladder is removed (radical cystectomy), a substitute arrangement may be surgically constructed using the intestinal tract. One method of construction is called the *ileal conduit* (Figure 10–19). A second design is the *continent urinary division*. In either case, the newly constructed design will allow storage and release of urine.

Urethritis

urethritis
(ū″-rē-thrī′-tĭs)

Any part of the urinary tract can become inflamed, and the urethra is no exception. This inflammation is called **urethritis.** In males, the infecting organism is usually a gonococcus, although other bacteria, viruses, or chemicals can cause this disease. The symptoms of urethritis include a discharge of pus from the urethra, an itching sensation at the opening of the urethra, and a burning sensation during urination. In females, urethritis frequently accompanies cystitis. An obstruction at the urinary opening is sometimes responsible for the inflammation in women.

➤ DIAGNOSTIC TESTS AND PROCEDURES

Kidney disease symptoms such as pain, dysuria (painful urination), blood or pus in the urine, or edema indicate that specific diagnostic tests should be performed. Edema is caused by the loss of protein from the blood, resulting in hypoproteinemia. Normally, these blood proteins have a water-holding power within the blood vessels. With their de-

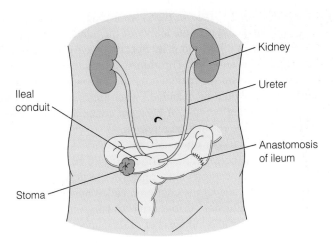

Figure 10–19

Ileal conduit. A segment of ileum is separated from the small intestine and formed into a tubular pouch with the open end brought to the skin surface to form a stoma. The ureters are connected to the pouch.

on the Practical Side

Urinary Incontinence

Lack of voluntary control over urination is normal in infants about 2 years old and younger because nerve control of the bladder is not completely developed. Training at the proper time overcomes the incontinence.

Involuntary urination or incontinence can occur in an adult as a result of damage to the spinal nerves controlling the bladder, unconsciousness, or disease of the urinary bladder. Irritation because of a urinary infection or irritating substance in the urine can also cause incontinence. The problem is often compounded by aging, because of the loss of muscle tone or lower hormone levels like estrogen.

Minor urinary incontinence may be relieved by exercising the pelvic muscles and the external bladder sphincter. These exercises are known as "Kegel" exercises. Another control mechanism is by injecting. Collagen into the neck of the bladder and urethral junction called the Marshall-Marchelli-Krantz (MMK) technique. These procedures reduce the need for adult diapers or incontinence pads.

pletion, fluid moves out of the capillaries and into the tissues, causing swelling or puffiness. Significant information can be obtained by a simple diagnostic procedure, a **urinalysis,** which examines a urine specimen physically, chemically, and microscopically. Physical observation gives the color, pH, and specific gravity of a urine specimen.

Chemical tests reveal the presence of abnormal substances: protein, specifically albumin, glucose, and blood. For microscopic examination a urine sample is centrifuged to obtain the sediment. Urine is normally yellow or amber, but hematuria (blood in the urine) can darken the color to a reddish brown. The degree of color depends on the amount of

urinalysis
(ū'-rĭ-năl'-ĭ-sĭs)

water the urine contains. Urine is pale in the case of diabetics, whose water output is large. In long-standing kidney diseases, the ability of the tubules to concentrate the urine is lost. As a result, the urine is dilute and pale. Specific gravity is low in this case.

The pH of urine has a broad range. The ability of the kidneys to excrete an acid or an alkaline urine is a mechanism for maintaining the narrow range of pH tolerated by the blood. Urine specimens should be examined when fresh as they tend to become alkaline (pH above 7) on standing because of bacterial contamination. Urine from a cystitic patient tends to be alkaline for the same reason.

Albuminuria indicates inflammation of the urinary tract, particularly of the glomeruli. The inflammation increases the permeability of blood vessels, allowing the protein, albumin, to enter the nephrons and appear in the urine. This loss reduces the level of protein in the blood, causing the condition called hypoproteinemia.

The presence of sugar (glucose) in the urine usually indicates diabetes mellitus. This is not a sign of a disease of the kidneys but of the endocrine areas of the pancreas. Diabetes over a period of time affects the kidneys adversely.

Hematuria may be obvious to the naked eye or require microscopic determination. Any serious disease of the urinary tract may give this symptom: glomerulonephritis, kidney stones, tuberculosis, cystitis, or tumors. If the passage of urine is accompanied by pain, a stone or tuberculosis may be the cause. Painless hematuria indicates the possibility of a malignant tumor in the urinary system.

Pyuria results from a suppurative inflammation caused by pyogenic bacteria, and pus causes the urine to appear cloudy. Microscopic examination of the urine reveals numerous pus cells, or polymorphs, engaged in fighting the infection. Diseases such as pyelonephritis, pyelitis, tuberculosis, and cystitis show pus in the urine.

Casts are cylindrical rods, molds of kidney tubules. They consist of coagulated protein, a substance not normally present in kidney tubules. Casts can include various kinds of blood cells, as well as epithelial cells from the lining of the urinary tract. Casts always indicate inflammation.

Microscopic examination determines the presence or absence of bacteria. Bacteria are found in tuberculosis of the kidney, pyelonephritis, and frequently, cystitis. For microscopic examinations, a urine sample may be removed from the bladder by catheterization to ensure that no external contamination occurs.

A cystoscopic examination enables the physician to view the inside of the bladder and urethra. The cystoscope is a long, lighted instrument resembling a hollow tube. Tumors, stones, or inflammations may be identified with this device. Using an additional instrument, small tumors may be removed or biopsied. Stones in the bladder can be crushed and removed.

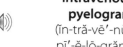

intravenous pyelogram

(ĭn-tră-vē′-nŭs pī′-ĕ-lō-grăm)

The **intravenous pyelogram** (IVP) allows the visualization of the urinary system by means of contrast dyes injected into the veins followed by x-ray examination. When these dyes concentrate in the urinary system, it is possible to note tumors, obstructions, or other deformities.

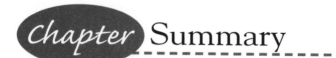

Chapter Summary

The importance of kidney function was reviewed to show the seriousness of kidney disease. Although acute glomerulonephritis generally has a good prognosis, repeated attacks can lead to chronic glomerulonephritis. This chronic disease, possibly persisting for many years, is one that often ends with kidney failure. Kidney failure can be acute caused by a newly developed condition. If the cause of the kidney failure is treated, renal function is restored to normal. Chronic renal failure does not respond to treatment and generally ends with uremia. Pyelonephritis is a destructive, suppurative inflammation of the kidney. Abscesses usually form, and pus appears in the urine. If not treated, renal failure results. Various other urinary tract infections were considered: cystitis, pyelitis, and urethritis. These infections frequently follow some obstruction of the flow of urine. Urinary calculi, tumors, and congenital anomalies can cause such blockages. Symptoms of kidney disease may include pain, painful urination, and blood or pus in the urine. Edema is also a sign of certain kidney diseases. An abnormal mass may be felt when a tumor of the kidney or bladder is large. This development is a late sign of malignancy, and metastases have probably already occurred. Interpretations of abnormal conditions of the urine were also discussed along with certain diagnostic procedures.

Diseases at a Glance: Urinary

Categories	* Disease ❏ Condition	Signs and Symptoms
Malignancies	* Hydronephroma	Painless hematuria early; later pain, loss of appetite, weight loss, anemia, elevated white blood count
	* Wilms' tumor	In young children, same signs and symptoms
Infections	* Pyelonephritis	Pyuria, chills, high fever, sudden back pain, dysuria, hematuria; eventually renal failure, uremia
	* Pyelitis	Dysuria, frequency, urgency
Inflammations	* Acute glomerulonephritis	Follows strep infection; chills, fever, loss of appetite, weakness, edema, albuminuria, hematuria, casts
	* Chronic glomerulonephritis	Remission and exacerbation of glomerulonephritis; may end with granular contracted kidneys, and uremia; specific gravity low and fixed in advanced cases
Other abnormal structure/function	❏ Acute Renal Failure	Sudden oliguria, may become anuria, headache, GI distress, odor of ammonia in breath, muscle weakness
	❏ Chronic Renal Failure	Slow development, urinary wastes increase in blood, nausea, vomiting, diarrhea, vision dim, CNS affected, convulsions, coma
	* Urinary calculi (kidney stones)	No symptoms until they block ureter, then intense pain radiating to groin
	❏ Hydronephrosis	Pain, hematuris, pyuria and fever if infection present
	❏ Polycystic kidney	Hypertension, eventual renal failure, uremia

Affected Organ/Body Region	Diagnostic Procedure	Treatment
Kidney	X-ray	Surgery
Kidney	X-ray	Surgery
Kidney and renal pelvis	Urinalysis, pus & blood in urine	Antibiotics
Renal pelvis	Urinalysis, numerous pus cells in urine	Antibiotics
Glomeruli and nephrons	Urinalysis, patient history	Antibiotics, steroids, immune suppression
Glomeruli and nephrons	Urinalysis, urine specific gravity low, patient history	Antibiotics, steroids, immune suppression
Nephrons	Patient history, blood and urinalysis	Drugs, fluid control, antibiotics, dialysis
Nephrons	Patient history, urinalysis, blood analysis	Dialysis, kidney transplant
Form in renal pelvis	Patient history, blood and urinalysis, x-ray	Lithotripsy, surgery
Ureters, kidneys	Urinalysis, IVP cystoscopic exam	Relief of obstruction, surgery
Abnormally developed nephrons	Urinalysis, IVP cystoscopic exam	Kidney transplant

Urinary Bladder and Urethra

Categories	* Disease ❑ Condition	Signs and Symptoms
Malignancies	* Carcinoma	Early asymptomatic, hematuria may occur, later pelvic pain and frequent urination
Infections	* Cystitis	Urinary frequency, urgency, burning sensation during urination, blood in urine
	* Urethritis	Burning sensation during urination, itching, pus discharge In females, accompanies cystitis
Other abnormal structure/function	❑ Incontinence	Involuntary loss of urine

Affected Organ/Body Region	Diagnostic Procedure	Treatment
Bladder	Cystoscopy	Surgery
Bladder	Microscopic exam of urine, may be diagnosed by patient's description of typical signs and symptoms	Antibiotics
Urethra	Microscopic exam of urine	Antibiotics
Nerve disease, sphincter muscle weakness, infection	Patient history	Exercises for muscles of pelvic floor, antibiotics for infection

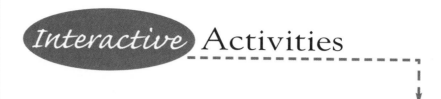

Interactive Activities

CASE FOR CRITICAL THINKING

Jill, a college sophomore, experienced painful urination and noticed blood in the urine. What is the likely scenario for this case?

Answer for Case Study:
Women having a relatively short urethra are prone to cystitis. The urinary bladder is a common site to be invaded whether one is sexually active or not. Painful urination (dysuria) would result with cystitis.

Sometimes blood may be present in the urine at the time of menses during the monthly cycle. If the menstrual cycle were not a factor, however, the blood plus the pain suggest a urinary bladder irritation.

MULTIMEDIA EXTENSION ACTIVITIES

www.prenhall.com/mulvihill
Use the above address to access the free, interactive companion Website created for this textbook. Included in the features of this site are chapter specific activities, internet links, and an audio-glossary.

Audio Glossary
Use the CD-ROM disk enclosed with your textbook to hear the pronunciation of the key terms in this chapter.

Diseases at a Glance: Urinary System

Use the chart on page(s) 192–195 to answer the following questions.

1. List 5 types of diseases or conditions that affect the urinary system.

2. What are the major signs and symptoms of the diseases or conditions you named?

Quick Self Study

MULTIPLE CHOICE

1. Which of the following would cause chronic uremia?
   - a. surgical shock
   - b. severe dehydration
   - c. complications of pregnancy
   - d. diabetes mellitus
   - e. severe burns

2. An inflammation of the interstitial tissue of the kidney is _____.
   - a. acute uremia
   - b. polycystic kidney
   - c. hydronephrosis
   - d. diabetic nephropathy
   - e. pyelonephritis

3. Inflammation of the renal pelvis is _____.
   - a. pyelonephritis
   - b. glomerulonephritis
   - c. pyelitis
   - d. congenital cystic kidney
   - e. tuberculosis

4. Breath has an ammonia-like odor of urine in _____.
   - a. glomerulonephritis
   - b. pyelonephritis
   - c. tuberculosis
   - d. uremia
   - e. cystitis

TRUE OR FALSE

_____ 1. A sudden drop in urine volume indicates chronic renal failure.

_____ 2. Glomerulonephritis is often an ascending infection.

_____ 3. In acute uremia, fluid intake should be decreased.

_____ 4. Albuminuria leads to hypoproteinemia.

_____ 5. Painful and frequent urination accompanies tuberculosis of the bladder.

_____ 6. Bacteria are not found in acute glomerulonephritis.

_____ 7. Pyelonephritis is a suppurative disease.

FILL-INS

1. _____ is an inflammation of the urinary bladder.

2. _____ _____ is a kidney disease resulting from diabetes mellitus.

3. Urinary calculi, or _____ _____, may be present and cause no symptoms until they become lodged in the ureter.

4. _____, the crushing of kidney stones, is now the preferable procedure to remove kidney stones, replacing the need for surgery.

5. _____ _____ is a congenital anomaly that usually involves both kidneys.

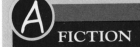

A FICTION

It is true that renal calculi may form anywhere within the urinary system, but they usually form in the renal pelvis or calyces of the kidney. Depending on the number and size of the stones, they may remain in the renal pelvis or travel into the ureter. Once in the ureter, stones may cause obstruction of urine flow and intense pain. Small stones may flush into the urinary bladders and settle or continue out of the urethra. Within the U.S. there is an area considered the "stone belt." The southeastern region of the country tends to have a greater proportion of persons with renal calculi, but the exact cause is unknown. Perhaps there is a tendency for dehydration because of the warmer climate, dietary habits may influence the development of renal calculi, or mineral factors in the soil or water that contribute to this problem.

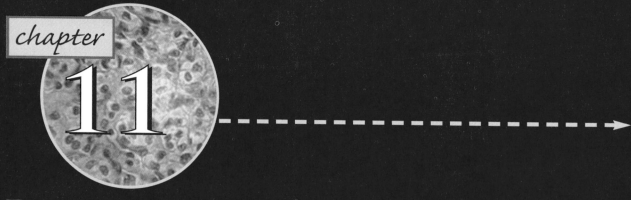

11

Diseases of the Digestive Tract

Food would be of no value to us if it were not broken down into units small enough to be absorbed from the gastrointestinal tract and into the bloodstream. The digestive system accomplishes this by breaking down carbohydrates to glucose and other simple sugars, proteins to amino acids, and lipids or fats to fatty acids and glycerides. Once these small units are absorbed by the blood, they are distributed to all the cells and tissues of the body. It is only in the cells that these units are metabolized—that is, used for production of energy—and converted into other material needed by the cells. Thus, nearly every cell of the body can be affected when disease interferes with the normal digestive process.

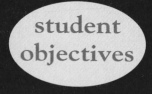

student objectives

After studying this chapter, students should be able to
➤ Describe the normal structure and function of the digestive tract
➤ Describe the key characteristics of major diseases of the digestive tract
➤ Name key diagnostic tests for selected digestive tract diseases
➤ Explain the cause of digestive tract diseases
➤ Name the treatment of digestive tract diseases
➤ Describe the general disorders and symptoms associated with digestive tract diseases

Key Terms

Achlorhydria

Adhesions

Anorexia

Atrophic

Barium

Cardiac sphincter

Chronic ulcerative colitis

Colostomy

Diverticula

Diverticulitis

Duodenal ulcers

Dysentery

Dysphagia

Endoscope

Esophagitis

Familial polyposis

Flatus

Gangrene

Gastric ulcers

Gastritis

Gastroscopy

Helicobacter pylori

Hematemesis

Hemorrhoids

Hiatal hernia

Intussusception

Irritable bowel

Lumen

Malabsorption

Melena

Mucosal

Occult blood

Organic obstructions

Paralytic obstruction

Peptic ulcers

Perforation

Peristalsis

Peritonitis

Pipe-stem colon

Proctoscope

Prolapse

Psychogenic factor

Pyloric sphincter

Reflux

Regional enteritis

Regurgitated

Spastic colon

Volvulus

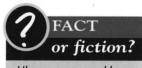

pyloric sphincter
(pī-lor'-ĭk sfĭngt'-ĕr)

peristalsis
(pĕr-ĭ-stăl-sĭs)

➤ THE DIGESTIVE PROCESS

The digestive system consists of a digestive tract, through which food passes, and of accessory organs that assist the digestive process. The digestive tract begins at the mouth and includes the pharynx, esophagus, stomach, small intestine, and large intestine. The accessory organs include the liver, gallbladder, and pancreas.

Digestion begins in the mouth with chewing, the mechanical breakdown of food. Salivation, the secretion of saliva, moistens the food and provides an enzyme for initial digestion of starch. The food is then swallowed and passes through the pharynx, or throat, and into the esophagus.

The moistened food moves down the esophagus to the stomach, where the digestion of proteins, large complex molecules, begins. A sphincter muscle at the juncture of the esophagus and stomach prevents regurgitation. The stomach secretes gastric juice that contains enzymes—biological catalysts—that act on protein. Gastric juice also contains hydrochloric acid, which activates these enzymes. The high acidity of gastric contents would be very irritating to the stomach lining if the lining were not protected by a thick covering of mucus. A great deal of moistening and mixing occurs within the stomach.

Food passes from the stomach into the small intestine through a sphincter muscle, the **pyloric sphincter.** This sphincter is closed until it receives nerve and hormonal signals to relax and open. The moistened food, referred to as chyme at this stage, is propelled along its course by rhythmical smooth muscle contractions called **peristalsis.**

The greatest amount of digestion occurs in the first part of the small intestine, the duodenum. Intestinal juice contains mucus and is rich in enzymes. Here digestive substances from other organs enter by means of ducts. The pancreas secretes enzymes for the digestion of protein, lipid, and carbohydrate. It also secretes an alkaline solution for the neutralization of acid carried into the small intestine from the stomach. This pancreatic juice enters the duodenum through the pancreatic duct.

Bile, secreted by the liver and stored in the gallbladder, enters the duodenum through the common bile duct. Bile is not an enzyme but an emulsifier, a substance that reduces large fat droplets into much smaller fat droplets. The action of bile enables the lipid enzymes to digest fat into small, absorbable units.

When digestion is complete, the nutrients are absorbed into blood capillaries and lymph vessels in the intestinal wall. The inner surface of the small intestine is arranged to provide the greatest amount of surface area possible for digestion and absorption. This mucosal surface contains numerous fingerlike projections called villi, each of which contains capillaries and lymph vessels for absorption (Figure 11–1).

Material not digested passes into the large intestine, or colon. The first part of the colon is a blind sac, the cecum, to which the appendix, a fingerlike mass of lymphatic tissue is attached. Water and minerals are absorbed from the large intestine, and the remaining matter is excreted as feces. Figure 11–2 illustrates the complete digestive system.

In this chapter, the diseases of each part of the digestive tract will be described. These include diseases of the mouth, esophagus, stomach, and small and large intestines. In the next chapter, diseases of the accessory organs of digestion—the pancreas, liver, and gallbladder—will be covered.

➤ DISEASES OF THE MOUTH

Complete coverage of oral pathology is beyond the scope of this book. This chapter will discuss the diseases directly affecting the digestive system. Diseases of the mouth can adversely affect the ability to taste, chew, moisten, and swallow food.

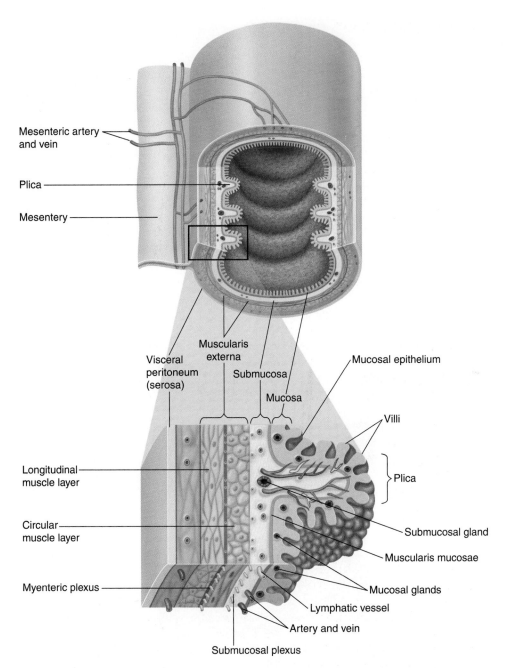

Figure 11–1
Mucosal surface of the small intestine.

Cancer of the Mouth

Neoplasms can develop in any part of the mouth: gums, cheeks, or palate. Mouth cancer remains among the top ten causes of cancer death worldwide. Tobacco (including smokeless tobacco) and alcohol use are major risk factors. A common malignant tumor is carcinoma of the lip. It occurs more often in men than in women and generally affects the lower lip. It may be related to pipe smoking. This malignancy may develop

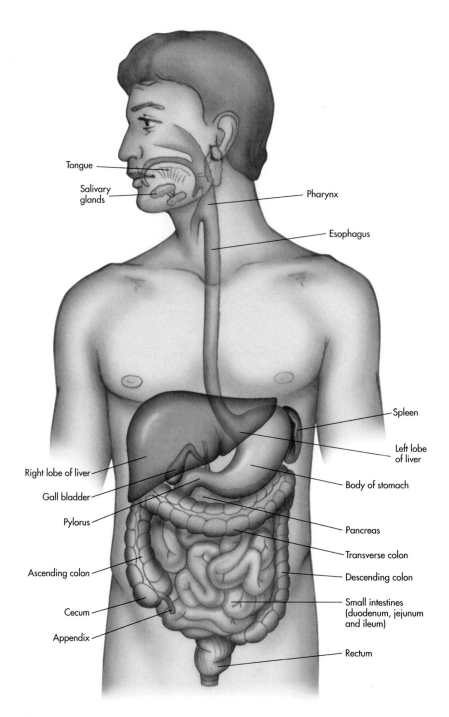

Figure 11–2
The digestive system.

from a chronic lesion, a sore or crack that does not heal. It is a type of cancer that responds well to treatment such as radiation or surgery. If not treated, it will spread.

A malignant tumor can develop on the tongue, usually at the edge. Carcinoma of the tongue may be caused by a chronic irritation from a tooth or denture. This cancer spreads rapidly and is more difficult to treat than cancer of the lip.

➤ DISEASES OF THE ESOPHAGUS

The function of the esophagus is the controlled passage of food to the stomach. Esophageal disease manifests itself as **dysphagia,** or difficult or painful swallowing.

dysphagia
(dĭs-fā'-jē-ă)

Cancer of the Esophagus

A malignant tumor of the esophagus narrows the lumen causing the principal symptom, dysphagia. The obstruction causes vomiting, and the person may experience a bad taste in his or her mouth or bad breath. There is accompanying weight loss because of the inability to eat.

The carcinoma spreads into adjacent organs and to remote sites through the lymph vessels. It frequently metastasizes before it is detected. Prognosis for cancer of the esophagus is poor. Like mouth cancer, tobacco and alcohol use, especially in combination, are major risk factors.

Esophageal Varices

Varicose veins sometimes develop in the esophagus and are called esophageal varices. They result from pressure within the veins. This pressure develops when venous return to the liver is obstructed. The veins appear very dilated and knotty. Esophageal varices are frequently a complication of cirrhosis of the liver. The destruction of liver tissue interferes with drainage of the portal vein. Congestion then builds within the veins, and those of the esophagus are unable to empty. The most serious danger in esophageal varices is hemorrhage.

Esophagitis

The most common cause of **esophagitis,** inflammation of the esophagus, is a **reflux**—a back-flow of the acid contents of the stomach. This is caused by an incompetent **cardiac sphincter.** The acid of the stomach is an irritant to the lining of the esophagus and stimulates an inflammatory response.

Esophagitis causes burning chest pains, which can resemble the pain of heart disease. The pain may follow eating or drinking, and some vomiting of blood may occur.

Treatment includes a nonirritating diet and antacids. Frequent small meals are recommended. Alcohol is an irritant to the inflamed mucosal lining and should be avoided.

esophagitis
(ē-sŏf-ă-jī'-tĭs)

reflux
(rē'-flŭks)

cardiac sphincter
(kar'-dĭ-ăk
sfĭngt'-ĕr)

Hiatal Hernia

A hernia is the protrusion of part of an organ through a muscular wall or body opening. A **hiatal hernia** is the protrusion of part of the stomach through the diaphragm at the point where the esophagus joins the stomach. Figure 11–3 shows this condition.

The person experiences indigestion and heartburn after eating and may feel short of breath. Avoidance of irritants such as spicy foods and caffeine and frequent small meals may be adequate treatment. If the person is obese, weight loss is recommended. Surgery is often required to correct the defect.

hiatal hernia
(hī-ĕ-t-al her'-nē-ā)

➤ DISEASES OF THE STOMACH

The stomach is well adapted for storing and mixing food with acid and enzymes. Alterations in the stomach lining or malignancies can cause painful and sometimes serious disease. Figures 11–4 and 11–5 show both a normal stomach and an ulcerated stomach.

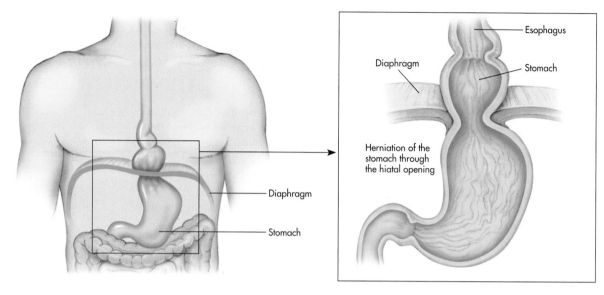

Figure 11–3
Hiatal hernia.

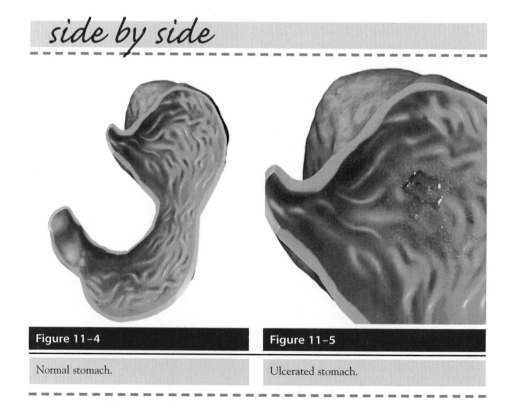

side by side

Figure 11–4

Normal stomach.

Figure 11–5

Ulcerated stomach.

Gastritis

Acute **gastritis** is an inflammation of the stomach caused by irritants such as aspirin, excessive coffee, tobacco, alcohol, or by an infection. Vomiting of blood frequently occurs as the principal symptom. **Gastroscopy** is extremely valuable in diagnosing this disease. A camera may be attached to the gastroscope, and the entire inner stomach is photographed. Although gastritis cannot be seen on an x-ray, it can be clearly viewed with this technique.

If bleeding of the mucous membrane is observed by gastroscopy, it can sometimes be stopped with the use of ice water, which constricts the small blood vessels. Acute alcoholism is a major cause of hemorrhagic gastritis. Alcohol stimulates acid secretion, which irritates the mucosa. If the bleeding cannot be controlled, surgery may be required.

gastritis
(găs-trī-tĭs)

gastroscopy
(găs-trŏs'-kă-pē)

Chronic Atrophic Gastritis

Lack of intrinsic factor as a cause of pernicious anemia was described in Chapter 7. In the absence of intrinsic factor, vitamin B_{12} cannot be absorbed. In cancer of the stomach neither intrinsic factor nor hydrochloric acid is secreted. This inability of the **mucosal** lining of the stomach to secrete its normal juices is due to chronic atrophic gastritis. Little can be done to treat the disease as the name, **atrophic** (wasting), suggests. It is a degenerative condition, and irritants such as alcohol, aspirin, and certain foods should be avoided.

mucosal
(mū-kō'-sal)

atrophic
(ă-trō'-fĭk)

Disease by the Numbers   x + ÷

EPIDEMIOLOGY

The old model for ulcer development: excess stomach acid eats through the stomach lining; the new model: *Helicobacter pylori* infects the stomach, secretes toxins that induce inflammation and damage the stomach lining. Which model is correct? Consider these numbers: patients who take H2-receptor blockers (drugs that inhibit acid production) to treat their ulcers face a 50% chance that the ulcer will recur when they stop taking the drugs; patients who take appropriate antibiotic therapy and eliminate the *H. pylori* infection experience no recurrence.

Peptic Ulcers

Ulcers are lesions of any body surface where necrotic tissue forms as a result of inflammation and is sloughed off, leaving a hole. Ulcers of the stomach and small intestine are termed **peptic ulcers.** They are due, in part, to the action of pepsin, a proteolytic enzyme secreted by the stomach. Figure 11–6 shows common sites of peptic ulcers.

Ulcer pain is caused by the action of hydrochloric acid on the raw surface of the lesion. Normally, the inner lining of the digestive tract is protected from the acid by a thick layer of mucus. The muscular contractions of peristalsis also intensify the pain.

Abdominal ulcer pain is relieved by antacids and temporarily by food, which acts as a protection from the acid. Ulcers of the stomach are called **gastric ulcers** and those of the small intestine are called **duodenal ulcers.** The person with a gastric ulcer experiences nausea, vomiting, and abdominal pain. The ulceration is thought to be caused by the hydrochloric acid and pepsin secretion of the stomach and by intestinal juice, including bile, that is regurgitated through the pyloric sphincter. The gastric mucosa becomes irritated by this bile-containing secretion, and the lesion develops.

peptic ulcers
(pĕp-tĭk ŭl'-sers)

gastric ulcers
(găs-trĭk ŭl'-sers)

duodenal ulcers
(dū"-ō-dē'-năl
ŭl'-sers)

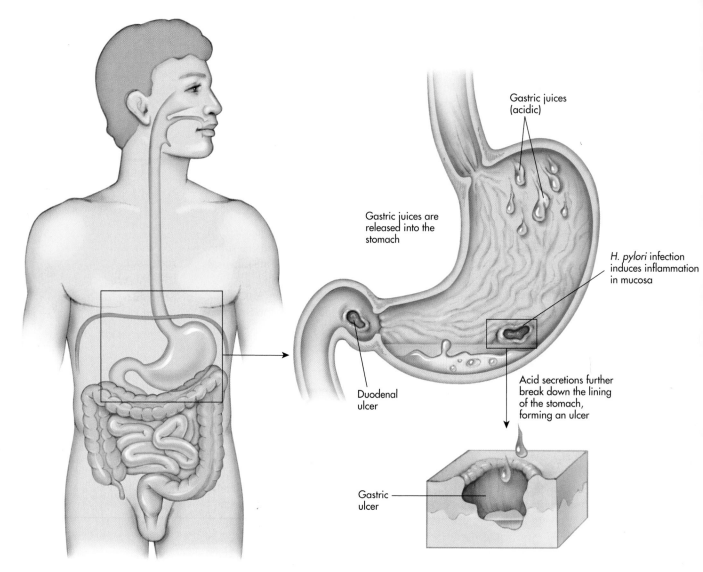

Figure 11–6
Peptic ulcer disease (PUD).

Duodenal ulcers are usually caused by an excessive secretion of hydrochloric acid. This acid secretion of the stomach is carried into the duodenum, where the ulceration develops. The mucous membrane becomes necrotic; the acid eats away the dead tissue, leaving a hole. The ulcer can erode through the pyloric sphincter, because hydrochloric acid secretion is under nerve and hormonal control, stressful situations can increase acid secretions.

Infection with the bacterium **Helicobacter pylori** is associated with ulcers. Treatment with antibiotics has been quite effective.

Several complications of a peptic ulcer are given in Figure 11–7. At times, bleeding from the ulcer occurs. A potential complication of any ulcer is hemorrhage; severe hemorrhage may lead to shock. It is possible for a large artery at the base of the ulcer to rupture as the erosion of the lesion goes deeper into underlying tissues. Bleeding

Helicobacter pylori
(hĕl″-ĭ-kō′-băk-ter pī-lŏr′-ĭ)

COMPLICATIONS OF PEPTIC ULCERS
Obstructions
Peritonitis
Hemorrhage/shock

Figure 11–7
Complications of peptic ulcers.

from the ulcer may appear as **hematemesis** or bloody vomitus. Blood from the upper part of the digestive tract gives the stools a dark, tarry appearance, which is referred to as **melena.**

A serious ulcer complication is **perforation.** If an ulcer perforates, that is, breaks through the intestinal or gastric wall, there is sudden and intense abdominal pain. Surgery is required immediately. **Peritonitis,** inflammation of the lining of the abdominal cavity, usually results when the digestive contents enter the cavity, because this material contains numerous bacteria.

Obstruction of the gastrointestinal tract can result from an ulcer and the scar tissue surrounding it. This is most likely to occur in a narrow area of the stomach, such as the area of the pyloric sphincter. The pain of the ulcer can cause the sphincter to go into spasm, also resulting in obstruction.

Treatment of ulcers is aimed at eliminating *H. pylori* infection and reducing gastric acidity to allow healing of the mucosal lining. Irritants such as aspirin, alcohol, and smoking tobacco should be avoided. Ulcers can usually be healed by medication, antacids, and proper diet, such as the avoidance of gas producers and fried foods. If the ulcer is stress- or tension-related, certain changes in the person's lifestyle might be advantageous. Even a change in the patient's psychological approach to the stressful situation can be beneficial.

Gastroenteritis and Food Poisoning

Gastroenteritis is an inflammation of the stomach and intestines. Symptoms include anorexia, nausea, vomiting, and diarrhea. The onset may be abrupt and violent with rapid loss of fluid and electrolytes.

Treatment replaces fluid and nutritional requirements including the lost salts. Antispasmodic medications can control the vomiting and diarrhea. Possible causes are bacterial or viral infection, chemical toxins, lactose intolerance, or other food allergy, although the actual cause is not always clear.

Food contaminated with human or animal feces may carry microorganisms that cause gastroenteritis and food poisoning. *Escherichia coli* is a common normal inhabitant of human or animal intestines. Certain strains may cause disease, like traveler's diarrhea, or more serious diseases, like hemolytic uremic syndrome, in which toxins cause potentially fatal shut-down of the kidneys. To prevent infection, cook meat thoroughly and practice good hygiene in the kitchen.

One of the most common forms of food poisoning is caused by the bacterium, *Salmonella.* These bacteria invade the intestinal mucosa and cause sudden, colicky abdominal pain, nausea, vomiting, and sometimes bloody diarrhea and fever that begins approximately 6 to 48 hours after eating contaminated food and lasts up to 2 weeks. A stool culture can identify the bacteria. *Salmonella* food poisoning (salmonellosis) is

hematemesis
(hē-mă-tĕm′-ĕh-sĭs)

melena
(mĕ-lĕ-nă)

perforation
(per″-fō-rā′-shŭn)

peritonitis
(pĕr″-ĭ-tō-nī′-tīs)

associated with contaminated eggs and poultry, but most any food may harbor the bacteria. Treatment usually consists of replenishing water, electrolytes, and nutrients. Elderly individuals, young children, and immunocompromised people are at risk of developing serious infection, and they may require more intervention.

Cancer of the Stomach

Pain is not an early sign of stomach cancer. Carcinoma of the stomach, which is more common in men than in women, may be very advanced before it is detected. It may even have spread to the liver and surrounding organs through the lymph and blood vessels. Early symptoms are vague; loss of appetite, heartburn, and general stomach distress. Blood may be vomited or appear in the feces. Pernicious anemia generally accompanies cancer of the stomach, because in both diseases the gastric mucosa fails to secrete intrinsic factor. Gastric analysis by means of a stomach tube demonstrates the absence of hydrochloric acid, or **achlorhydria.** Biopsy of any lesions seen through the gastroscope is an essential diagnostic procedure for carcinoma of the stomach.

 achlorhydria
(ă″-klor-hĭ-drē-ă)

The malignancy may be a large mass projecting into the lumen of the stomach or it may invade the stomach wall, causing it to thicken. As the tumor grows, the lumen is narrowed to the point of obstruction. The remainder of the stomach becomes extremely dilated due to the blockage, and pain is experienced from the pressure on nerve endings. Infection frequently accompanies cancer, which causes additional pain.

The etiology of this malignancy is not known, but current research suggests an association with the consumption of preserved, salted, cured foods, and a diet low in fresh fruits and vegetables. *H. pylori* infection appears to increase the risk for stomach cancer, probably through its damaging effects on the mucosal cells. Good prognosis for this disease depends on early detection and treatment.

➤ DISEASES OF THE INTESTINES

The small intestine is the site of most of the digestion and absorption that occurs in the digestive tract, while the large intestine absorbs remaining water and stores and concentrates the feces. Diseases in these areas may manifest themselves as diarrhea, constipation, changes in stool characteristics, or in secondary diseases that arise as a result of poor nutrition.

Appendicitis

Appendicitis is an acute inflammation of the appendix usually caused by infection or obstruction. The wormlike shape of the appendix and its location on the cecum make it a trap for fecal material, which contains bacteria, particularly *Escherichia coli*. Figure 11–8 illustrates this potential site of infection.

The pain of appendicitis is not always typical. It often begins in the middle of the abdomen and shifts to the lower right quadrant. Nausea, vomiting, and fever are often symptoms. Leukocytosis is indicative of the inflammation. Perforated ulcer, kidney stones, pancreatitis, and other diseases have similar symptoms, making diagnosis difficult.

The inflamed appendix becomes swollen, red, and covered with an inflammatory exudate. Because the swelling interferes with circulation, it is possible for **gangrene** to develop. The appendix then becomes green and black.

gangrene
(găng′-grēn)

The wall of the appendix can become thin and rupture. Fecal material then spills out into the peritoneal cavity, causing peritonitis. Before antibiotic treatment, peritoni-

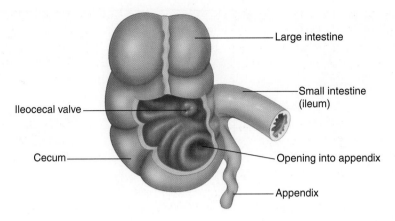

Large intestine

Small intestine (ileum)

Ileocecal valve

Opening into appendix

Cecum

Appendix

Figure 11–8
Appendix attached to cecum, into which the small intestine empties.

tis was almost always fatal. Rupture of the appendix tends to give relief from the pain, which is very misleading. Surgery should be performed before rupture occurs.

Malabsorption Syndrome

A person unable to absorb fat or some other substance from the small intestine is said to have **malabsorption** syndrome. Defective mucosal cells can account for this abnormality. Because fat cannot be absorbed from the intestine it passes into the feces, and the result is unformed, fatty, pale stools that have a foul odor. The fat content causes the stools to float.

Many other diseases cause secondary malabsorption syndrome. A diseased pancreas or blocked pancreatic duct deprives the small intestine of lipases. In the absence of the enzymes, fat is not digested and cannot be absorbed.

Inadequate bile secretion, due to liver disease or a blocked bile duct, will also prevent lipid digestion and cause secondary malabsorption. One of the complications of the malabsorption syndrome is a bleeding tendency. Vitamin K, a fat-soluble vitamin that is essential to the blood-clotting mechanism, cannot be absorbed.

Treatment for malabsorption syndrome depends on its cause, and diet is carefully controlled. Supplements are administered, such as the fat-soluble vitamins A, D, E, and K, which are not being absorbed.

malabsorption
(măl-ăb-sorp′-shŭn)

Diverticulitis

Diverticula are little pouches or sacs formed when the mucosal lining pushes through the underlying muscle layer. These may cause no harm themselves.

Diverticulitis is an inflammation of the diverticula. This may occur in the colon or in the small intestines. The inflammation occurs when the sacs become impacted with fecal material and bacteria. The patient experiences low cramplike pain, usually on the left side of the abdomen. As inflammation spreads, the lumen of the intestine is narrowed and an obstruction can develop. Abscesses frequently form. Antibiotic therapy, together with a controlled diet, is usually effective. Figure 11–9 shows an example of diverticulitis.

diverticula
(dī″-vĕr-tĭk″-ū-lŭ)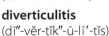

diverticulitis
(dī″-vĕr-tĭk″-ū-lī′-tĭs)

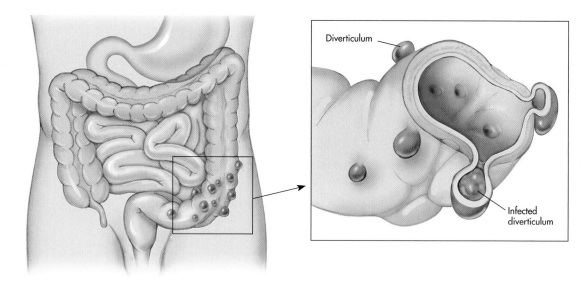

Figure 11–9
Diverticulitis.

Regional Enteritis (Crohn's Disease)

regional enteritis
(rē′-jŭ-nŭl
ĕn″-tĕr-ī′-tĭs)

Regional enteritis is an inflammatory disease of the intestine that most frequently affects young adults, particularly females. The intestinal walls become thick and rigid. As the wall thickens with the formation of fibrous tissue, the lumen is narrowed and a chronic obstruction can develop.

The cause of regional enteritis is not known, but there seems to be a psychogenic element involved; stress or emotional upsets can trigger relapses.

The pain of regional enteritis resembles that of appendicitis; it is in the lower right quadrant of the abdomen. A tender mass may be felt in this area, and there is frequently an alternation between diarrhea and constipation. Melena, dark stools containing blood pigments, is common. The severe diarrhea can cause an electrolyte imbalance because of the large amount of water and salt lost in the stools.

anorexia
(ăn″-ō-rĕks′-ĭ-ă)

Anorexia, nausea, and vomiting lead to a loss of weight. Periods of exacerbation, remission, and relapse are common. In severe cases, hemorrhage or perforation is a threat.

Regional enteritis is usually treated with medication, such as corticosteroids, which reduces the inflammation. Surgery is not performed unless complications demand it.

Chronic Ulcerative Colitis

chronic
ulcerative
colitis
(krŏn′-ĭk ŭl′-sĕr-ă-tĭv
kō-lī′-tĭs)

psychogenic
factor
(sī-kō-jĕn′-ĭk făk′-tor)

Chronic ulcerative colitis is a serious inflammation of the colon, the origin of which is unknown. A **psychogenic factor** may be involved, as the condition is often aggravated by stress. Persons of high-strung temperament are most prone to the disease. Hypersensitivity to certain foods may play a part in the course of the disease. Chronic ulcerative colitis may be an autoimmune disease in which the person's antibodies destroy the body's own tissue. Periods of remission and exacerbation are characteristic of ulcerative colitis.

There is extensive ulceration of the colon and rectum. Diarrhea with pus, blood, and mucus in the stools is the typical symptom. Cramplike pain is experienced in the lower abdomen. Anemia often accompanies ulcerative colitis because of the chronic blood loss through the rectum.

The colon with chronic ulcerative colitis has a characteristic appearance on x-ray examination. The normal pouchlike markings of the colon, the haustra, are lacking. The colon appears straight and rigid, and it is referred to as a **"pipe-stem" colon** (Figure 11–10).

There is a high risk of a colon malignancy developing as a complication of long-standing ulcerative colitis.

pipe-stem colon
(pīp-stĕm kō'-lĕn)

on the Practical Side

Bacteria, Coolers, and Food Poisoning

Refrigeration and freezing do not kill bacteria. They are only inhibited until warmer temperatures allow them to grow. Bacteria can multiply rapidly; under optimum conditions they may double their numbers every 30 minutes. So, a contaminated potato salad may be safe to eat right out of the refrigerator, but it may become the source of a serious infection if brought to a picnic and left to stand at air temperature for a couple of hours. In other words, it is a good idea to keep the potato salad in the cooler while you are playing softball at your next picnic!

Treatment of any chronic disease is limited, but the symptoms of chronic ulcerative colitis may be alleviated if certain stressful conditions are removed. Foods found to aggravate the disease should be avoided. If the person is of a nervous temperament, mild sedation may be helpful. Corticosteroids are sometimes administered to control autoimmunity.

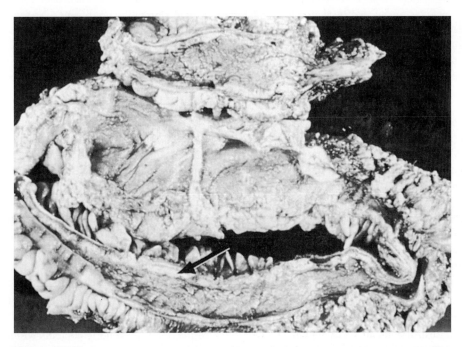

Figure 11–10
Chronic ulcerative colitis. Arrow indicates the thickened rigid wall referred to as a "pipe-stem" colon. (*Courtesy of Dr. David R. Duffell.*)

colostomy
(kō-lŏs′-tō-mē)

If the person does not respond to these treatments, surgery may be necessary, occasionally requiring a colostomy. A **colostomy** is an artificial opening in the abdominal wall with a segment of the large intestine attached. Evacuation of the feces is through this opening. A colostomy may be temporary or permanent depending on the nature of the colon surgery.

Carcinoma of the Colon and Rectum

Carcinoma of the colon and rectum is a leading cause of death from cancer in the United States, yet it can be more easily diagnosed than many other cancers. The mass is often felt by rectal examination or seen with the protoscope or colonoscope, endoscopes used for viewing the rectum and colon. If detected early, it responds well to surgical treatment.

The symptoms vary according to the site of the malignancy. A change in bowel habits—diarrhea or constipation—is symptomatic. As the tumor grows, there may be abdominal discomfort and pressure. Blood often appears in the stools, and continuous blood loss from the malignant tumor causes anemia.

PREVENTION *PLUS!*

Cancer Prevention through Detection

Early detection of colorectal cancer is the key to survival. Death rates are low for patients whose colorectal cancer is detected at an early localized stage: about 9% die within 5 years. Death rates are much higher, however, when the diagnosis occurs at an advanced stage: about 92% die within 5 years. Screening is underused even though its benefits seem clear. Regular screening should be done for adults aged 50 years and over. This includes an annual fecal occult blood test, a flexible sigmoidoscopy every 5 years, and a colonoscopy every 10 years. These tests could identify precancerous polyps that can be removed, or they can detect cancer in the early localized stage, which can be treated before the cancer has a chance to spread.

lumen
(loo′-mŭn)

The mass can partially or completely obstruct the **lumen** of the colon. As the tumor invades underlying tissue, the cancer cells spread through the lymph vessels and veins.

As in all cancers, early detection and treatment are essential to prevent its spread. Most malignancies of the large intestine are in the rectum or the sigmoid colon. This makes their detection and removal easier than malignant tumors in other areas of the digestive tract. A colostomy may be necessary.

There are two diseases that predispose to cancer of the colon: long-standing ulcerative colitis, which has been described, and familial polyposis of the colon. **Familial polyposis** is a hereditary disease in which numerous polyps develop in the intestinal tract. The polyps usually give no symptoms unless a malignancy develops. Another factor that is associated with risk for colon cancer is a diet high in red meat and low in food sources of fiber, such as vegetables, legumes, and whole grain cereals.

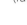

familial polyposis
(famĭl′-yul pŏl″-ē-pō-sĭs)

organic obstructions
(or-găn′-ĭk obs-trŭk-shŭns)

paralytic obstruction
(păr″-ă-lĭt′-ĭk obs-trŭk-shŭn)

Intestinal Obstructions

An obstruction can occur anywhere along the intestinal tract, preventing contents within the tract from moving forward. **Obstructions** are classed as **organic** when there is some material blockage, or as **paralytic,** in which case there is a decrease in peristalsis preventing the propulsion of intestinal contents.

Disease by the Numbers x + ÷

EPIDEMIOLOGY
Cancer of the colon or rectum is the second leading cause of cancer-related death in the United States. The American Cancer Society estimates that 56,000 Americans will have died of colorectal cancer in 1999.

Tumors and hernias, both hiatal and inguinal, can cause organic obstructions. The intestine may be twisted on itself, a condition known as **volvulus** that may be unwound surgically (Figure 11–11). The intestine may be kinked, allowing nothing to pass. **Adhesions,** the linking together of two surfaces normally separate, can distort the tract. Abdominal adhesions sometimes follow surgery, when fibrous connective tissue grows around the incision. Adhesions also develop as a result of inflammation. Another type of organic obstruction is **intussusception,** in which a segment of intestine telescopes into the part forward to it. This occurs more often in children than in adults. Figure 11–12 shows various types of organic obstructions.

A paralytic obstruction can result from peritonitis. If a loop of small intestine is surrounded by pus from the infection, the smooth muscle of the intestinal wall cannot contract. Sphincters can go into spasm and fail to open as a result of intense pain.

An acute organic obstruction causes severe pain. The abdomen is distended and vomiting occurs. There is complete constipation; not even gas (**flatus**) is passed. Sometimes the obstruction can be relieved by means of a suction tube, but frequently surgery is required. If the obstruction is a strangulated hernia, a protrusion of intestine through the abdominal wall, surgery is required as the blood supply is cut off to the strangulated segment, and it can become gangrenous.

volvulus
(vŏl'-vū-lŭs)

adhesions
(ăd'-hē-zhŭns)

intussusception
(ĭn-tŭs-sŭs-sĕp'-shūn)

flatus
(flā'-tŭs)

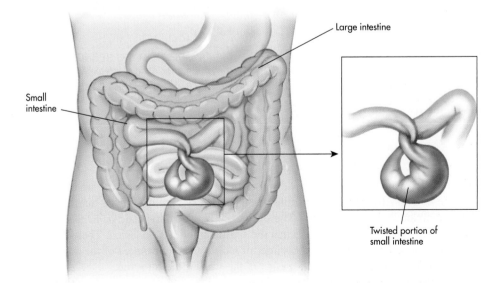

Figure 11–11
Volvulus.

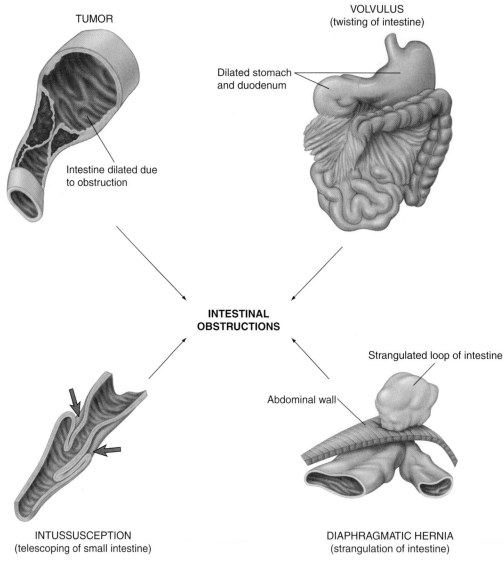

Figure 11–12
Organic obstructions of the intestinal tract.

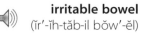

Spastic Colon (Irritable Bowel Syndrome)

Many of the symptoms described for diseases of the lower intestinal tract are also characteristic of a **spastic colon** or **irritable bowel.** These symptoms include diarrhea, constipation, abdominal pain, and gas. The difference between a spastic or irritable colon and the diseases already discussed is that the spastic colon has no lesion. There is no tumor or ulceration. It is a functional disorder of motility, the movement of the colon. The pain is probably caused by muscle spasms in the wall of the intestine.

Certain foods and beverages, particularly caffeine, alcohol, spicy foods, fatty foods, and concentrated orange juice, can irritate the bowel, and should be avoided. Laxatives should not be used; adding fiber to the diet helps prevent constipation.

spastic colon
(spăs-tĭk′ kō′-lĕn)

irritable bowel
(ĭr′-ĭh-tăb-il bŏw′-ĕl)

Emotional stress has an adverse effect on the digestive system, because digestion is affected by the nerves of the autonomic nervous system. If stressful situations can be alleviated, the colon will function more normally. Tension-relieving activities, sports, hobbies, or regular exercise (see Chapter 19) may help.

Dysentery

People often use the terms dysentery and diarrhea interchangeably, which is not accurate. Dysentery is a disease; diarrhea is a symptom. **Dysentery** is an acute inflammation of the colon, a colitis. It can be caused by bacteria, parasitic worms, and other microorganisms. A major cause is the protozoan, *Entamoeba histolytica,* which is transmitted in feces-contaminated food and water. The major symptom of dysentery is diarrhea in which the stools contain pus, blood, and mucus. Severe abdominal pain accompanies the diarrhea. Organisms invade the wall of the colon and cause numerous ulcerations, which account for the pus and blood in the stools. Antibiotics can be effective for bacterial dysentery, and other medications are used for amoebic dysentery.

dysentery
(dĭs'-ĕn-tĕr"-ē)

➤ GENERAL DISORDERS OF THE DIGESTIVE TRACT

The symptoms describing the diseases of the digestive system are common phenomena. Vomiting, diarrhea, and constipation are some of these symptoms. The physiologic basis of each symptom will be described briefly.

Vomiting

Vomiting is a protective mechanism, a means of ridding the digestive tract of an irritant or of alleviating overdistention. Sensory nerve fibers are stimulated by the irritant, and the message is conveyed to the vomiting center in the medulla of the brain. Motor impulses then stimulate the diaphragm and abdominal muscles. Contraction of these muscles squeezes the stomach. The sphincter at the base of the esophagus is opened, and the gastric contents are **regurgitated.**

A feeling of nausea often precedes vomiting. The cause of the nausea may be nerve factors other than a gastric or intestinal irritant. Motion sickness produces this effect. A very unpleasant smell or sight can cause nausea with possible subsequent vomiting.

regurgitated
(rē-gŭr'-jŭ-tā"-ĕd)

Diarrhea

Diarrhea results when the fluid contents of the small intestine are rushed through the large intestine, causing watery stools. It was stated earlier that the main function of the large intestine is to reabsorb water and minerals. In an attack of diarrhea, there is no time for this reabsorption. The smooth muscle in the walls of the intestine is so stimulated that peristalsis is intensified.

Nervous states can cause this increased motility of the large intestine. An intestinal infection or food poisoning can cause diarrhea through toxins that increase intestinal motility or impair water absorption by mucosal cells.

Constipation

Constipation results when feces remain in the colon too long, with excessive reabsorption of water; they then become hard and dry. Poor habits of elimination are a cause of constipation. Defecation should be allowed to occur when the defecation reflexes are strong. A proper diet is also important, one that contains adequate amounts of fiber. Fiber is obtained from fresh fruits, vegetables, and cereals. Various disorders of the digestive system cause constipation. Any obstruction of the lumen or interference with motility will result in this condition.

Hemorrhoids

proctoscope
(prŏk'-tă-skōp)

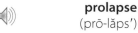

prolapse
(prō-lăps')

Hemorrhoids, also called "piles," are enlarged (varicosed) veins in the lining of the rectum near the anus. Hemorrhoids may be internal or external. A physician can observe internal hemorrhoids with a **proctoscope,** a hollow tube with a lighted end. Straining to have a bowel movement can cause bleeding or cause the hemorrhoid to **prolapse,** i.e., come through the anal opening. External hemorrhoids can be seen with a hand-held mirror and appear blue because of decreased circulation. They can become red and tender if inflamed.

Causes of hemorrhoids include heredity, poor dietary habits, inadequate fiber, overuse of laxatives, and lack of exercise. Hemorrhoids frequently develop during pregnancy because of pressure from an enlarged uterus.

Treatment includes adding fiber and water to the diet to soften the stools and the use of medicated suppositories or anorectal creams.

➤ DIAGNOSTIC PROCEDURES FOR THE DIGESTIVE TRACT

A combination of procedures enables the physician to view the inside of the digestive tract for malignancies, polyps, diverticulitis, bleeding, and inflammatory bowel disease. To visualize the upper gastrointestinal (GI) tract, esophagus, stomach, and small intestines under fluoroscopy, the patient swallows barium sulfate. The lumen and mucosa of the colon can be studied through x-ray after a barium or barium and air enema (Figure 11–13).

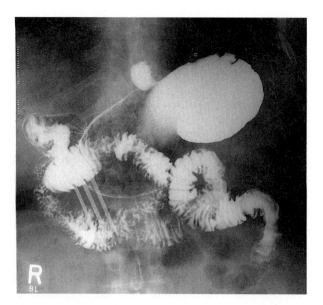

Figure 11–13
Upper GI series (*Courtesy of Teresa Resch*).

Barium is opaque to x-rays, so the rays do not pass through it. The silhouette produced shows tumors, malformations, or other obstructions that may be present. Motion pictures can even be taken of the movement of barium through the gastrointestinal tract. These pictures can show abnormalities of smooth muscle action or improperly functioning sphincters.

Certain lesions of the inner wall of the digestive tract do not show up on x-ray examination. To view this inner surface an instrument called an **endoscope** is used. It is a hollow tube with a lens and light system. There is an endoscope designed specially for each part of the digestive tract. It is possible with this technique to take a biopsy of a suspected malignant lesion. Gastric analysis is performed to determine if the patient is able to secrete acid and the rate of gastric secretion. Lack of gastric juice is significant in diagnosing pernicious anemia whereas a high rate of secretion suggests active peptic ulcer disease.

barium
(ba'-rē-ŭm)

endoscope
(en'-dăs-kōp)

➤ DISEASES INDICATED BY STOOL CHARACTERISTICS

Microscopic examination of stool may identify the cause of food poisoning, gastroenteritis, or dysentery. Other information can also be obtained from stool samples. Signs of several of the diseases discussed include blood in the stools. Blood appears differently, however, depending upon the site of bleeding.

Streaks of red blood can indicate bleeding hemorrhoids. **Hemorrhoids** are varicose veins of the rectum or anus. If the blood in the stools is bright red, the bleeding is from the distal end of the colon, the rectum. This symptom can indicate cancer of the rectum.

Dark blood may appear in the stools giving them a dark, tarry appearance; the condition of melena. This blood was altered as it passed through the digestive tract, so it is from the stomach or duodenum. A bleeding ulcer or cancer of the stomach may be indicated by melena. Certain medications, those containing iron, for instance, can also give this tarry appearance to the stools.

Blood may not be apparent to the naked eye, but a chemical test can show its presence. This is referred to as **occult blood.** It can indicate bleeding ulcers or a malignancy in the digestive tract.

If the stools are large and pale, appear greasy, and float on water, they contain fat. This is a symptom of malabsorption syndrome. It may also indicate a diseased liver, gallbladder, or pancreas. Diseases of these organs will be discussed in the next chapter.

hemorrhoids
(hĕm'-ō-roydz)

occult blood
(u-kŭlt'blud)

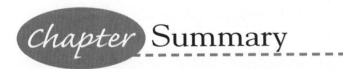 *Chapter* Summary

The structure and function of the digestive system was reviewed, emphasizing the normal digestive process. Diseases of the digestive tract were discussed. These included malignancies (mouth, esophagus, stomach, colon), infections (gastroenteritis, food poisoning, dysentery, ulcers), abnormal structure and function (herniations, obstructions), and inflammatory/immune disorders (gastritis, ulcerative colitis, Crohn's disease). General conditions like diarrhea, constipation, and vomiting were explained and related to diseases. Certain diagnostic tools such as endoscopy, barium x-rays, stool analysis, and biopsy were also discussed.

Diseases at a Glance: Digestive Tract

Categories	* Disease ■ Disorder ✓ Stress-related	Signs and Symptoms
Malignancies	* Carcinoma of lip, tongue	Abnormal growths or lesions that don't heal
	* Cancer of esophagus	Dysphagia, obstruction
	* Stomach cancer	Appetite loss, discomfort, hematemesis, blood in stool, and pain late
	* Colon cancer	Change in bowel habits, diarrhea or constipation, blood in stool
Infections	* Gastroenteritis	Nausea, vomiting, diarrhea, abdominal discomfort
	* Gastric/duodenal ulcer	Upper abdominal pain, hemorrhage, blood in stool
	* Salmonellosis	Abdominal pain, nausea, vomiting, fever, diarrhea
	* Dysentery	Abdominal pain, bloody diarrhea with pus and mucus
Inflammations	* Esophagitis	Burning chest pain (heartburn), especially after eating
	* Gastritis	Stomach pain, hematemesis
	* Chronic atrophic gastritis	Gastritis with poor digestion and absorption
	✓ Gastric/duodenal stress ulcer	Upper abdominal pain, hemorrhage, blood in stool
	* Appendicitis	Lower right abdominal pain, nausea, fever
	* Diverticulitis	Cramping, pain in lower abdomen
	✓* Regional enteritis (Crohn's disease)	Lower right pain, diarrhea and constipation, local thickening of intestinal wall, melena
	✓ Chronic ulcerative colitis	Diarrhea, pus, blood, mucus in stool, diffuse ulcerations of intestinal lining
Other Vascular Diseases	* Esophageal varices	Swollen, dilated esophageal veins, hematemesis, anemia
	* Hemorrhoids	Swollen, painful veins in and around anus, burning itchy, sometimes bleeding

Affected Organ/Body Region	Diagnostic Procedures	Treatment
Mouth	Physical exams, biopsies	Radiation, surgery
Esophagus	Endoscopy, esophageal washings	Radiation, surgery, chemotherapy
Stomach	Gastroscopy, biopsy, gastric fluid analysis, barium x-ray	Surgery, chemotherapy
Colon/rectum	Endoscopy, biopsy, barium x-ray, stool analysis	Surgery, radiation, chemotherapy
Stomach, intestines	Stool analysis	Fluid and nutrient replacement, antispasmodic medication
Stomach, intestines	Gastroscopy, gastric washings, barium x-ray	Antibiotics
Intestines	Stool analysis	Replenishing water, electrolytes, nutrients
Intestines	Stool analysis	Antibiotics
Esophagus	Physical examination	Nonirritating diet, antacids, avoid alcohol
Stomach	Gastroscopy	Ice water, surgery, avoid alcohol
Stomach	Analysis of gastric secretions	Avoid aspirin, alcohol, irritant food
Stomach, duodenum	Gastroscopy, gastric washings, barium x-ray	Medication, antacids, dietary change, reduce stress
Appendix	Blood count, physical examination	Surgery
Intestines	Endoscopy	Antibiotics, controlled diet
Intestines	Stool analysis	Corticosteroids, and rarely, surgery
Colon	Endoscopy, x-ray, "pipe-stem" colon	Reduce stress, dietary changes, sedatives, corticosteroids, colostomy
Esophagus	Endoscopy, physical examination, associated with alcoholism	Compression via inflatable tubes, sclerosing agent, rarely surgery
Rectum, anus	Proctoscope, stool analysis	Increase fiber and water in diet, medicated suppositories, anorectal creams

Digestive Tract (continued)

Categories	* Disease ■ Disorder ✓ Stress-related	Signs and Symptoms
Anatomic Abnormalities	* Hiatal hernia	Indigestion, heartburn after eating, esophageal reflux

	* Organic obstructions
	  Volvulus
	  Intussusception
	  Adhesions
		Complete constipation, severe pain, distension of abdomen, vomiting

Abnormal Function	* Paralytic obstructions	Complete constipation, severe pain, distension of abdomen, vomiting
	✓■ Spastic colon	Diarrhea, pain, gas, constipation
	* Malabsorption syndrome (often secondary to other disease)	Malnutrition, failure to absorb fats, fatty, pale, floating stools, bad odor

Affected Organ/Body Region	Diagnostic Procedures	Treatment
Stomach	X-ray	Avoid irritating foods, frequent small meals, surgery
Intestines	Physical examination, x-ray	Suction tube, surgery
Intestines	Physical examination, x-ray	Suction tube
Colon	No lesions present	Avoid caffeine, alcohol, spicy food, fats, increase fiber in diet
Intestines	Stool analysis	Control of diet, vitamin supplements

Interactive Activities

CASE FOR CRITICAL THINKING

A 45-year-old woman experiences frequent heartburn, occasional swallowing difficulty, and sharp pains below her sternum. Sometimes at night she experiences gastric reflux, or a regurgitation of stomach acid into the esophagus, a condition that is extremely painful. What could produce these symptoms? What diagnostic procedures could be used? How should she be treated?

MULTIMEDIA EXTENSION ACTIVITIES

www.prenhall.com/mulvihill
Use the above address to access the free, interactive companion Website created for this textbook. Included in the features of this site are chapter specific activities, internet links, and an audio-glossary.

Audio Glossary
Use the CD-ROM disk enclosed with your textbook to hear the pronunciation of the key terms in this chapter.

Diseases at a Glance: Digestive Tract

Use the chart on page(s) 218–221 to answer the following questions.

1. List 5 types of diseases or conditions that affect the digestive tract.

2. What are the major signs and symptoms of the diseases or conditions you named?

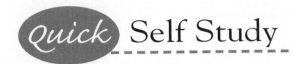 Self Study

MULTIPLE CHOICE

1. Which of the following occurs in gastritis?
   a. loss of stomach muscle tone
   b. inflammation of stomach mucosa
   c. stomach unable to secrete acid
   d. bloody diarrhea

2. Recurrent bloody diarrhea may be a symptom of _____.
   a. gastric ulcer
   b. ulcerative colitis
   c. hiatal hernia
   d. esophagitis

3. Which disease is characterized by the destruction of intestinal villi, leading to inability to absorb fats and other nutrients?
   a. ulcerative colitis
   b. celiac disease/malabsorption syndrome
   c. Crohn's disease
   d. peptic ulcer

4. Small pouches of the large intestine become inflamed during this disease:
   a. Crohn's disease
   b. gastritis
   c. hemorrhoids
   d. diverticulitis

TRUE/FALSE

____F____ 1. Hemorrhoids are caused by infection with *E. coli*.

____T____ 2. Oral and esophageal cancers are linked to tobacco and alcohol use.

____F____ 3. Drinking too much water causes diarrhea.

____T____ 4. Dark stools are known as melena.

FILL-INS

1. *Entamoeba histolytica* is the cause of _____ ameobaic dysentery _____

2. Thickened intestinal walls, leading to obstruction and abdominal pain, are found in _____ Chron's disease _____.

3. An abdominal _____ hernia _____ is protrusion of an organ through abdominal wall muscles.

4. An instrument called a(n) _____ endoscope _____ is used to view the lining of the esophagus or other organs of the digestive tract.

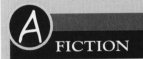

FICTION

The bacterium Helicobacter pylori is now known to be responsible for many stomach ulcers.

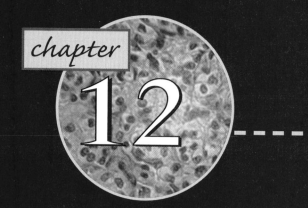
Diseases of the Liver, Gallbladder, and Pancreas

The liver, gallbladder, and pancreas have been called accessory organs of the digestive system. Yet they are crucial to the normal digestive process: they enable the digestive tract to digest, absorb, and process nutrients. How would the body be affected if disease interfered with the normal functions of these accessory organs?

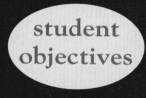

student objectives

After studying this chapter, students should be able to

➤ Describe the normal functions of the liver, gallbladder, and pancreas
➤ Describe the key characteristics of major diseases of the liver, gallbladder, and pancreas
➤ Name the causes of diseases of the liver, gallbladder, and pancreas
➤ Name the diagnostic procedures for diseases of the liver, gallbladder, and pancreas
➤ Describe the treatment options for diseases of the liver, gallbladder, and pancreas

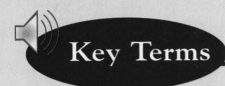

Key Terms

Adenocarcinoma	Glycogen
Amylase	Gynecomastia
Ascites	Hematemesis
Bile	Hepatic coma
Biliary calculi	Hepatocarcinoma
Biliary cirrhosis	Hypoalbuminemia
Cholecystectomy	Immunoglobulin
Cholecystitis	Jaundice
Cholelithiasis	Kuppfer's cells
Chymotrypsin	Lipase
Cirrhosis	Pancreatitis
Fulminating	

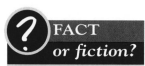

glycogen
(glī'-kŏ-jĕn)

Kuppfer's cells
(Koop'-fĕrz sĕlz)

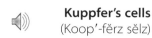

bile
(bīl)

➤ FUNCTIONS OF THE LIVER AND THE GALLBLADDER

The liver is located below the diaphragm, in the upper right quadrant of the abdominal region. The liver is the largest glandular organ of the body, and it is unique in that it has great powers of regeneration; it can replace damaged or diseased cells. Still, chronic liver disease may cause irreversible damage and loss of function.

The liver has a dual blood supply: It receives oxygenated blood from the hepatic artery and blood rich in nutrients from the portal vein. The blood reaching the liver through the portal vein comes from the stomach, intestines, spleen, and pancreas. Blood from the small intestines carries absorbed nutrients such as simple sugars and amino acids. One of the functions of the liver is to store any of these substances that are in excess. The liver plays an important role in maintaining the proper level of glucose in the blood. It acts as a buffer, taking up excess glucose and storing it as **glycogen.** When the level of circulating glucose falls below normal, the liver converts glycogen into glucose, which is then released into the blood. Iron and vitamins are also stored by the liver.

Another function of the liver is to synthesize various proteins, including enzymes necessary for cellular activities. One means of evaluating liver function is to determine the level of these enzymes in the blood. The liver also synthesizes plasma proteins. Albumin is the plasma protein that has a water-holding power within the blood vessels. If the albumin level is too low, plasma seeps out of the blood vessels and into the tissue spaces, causing edema. Other essential plasma proteins synthesized by the liver are those required for blood clotting, fibrinogen and prothrombin. If the liver is seriously diseased or injured and is unable to make these proteins, hemorrhaging may occur.

The liver can detoxify various substances, i.e., make poisonous substances harmless. Ammonia, which results from amino acid metabolism, is converted to urea by the liver. The urea then enters the bloodstream and is excreted by the kidneys. Certain drugs and chemicals are also detoxified by the liver. Specialized cells called **Kuppfer's cells** line the blood spaces within the liver. These cells engulf and digest bacteria and other foreign substances, thus cleansing the blood.

Bile, necessary for fat digestion, is secreted by the liver. As mentioned in the previous chapter, bile is an emulsifier, acting on fat in such a way that the lipid enzymes can digest it. The end product of lipid digestion can then be absorbed by the walls of the small intestine. In the absence of bile, the fat-soluble vitamins A, D, E, and K cannot be absorbed. Various functions of the liver are shown in Figure 12–1.

LIVER FUNCTIONS

Secrete bile
Store nutrients, glucose, amino acids, iron
Remove nitrogenous waste from blood
Inactivate ingested toxins
Remove dead blood cells, cell debris, and bacteria from blood
Synthesize enzymes and plasma proteins

Figure 12–1
Functions of the liver.

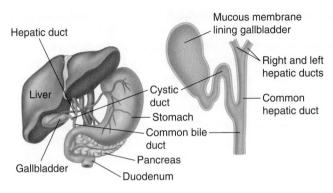

Figure 12–2
Bile duct system of the liver and gallbladder.

Bile consists of water, bile salts, cholesterol, and bilirubin, which is a colored substance resulting from the breakdown of hemoglobin. It is bilirubin that gives bile its characteristic color of yellow or orange.

The gallbladder is a small sac-like structure on the underside of the liver. Bile is secreted continuously by the liver into the hepatic duct, which carries bile to the gallbladder for storage and concentration (Figure 12–2). The gallbladder releases the bile through the cystic duct to the common hepatic duct, which carries the bile to the duodenum. Release of bile is coordinated with the appearance of fats in the duodenum.

➤ DISEASES OF THE LIVER

Liver disease manifests itself when chronic damage to liver cells cannot be repaired. When fibrous tissue replaces liver cells, the normal functions of the liver become impaired.

Jaundice

One sign frequently associated with liver disease is jaundice. **Jaundice** is a yellow or orange discoloration of the skin, tissues, and the whites of the eyes. It is caused by a build-up of bilirubin, a pigment which is normally secreted in the bile and removed from the body in the feces.

jaundice
(jawn′-dĭs)

Causes of Jaundice   The normal flow of bile from the gallbladder to the duodenum may be obstructed. The obstruction might be a tumor, a gallstone in the duct system, or a congenital defect. Because the bile cannot move forward, it leaks into the blood, with bilirubin coloring the plasma. When the blood reaches the kidneys, the bile appears in

on the Practical Side

Neonatal Jaundice
Newborns may exhibit jaundice shortly after birth, but this may not be a sign of a serious illness. The liver of newborns often is not mature, so bilirubin builds up in the tissues. Normally, however, within a few days, the newborn's liver processes the bilirubin and jaundice subsides.

the urine, giving it a dark color. Inasmuch as the bile is unable to reach the duodenum, the stools are light in color. They are usually described as clay-colored.

Complications can result from this blockage to bile flow. Infection or inflammation of the gallbladder or bile ducts could occur. Lack of bile interferes with fat digestion and absorption, which means that the fat-soluble vitamins are not being absorbed. In the absence of vitamin K, bleeding tendencies may develop. The obstruction can also cause liver damage.

Jaundice can also indicate liver disease, such as hepatitis or cirrhosis.

Hemolytic jaundice has an entirely different etiology. This type of jaundice accompanies the hemolytic anemias explained in Chapter 7. In these anemias, the red blood cells hemolyze, and an excess of bilirubin results from the breakdown of released hemoglobin. Abnormal discoloration follows. Figure 12–3 illustrates the causes of jaundice.

PREVENTION *PLUS!*

Know Your Viruses

The more you know about how a virus is transmitted, the better prepared you can be to prevent infection. Hepatitis A is transmitted primarily through contaminated food and water. Workers in the food service industry must use sanitary procedures when handling food—including the simple task of washing their hands. You can protect yourself at home by thoroughly cooking meat and seafood. Hepatitis B and C are transmitted through blood transfusions. Healthcare workers receive vaccination against hepatitis B, and blood is screened for contamination by hepatitis B and C.

Viral Hepatitis

Hepatitis, or inflammation of the liver, is caused by a number of factors. Several viruses have been identified as causing hepatitis. Three important causes are hepatitis virus type A, hepatitis virus type B, and hepatitis virus type C.

Hepatitis virus type A, formerly called *infectious hepatitis,* is the least serious form and can develop as an isolated case or in an epidemic. The incubation period, the time from exposure to the development of symptoms, is from 2 to 6 weeks. The symptoms include anorexia, nausea, and mild fever. The urine becomes dark in color, and jaundice appears in some cases. On examination, the liver may be found to be enlarged and tender. Contaminated water or food is the usual source of the infection, which spreads under conditions of poor sanitation. The virus is excreted in the stools and urine, infecting soil and water.

Hepatitis virus type A is usually mild in children; it is sometimes more severe in adults. Prognosis is usually good, with no permanent liver damage resulting. **Immuno-**

immunoglobulin
(ĭm″-ū-nō-glŏb′-ū-lĭn)

CAUSES OF JAUNDICE

| Obstruction of bile ducts |
| Hepatitis |
| Cirrhosis |
| Hemolytic anemia |

Figure 12–3
Causes of jaundice.

globulin injections provide temporary protection against hepatitis virus type A for people exposed to it. Once a person has had either type of hepatitis, he or she is immune to that particular type for life.

Hepatitis virus type B, formerly called *serum hepatitis,* is a more serious disease. It can lead to chronic hepatitis or cirrhosis of the liver. Occasionally, a **fulminating** case of hepatitis virus type B develops, and it is fatal. This form has a sudden onset and progresses rapidly. The person becomes delirious, then becomes comatose, and dies. Hepatitis virus type B can be transmitted by blood or serum transfusions in which the donated blood contains the virus. It also is transmitted through the use of contaminated needles or syringes used by drug addicts and as a sexually transmitted disease.

The symptoms are similar to those of hepatitis virus type A but develop more slowly. The incubation period is long, lasting from 2 to 6 months. The severity of the disease varies greatly. A person's physical condition at the onset of the disease makes a difference in the seriousness of the infection. A person with poor nutritional status, for example, will be more adversely affected by hepatitis.

Blood and plasma are screened for hepatitis, but hospital personnel still must be well informed of the hazards that can lead to acquiring hepatitis. Precautions must be taken by nurses, laboratory technicians, dialysis workers, and blood bank personnel to prevent becoming infected. Vaccination provides immunity to the virus, and it should be considered by any personnel that handle or come in close contact with blood or other bodily fluids. (See Precautions for Health Care Providers, Chapter 2, under AIDS).

fulminating
(fŭl-mĭ-nă-tĭng)

Disease by the Numbers x + ÷

EPIDEMIOLOGY

Nearly 2 of every 100 adults in the U.S. are infected with hepatitis C virus. About 9000 people die per year from complications of this disease, a number that is expected to triple by 2010.

Hepatitis C is emerging as one of the major causes of chronic liver disease, and is now the most common reason for liver transplants. The virus is transmitted mostly through blood transfusions, although transmission has been traced to intravenous drug use, and epidemiologic studies show a risk associated with sexual contact with someone with hepatitis and with having had more than one sex partner in a year. The initial symptoms are nonspecific and similar to those of hepatitis A or B, but the disease persists for months, even years. About 20% of infected persons develop cirrhosis, and a number of these can lead to end-stage liver disease. Treatments of hepatitis C include interferon injections and oral ribavirin. Treatment for end-stage cirrhosis may include liver transplant.

Cirrhosis of the Liver

Cirrhosis of the liver is a very serious disease. There are several types of cirrhosis, but the symptoms for each are similar. Most people associate cirrhosis of the liver with chronic alcoholism, which is the leading cause, but severe chronic hepatitis can develop into cirrhosis. A chronic inflammation of the bile ducts can also lead to cirrhosis. Certain drugs and toxins can cause necrosis of the liver cells, which is the first step in the development of cirrhosis.

Cirrhosis is chronic destruction of liver cells and tissues with a nodular, bumpy regeneration. In the normal liver, there is a highly organized arrangement of cells, blood

cirrhosis
(sĭ-rŏ-sĭs)

vessels, and bile ducts. A cirrhotic liver loses this organization and, as a result, the liver cannot function. (Figures 12–4 and 12–5)

As the liver cells are damaged by excessive alcohol, drugs, or viral infection, they die and are replaced by fibrous connective tissue and scar tissue. This tissue has none of the liver cell functions. At first, the liver is generally enlarged due to regeneration but then becomes smaller as the fibrous connective tissue contracts. The surface acquires a nodular appearance. This liver, sometimes referred to as a "hobnailed" liver, is pictured in Figure 12–6.

Alcoholic cirrhosis, the most common type of cirrhosis, will be described in detail. This disease is also called portal, Laennec's, or fatty nutritional cirrhosis (an accumulation of fat often develops within the liver). Cirrhosis is more common in males than in females. The exact effect of excessive alcohol on the liver is not known, but it may be related to the malnutrition that frequently accompanies chronic alcoholism, or the alcohol itself may be toxic.

In cirrhosis, circulation through the liver is impaired. As a result, high pressure builds in vessels of the abdomen and in other areas. The esophageal veins swell, forming esophageal varices (Chapter 9). Abdominal organs like the spleen, pancreas, and stomach also swell. These organs and vessels may hemorrhage, causing hemorrhagic shock. Hemorrhage of vessels in the stomach or intestines may cause vomiting of blood, **hematemesis.**

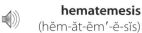

hematemesis
(hĕm-ăt-ĕm′-ĕ-sĭs)

ascites
(ă-sī′-tez)

A characteristic symptom of cirrhosis is distention of the abdomen caused by the accumulation of fluid in the peritoneal cavity. This fluid is called **ascites** and develops as a result of liver failure. The pressure within the obstructed veins forces plasma into the abdominal cavity. This fluid often has to be drained.

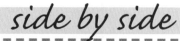

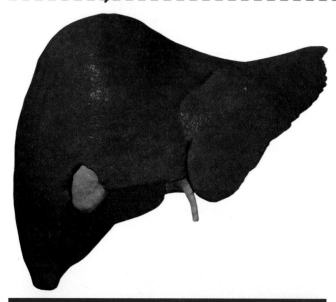

Figure 12–4

Normal liver.

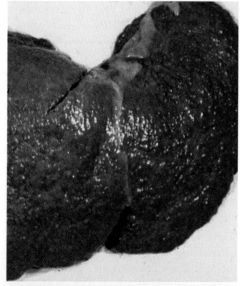

Figure 12–5

Cirrhotic liver.

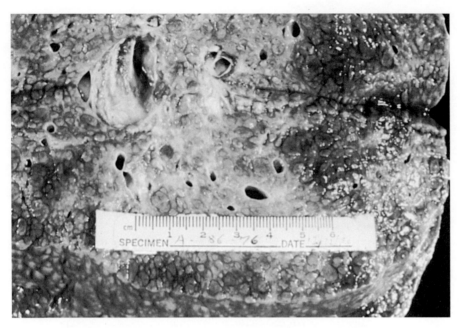

Figure 12–6
Typical "hobnailed" appearance of a liver affected by cirrhosis. (*Courtesy of Dr. David R. Duffell.*)

When the liver fails to produce adequate amounts of albumin, an albumin deficiency **(hypoalbuminemia)** develops and fluid leaks out of the blood vessels, causing edema. Because the necrotic cells of the cirrhotic patient fail to produce albumin, ascitic fluid develops, as does edema, particularly in the ankles and legs.

Blockage of the bile ducts, like that of the blood vessels, follows the disorganization of the liver. Bile accumulates in the blood, leading to jaundice and, because bile is not secreted into the duodenum, stools are clay-colored. The excess of bile, carried by the blood to the kidneys, gives a dark color to urine.

Other signs are related to the fact that the diseased liver cannot perform its usual biochemical activities. Normally, the liver inactivates small amounts of female sex hormones secreted by the adrenal glands in both males and females. Estrogens then have no effect on the male, but the cirrhotic liver does not inactivate estrogens. They accumulate and have a feminizing effect on males. The breasts enlarge, a condition known as **gynecomastia,** and the palms of the hand are red because of the estrogen level. Hair on the chest is lost, and a female-type distribution of hair develops. Atrophy of the testicles can also occur.

The damaged liver cells are unable to carry out their normal function of detoxification, so ammonia and other poisonous substances accumulate in the blood and affect the brain, causing various neurologic disorders. The person becomes confused and disoriented, even to the point of stupor, and a characteristic tremor or shaking develops. This shaking, is referred to as "liver flap." Somnolence or abnormal sleepiness are symptoms of cirrhosis. **Hepatic coma** is a possible cause of death in cirrhosis. The typical signs of cirrhosis are shown in Figure 12–7.

Carcinoma of the Liver

Hepatocarcinoma, or cancer of the liver, is sometimes a complication of cirrhosis. This is a primary malignancy of the liver, which is rare. More often, cancer detected in the

hypoalbuminemia
(hī″pō-ăl-bū″-mĭn-ē′-mē-ă)

gynecomastia
(jī″-nĕ-kō-măs′-tĭ-ă)

hepatic coma
(hĕ-păt′-ik kō-mă)

hepatocarcinoma
(hĕp″-ă-tŏ-kăr″-sĭn-ō-mă)

SIGNS OF ADVANCED CIRRHOSIS

Neurologic manifestations: Somnolence, mental confusion, flapping tremor, coma
Loss of chest hair
Severe liver damage, "hobnailed" liver
Ascitic fluid
Red palms
Testicular atrophy
Tendency to hemorrhage
Edema in ankles
Female distribution of hair
Dilated abdominal veins
Enlarged spleen
Gynecomastia
Esophageal varices

Figure 12–7
Signs of advanced cirrhosis.

liver is a result of metastasis from other organs, such as the breast, the colon, or the pancreas. These tumors are secondary carcinomas.

As mentioned in the chapter on neoplasia (Chapter 4), cancer spreads by way of the blood vessels and lymphatics. Because of the arrangement of these vessels through the liver, it is a frequent site of metastases. A high percentage of people who die of cancer are found to have had liver metastases. Cancer also spreads by invading surrounding tissue. A malignancy of the gallbladder or pancreas can grow into the liver.

The symptoms of hepatocarcinoma vary according to the site of the tumor. If the tumor is obstructing the portal vein, ascites develops in the abdominal cavity, as it does in cirrhosis. If the fluid is found to contain blood, a malignancy is indicated. A tumor blocking the bile duct will cause jaundice. General symptoms may include loss of weight, an abdominal mass, and pain in the upper right quadrant of the abdomen.

Prognosis for cancer of the liver is poor. Usually, the malignancy has developed elsewhere and has spread to the liver. Techniques such as the liver scan and needle biopsy are used in diagnosing the condition.

➤ DISEASES OF THE GALLBLADDER

The function of the gallbladder is to store and concentrate bile. Gallbladder disease will impair the storage and delivery of bile to the duodenum.

Cholecystitis

Cholecystitis is an inflammation of the gallbladder. The root word *chole* always refers to bile. A cyst is a sac. The gallbladder is a sac containing bile. The suffix, *itis,* indicates inflammation.

Cholecystitis is usually caused by an obstruction, a gallstone or tumor. Because of the blockage, bile cannot leave the gallbladder. The bile becomes more concentrated and irritates the walls of the gallbladder. The typical inflammatory response occurs, and the gallbladder becomes extremely swollen. Pain is experienced under the right rib cage and radiates to the right shoulder. At this point, the gallbladder can usually be felt (palpated). The person experiences chills and fever; nausea and vomiting are also common symptoms.

Serious complications can result from cholecystitis. Lack of blood flow because of the obstruction brought about by the swelling can cause an infarction. With the death of the tissues, gangrene can set in. The acutely inflamed gallbladder, like an inflamed appendix, may rupture, causing peritonitis. A complication of chronic cholecystitis is that bile accumulates in the bile ducts of the liver. This causes necrosis and fibrosis of the liver cells lining the ducts. This is another form of cirrhosis, **biliary** (bile) **cirrhosis.** Possible complications of bile duct obstruction are summarized in Figure 12–8.

A person with chronic cholecystitis experiences distress after eating fatty foods. The presence of fat in the duodenum stimulates the gallbladder to contract and release bile, and the contraction of the inflamed gallbladder causes pain. Nausea and indigestion, accompanied by belching, follow eating a heavy meal.

Prolonged inflammation causes the gallbladder to lose its ability to concentrate bile. The walls of the gallbladder may thicken, making it impossible for the gallbladder to contract properly.

Gallstones (Cholelithiasis)

Gallstones, also called **biliary calculi,** may be present in the gallbladder and give no symptoms. There may be one gallstone present or several hundred, which can be large or small. Small stones, referred to as gravel, are the ones that enter the cystic duct and cause an obstruction with excruciating pain. The formation or presence of gallstones is called **cholelithiasis;** the word element *lith(o)* refers to a stone.

Gallstones form when substances that are normally soluble precipitate out of solution. The stones consist principally of cholesterol, bilirubin, and calcium when in excess. Certain factors tend to stimulate gallstone formation, such as obesity and pregnancy (because of an increased cholesterol level). The incidence of gallstones is higher in women.

cholecystitis
(kō″-lē-sĭs′-tī-tĭs)

biliary cirrhosis
(bĭl′-ē-ār-ē sĭ-rŏ-sīs)

biliary calculi
(bil′-e-ar-e kăl′kyu-lī)

cholelithiasis
(kō″-lē-lĭ-thī′-ă-sĭs)

COMPLICATIONS OF BILE DUCT OBSTRUCTION

Rupture and peritonitis
Impaired lipid digestion and absorption
Impaired circulation and necrosis
Biliary cirrhosis

Figure 12–8
Complications of bile duct obstruction.

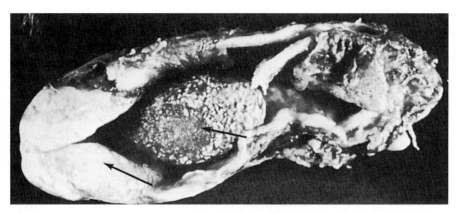

Figure 12–9
Gallbladder with chronic cholecystitis. *Center arrow* illustrates the gallstone. Left arrow points to the thickened inflamed wall. (*Courtesy of Dr. David R. Duffell.*)

The danger of gallstones is obstruction of the bile ducts, which causes inflammation. The converse is also true; inflammation of the gallbladder causes gallstone formation. Figure 12–9 shows a gallbladder with chronic cholecystitis and cholelithiasis. Stones can sometimes be dissolved by medication, depending on their chemical composition.

Extracorporeal shockwave lithotripsy (ESWL) shatters gallstones for removal without surgery. Lithotripsy was described in Chapter 10 for the removal of kidney stones. The position of the stones is one significant factor in determining feasibility of the procedure.

Gallstones can be located by sonography and x-ray. The usual treatment for cholecystitis and cholelithiasis is surgical removal of the gallbladder, a **cholecystectomy.** The cystic duct is then ligated, and the common bile duct examined for stones. Occasionally, undetected cholesterol stones are retained in the common bile duct after surgery. These stones have been successfully dissolved by administering a solubilizing agent through a catheter into the bile duct. This prevents the necessity of repeated surgery.

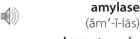 **cholecystectomy**
(kō-lē-sĭs-tĕk′-tō-mē)

➤ STRUCTURE AND FUNCTION OF THE PANCREAS

The pancreas is a fish-shaped organ extending across the abdomen behind the stomach. The head fits into the curve of the duodenum, and it is here the pancreatic duct empties. The duct carries digestive enzymes from the pancreas to the duodenum. These enzymes include **amylase,** which breaks down carbohydrates, trypsin and **chymotrypsin,** which digest protein, and **lipase,** which breaks down lipid or fat.

Diseases of the pancreas severely interfere with the digestive process. The many digestive enzymes contained within the pancreas make it a threat to itself, as will be explained in a particular disease condition. Figure 12–10 shows the structure of the pancreas. Figure 12–11 shows the relationship between the pancreas and other digestive organs.

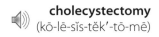 **amylase**
(ăm′-ĭ-lās)

chymotrypsin
(kī″-mō-trĭp′-sĭn)

lipase
(lĭ′-păs)

➤ DISEASES OF THE PANCREAS

Pancreatitis

Acute **pancreatitis** is a serious inflammation of the pancreas that can result in death. For some reason, the protein- and lipid-digesting enzymes become activated within the pancreas and begin to digest the organ itself. Severe necrosis and edema of the pancreas

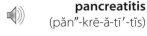 **pancreatitis**
(păn″-krē-ă-tī′-tĭs)

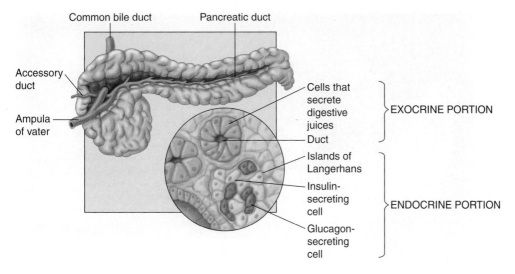

Figure 12–10
The pancreas—an endocrine and exocrine gland.

result. The digestion can extend into blood vessels, which, of course, causes bleeding; if hemorrhaging occurs, the person may go into shock. When the condition becomes this severe, it is called acute hemorrhagic pancreatitis. This is shown in Figure 12–12.

Severe, steady abdominal pain of sudden onset is the first symptom. The intense pain radiates to the back, and it can resemble the sharp pain of a perforated ulcer. Drawing up the knees or assuming a sitting position may provide some relief. There may also be nausea and vomiting. Jaundice sometimes develops if the swelling of inflammation blocks the common bile duct.

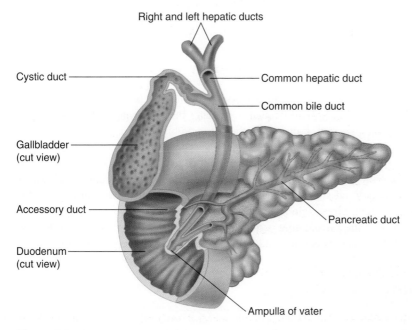

Figure 12–11
Relationship between pancreas and other digestive organs.

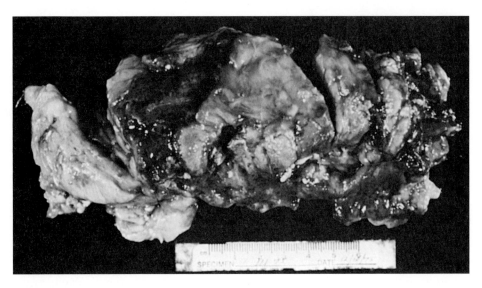

Figure 12–12
Acute hemorrhagic pancreatis. (*Courtesy of Dr. David R. Duffell.*)

Several factors can cause pancreatitis, but the most common one is excessive alcohol consumption. Inflammation of pancreatic ducts caused by the presence of gallstones is another possible cause. Many cases of pancreatitis cannot be attributed to either of these causes. The etiology is said to be idiopathic, its cause is unknown. Pancreatitis is more common in women than in men and usually occurs after age 40.

If a large area of the pancreas is affected, both endocrine and digestive functions of the gland become inadequate. In the absence of lipid enzymes from the pancreas, fat cannot be digested. Stools are then greasy and have a foul odor. Secondary malabsorption syndrome develops, because fat that is not digested cannot be absorbed.

The most significant diagnostic procedures for pancreatitis are blood tests and urine tests. High levels of pancreatic enzymes, particularly amylase, confirm the diagnosis of pancreatitis.

Cancer of the Pancreas

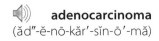

adenocarcinoma
(ăd″-ĕ-nō-kăr′-sĭn-ō′-mă)

Cancer of the pancreas, an **adenocarcinoma** because the pancreas is a gland, has a high mortality rate. It occurs more frequently in males than in females. If the malignancy is in the head of the pancreas, it can block the common bile duct. This will give earlier symptoms than cancer in the body or tail, which can be very advanced before it is discovered.

Obstruction of the bile duct causes jaundice and digestion is impaired because the pancreatic enzymes and bile cannot enter the duodenum. This causes malabsorption of fat and clay-colored stools. The person cannot absorb sufficient nutrients and calories and loses weight. Great pain is experienced as the tumor grows, and the cancer usually metastasizes to the surrounding organs: the duodenum, stomach, and liver. Prognosis for cancer of the pancreas is poor, and death occurs in a relatively short time.

➤ DIAGNOSTIC TESTS

Liver function tests include those for serum and urine bilirubin, and serum enzyme assays. Ultrasound is used to evaluate the liver, biliary system, including the gallbladder and pancreas. High-frequency sound waves are directed into the area to be examined. Through echoes converted into electrical energy, a pattern of spikes and dots appearing on an oscilloscope can depict organ size, shape, and position. Ultrasound has generally replaced the cholecystogram and cholangiogram, which are x-rays used in combination with radiopaque dyes to show the presence of gallstones, tumors, or a malfunctioning gallbladder. Computed tomography (CT) scans of the abdomen and pelvis visualize the liver, biliary system, and pancreas. This is a very significant test in diagnosing acute pancreatitis and cancer of the pancreas.

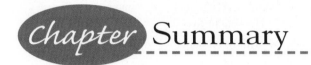 ## *Chapter* Summary

The normal functions of the liver were reviewed, so that symptoms of liver disease would be meaningful. Liver cells become necrotic when injured, but the liver is able to regenerate new cells if the injury is slight. If the liver damage is extensive and liver cells are replaced by fibrous scar tissue, liver function fails.

Jaundice is frequently associated with liver disease because of abnormal bile production or release. Bile deficiency impairs digestion of fat and absorption of fat-soluble vitamins. In the absence of vitamin K, bleeding tendencies develop.

Hepatitis and cirrhosis are the serious liver diseases that were considered. Chronic hepatitis can lead to cirrhosis, but the most common cause of cirrhosis is alcoholism.

Cholecystitis, inflammation of the gallbladder, can cause gallstone formation, which, in turn, can cause inflammation. The most serious complication of gallstones is obstruction of the bile duct.

Inflammation of the pancreas, pancreatitis, is a serious disease in which enzymes intended for the digestive tract digest the pancreas itself. Carcinoma of the pancreas is a malignancy with a very poor prognosis.

Diseases at a Glance:
Liver, Gallbladder, and Pancreas

Categories	* Disease ❑ Condition ● Disorder	Signs and Symptoms
Malignancy	* Liver cancer	Usually metastatic, occasionally primary, bile duct obstruction, jaundice, impaired clotting, ascites, weight loss
	* Pancreatic cancer	Malabsorption, jaundice, upper abdominal pain
Infections	* Hepatitis Type A Type B Type C	Jaundice, anorexia, weakness, weight loss, mild fever, enlarged tender liver, progression to cirrhosis in some cases
Inflammations and Degenerative Disorders	* Cirrhosis	Jaundice, abdominal distension due to ascites, bleeding tendencies, edema malabsorption of fats, gynecomastia, delerium tremens, hepatic coma
	* Cholecystitis	Upper right abdominal pain especially after eating fatty food, nausea, indigestion, belching
	* Acute pancreatitis	Severe, sharp, radiating abdominal pain, risk of hemorrhage, jaundice, vomiting, secondary malabsorption
Other abnormal structure/function	* Cholelithiasis (gallstones)	None, or upper right abdominal pain especially after eating

Affected Organ/ Body Region	Diagnostic Procedures	Treatment
Liver	Ultrasound, CT scan, needle biopsy	Chemotherapy (prognosis poor)
Pancreas	Ultrasound, CT scan, needle biopsy	Chemotherapy (prognosis poor)
Liver	Blood test for virus	Interferon injection, oral ribovarin, liver transplant
Liver	Patient history, serum enzymes	No specific treatment; improved diet, liver transplant
Gallbladder	Ultrasound scan, CT scan, fecal fat test	Cholecystectomy
Pancreas	Ultrasound scan, CT scan, serum enzymes	Pain relief, gastric suction, fluid replacement, IV nutrients
Gallbladder	Ultrasound scan, CT scan, x-ray, fecal fat test	Cholecystectomy ESWL (extracorporeal shockwave lithotripsy)

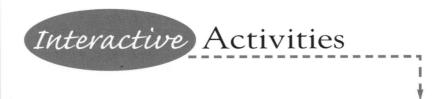

Interactive Activities

CASE FOR CRITICAL THINKING

T. W. experiences sharp pain in his upper right abdomen after eating a high-fat meal. Also, he has noted that his feces are grayish white instead of brown. What disease is the likely cause of his symptoms? Explain why each of these symptoms occurs with this disease.

MULTIMEDIA EXTENSION ACTIVITIES

www.prenhall.com/mulvihill
Use the above address to access the free, interactive companion Website created for this textbook. Included in the features of this site are chapter specific activities, internet links, and an audio-glossary.

Audio Glossary
Use the CD-ROM disk enclosed with your textbook to hear the pronunciation of the key terms in this chapter.

Diseases at a Glance: Liver, Gallbladder, and Pancreas

Use the chart on page(s) 238–239 to answer the following questions.

1. List 5 types of diseases or conditions that affect the liver, gallbladder, and pancreas.

2. What are the major signs and symptoms of the diseases or conditions you named?

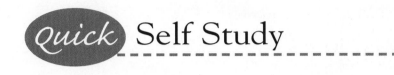

Quick Self Study

MULTIPLE CHOICE

1. Which is FALSE about pancreatic cancer?
   a. characterized by abdominal pain, weakness, weight loss
   b. higher incidence with age
   c. most are diagnosed after the cancer has metastasized
   d. prognosis is good with an 85% cure rate

2. Which is FALSE about cirrhosis?
   a. irreversible degenerative changes in liver
   b. normal liver replaced with fibrous scar tissue
   c. most often caused by diabetes
   d. esophageal varices (varicose veins) are a sign of cirrhosis

3. Acute pancreatitis is most closely associated with _____.
   a. hepatitis C virus infection   b. chronic alcoholism
   c. bile duct obstruction   d. complication of cirrhosis

4. Esophageal varices arise in which disease?
   a. cirrhosis   b. pancreatic cancer
   c. cholecystitis   d. cholelithiasis

TRUE/FALSE

_____T_____ 1. Neurologic disorders can accompany liver disease.

_____F_____ 2. Hepatitis A is acquired through blood products.

_____F_____ 3. Most cancer in the liver is primary liver cancer.

_____F_____ 4. Gallstones are made of undigested food particles too large to pass.

FILL-INS

1. Hepatitis type _____C_____ is the major viral cause of cirrhosis.
2. Extra corporeal shockwave lithotripsy is used to treat ___gall stones___.
3. Biliary cirrhosis arises if there is obstruction of the ___bile duct___.
4. Accumulation of fluid in the abdomen is called ___ascites___.

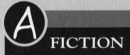

FICTION

Although it is correct that the liver is large and has great capacity to rebound from injury, chronic disease can cause it to lose function and can lead to cirrhosis and liver failure.

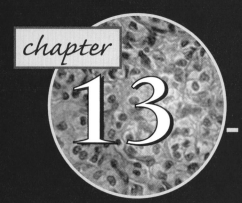

13

Diseases of the Respiratory System

We often use the familiar phrase "breath of life." What does this really mean? Every cell of the body is dependent on a fresh oxygen supply to utilize nutrients and obtain energy.

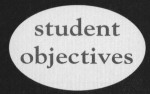

student objectives

After studying this chapter, students should be able to

➤ Describe the normal functions of the respiratory organs
➤ Describe the key characteristics of major diseases of the respiratory system
➤ Name the major causes of common diseases of the respiratory system
➤ Name the common diagnostic procedures for diseases of the respiratory system
➤ Name the common treatment options for diseases of the respiratory system

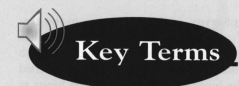

Key Terms

Abdominal	Larynx
Antihistamine	Legionnaire's disease
Alveoli	Lower respiratory diseases
Bronchi	
Bronchogenic carcinoma	Mucus
	Mucosa
Bronchopneumonia	Pharynx
Bronchioles	Pleura
Bronchitis	Pleural cavity
Caseous	Pleurisy
Chronic obstructive pulmonary disease	Pneumonia
	Primary atypical pneumonia
Cilia	
Cyanosis	Rales
Cystic fibrosis	Respiratory epithelium
Desensitize	Secondary pneumonia
Diaphragm	Spirometer
Dyspnea	Spirometry
Emphysema	Status asthmaticus
Epinephrine	Tubercles
Exocrine glands	Tuberculosis
External intercostals	Trachea
Fluoroscopy	Tracheotomy
Hypoxia	Upper respiratory diseases
Influenza	
Internal intercostal muscles	Wheezing

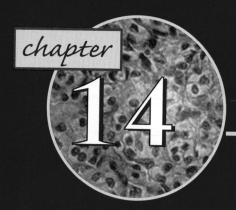
Diseases of the Endocrine System

The functions of the endocrine system cover a broad range of action. Endocrine activity affects the entire body: growth and development, metabolism, sexual activity, and even mental ability and emotions. The endocrine system is a means of communication between one body part and another.

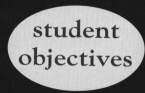

student objectives

After studying this chapter, students should be able to

➤ Describe the normal structure and functions of the endocrine glands

➤ Name the hormones secreted from each endocrine gland

➤ Describe the normal functions of hormones secreted from the endocrine glands

➤ Identify diseases of the anterior and posterior pituitary glands

➤ Describe the consequences of hyposecretion and hypersecretion of the anterior pituitary

➤ Describe the consequences of hyposecretion of the posterior pituitary

➤ Define the causes and consequences of goiter, hyperthyroid, and hypothyroid

➤ Identify and describe diseases of the adrenal cortex and the adrenal medulla

➤ Describe the effects of excessive parathormone and deficiency of parathormone

➤ Describe the regulatory function of insulin and glucagon

➤ Differentiate between Type I and Type II diabetes

➤ Identify the warning signs of diabetes

➤ Describe the complications associated with diabetes

➤ Distinguish between diabetic coma and insulin shock

➤ Identify and describe the various diagnostic procedures and tests for adrenal gland function

Key Terms

Acidosis

Acromegaly

Adenohypophysis

Adenoma

Adrenocorticotropic hormone

Aldosterone

Androgens

Androgenital syndrome

Antidiuretic hormone

Aspermia

Cortisol

Cortisone

Cretinism

Cushing's syndrome

Diabetes insipidus

Diabetes mellitus

Epinephrine

Estrogen

Exopthalmos

Gigantism

Glucagon

Glucocorticoids

Glycosuria

Goiter

Gonadotropins

Hirsutism

Hyperactive

Hypercalcemia

Hyperglycemia

Hyperparathyroidism

Hyperpituitarism

Hyperthyroidism

Hypoactive

Hypophysis

Hypothalamus

Insulin

Ketone bodies

Lethargy

Mineralocorticoids

Myxedema

Osteoblasts

Osteoclasts

Oxytocin

Parathormone

Polydipsia

Polyuria

Tetany

Thyroxine

Tremors

Triiodothyronine

Vasopressin

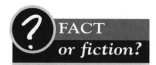

➤ FUNCTIONS OF THE ENDOCRINE GLANDS

The endocrine system consists of a group of organs of internal secretion. These glands secrete hormones, or chemical messengers directly into the bloodstream. The major organs of the endocrine system are the hypothalamus, the pituitary gland, the thyroid gland, the parathyroid glands, the pancreatic islets, the adrenal glands, the testes, and the ovaries. The sex glands—the ovaries and testes—will be studied with the Reproductive System in Chapter 15. Figure 14–1 shows the location of the endocrine glands.

Hormones are released from endocrine glands into the bloodstream where they affect activity in cells at distant sites. Some hormones affect the whole body whereas others act only on target or distant organs. Most hormones are composed of proteins or chains of amino acids; others are steroids or fatty substances derived from cholesterol.

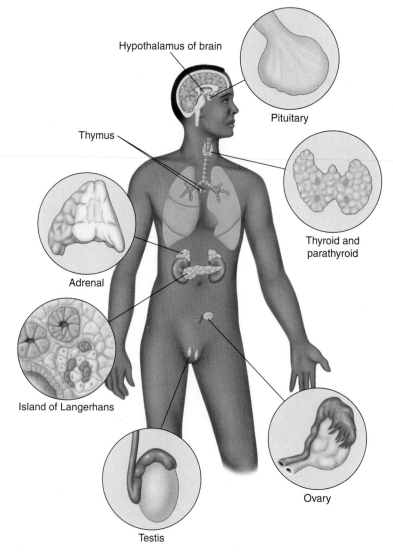

Figure 14–1
The endocrine glands.

Most glandular activity is controlled by the pituitary, which is sometimes called the *master gland*. The pituitary itself is controlled by the *hypothalamus*.

The body is conservative and secretes hormones only as needed. For example, **insulin** is secreted when the blood sugar level rises. Another hormone, **glucagon,** works antagonistically to insulin and is released when the blood sugar level falls below normal. Hormones are potent chemicals, so their circulating levels must be carefully controlled. When the level of a hormone is adequate, its further release is stopped. This type of control is called a negative feedback mechanism. Its importance will become clearer as specific diseases of the endocrine system are considered.

Overactivity or underactivity of a gland is the malfunction that most commonly causes endocrine diseases. If a gland secretes an excessive amount of its hormone, it is **hyperactive.** This condition is sometimes caused by a hypertrophied gland or by a glandular tumor.

A gland that fails to secrete its hormone or secretes an inadequate amount is **hypoactive.** The gland may be diseased, tumorous, or it may have been adversely affected by trauma, surgery, or radiation. A gland that has decreased in size and consequently is secreting inadequately is said to be atrophied. Each endocrine gland will be discussed with an emphasis on normal function and importance. The diseases caused by hypoactivity and hyperactivity of each gland will then be explained.

insulin
(ĭn′-sū-lĭn)

glucagon,
(gloo′-kă-gŏn)

hyperactive
(hī″-pĕr-ăk′-tĭv)

hypoactive
(hī″-pō-ak′-tĭv)

PREVENTION *PLUS!*

Overweight children are not gluttonous or lazy. Tests of endocrine function are recommended for children who are overweight and lower in stature than normal. Obese children without endocrine abnormalities actually expend more energy than their nonobese counterparts. Obese children need less food and more activity than their peers do.

➤ STRUCTURE AND FUNCTION OF THE PITUITARY GLAND

The wonder of the pituitary gland is its tiny size and yet its tremendous functions. It is only the size of a pea suspended from the base of the brain by a small stalk. The pituitary gland fits into a bony depression in one of the skull bones that carefully protects it from injury. The pituitary gland is illustrated in Figure 14–2.

Another name for the pituitary gland is the **hypophysis.** The hypophysis has two parts to it, each of which acts as a separate gland. Each part is stimulated differently to cause secretion, and each secretes entirely different hormones.

The anterior and larger portion of the hypophysis is the **adenohypophysis.** *Adeno* means gland, and this part is truly glandular. It is in direct communication with the **hypothalamus** of the brain. Portal blood vessels extending through the stalk connect the two. The hypothalamus is an extremely important coordinating center for the brain. It directs which hormones the anterior pituitary gland should secrete at a particular time. It does this by sending substances called releasing factors to the anterior pituitary through the connecting blood vessels. The pituitary then secretes the proper hormone.

The posterior pituitary, or neurohypophysis works differently. It receives hormones secreted by the hypothalamus and stores them for subsequent release. These hormones

hypophysis
(hī-pŏf′-ĭ-sĭs)

adenohypophysis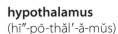
(ăd″-ĕ-nō-hī-pŏf′-ĭ sĭs)

hypothalamus
(hī″-pō-thăl′-ă-mŭs)

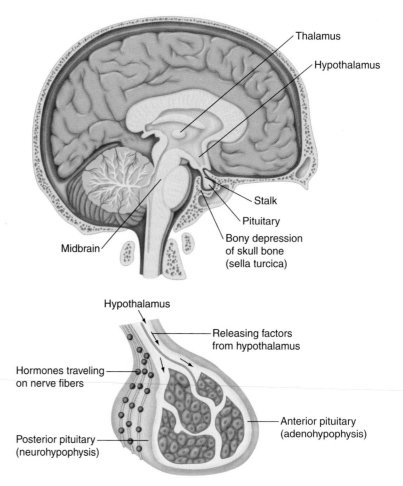

Figure 14-2
The pituitary gland and its relation to the brain.

travel over nerve fibers from the hypothalamus to the neurohypophysis. It is because of the neural connection with the hypothalamus that the posterior portion of the pituitary gland is called the neurohypophysis.

What can this little pea-sized structure control that makes it the master gland? The anterior pituitary, the adenohypophysis, secretes six hormones called *tropic hormones*. The word element *tropic* means going toward. That is what these six hormones do. They go toward a particular target organ.

Hormones of the Anterior Pituitary Gland

Growth hormone (GH; also called somatotropin) affects all parts of the body by promoting growth and development of the tissues. Before puberty, it stimulates the growth of long bones, increasing the child's height. Soft tissues—organs such as the liver, heart, and kidneys—also increase in size and develop under the influence of growth hormone. After adolescence, growth hormone is secreted in lesser amounts but continues to function in promoting tissue replacement and repair.

The thyroid gland regulates metabolism, the rate at which the body produces and uses energy. Secretion of thyroid hormone is controlled by the anterior pituitary. The pituitary hormone that stimulates the thyroid gland is *thyroid stimulating hormone* (TSH; also called thyrotropin). In the absence of TSH, the thyroid gland stops functioning.

The adrenal glands are also regulated by the anterior pituitary. The adrenal glands have an inner part, the medulla, and an outer portion, the cortex. It is the cortex that is controlled by the anterior pituitary. The tropic hormone affecting the adrenal cortex is **adrenocorticotropic hormone** (ACTH).

The anterior pituitary regulates sexual development and function by means of hormones known as the **gonadotropins.** These are not sex hormones, but they affect the sex organs, the gonads. They are follicle-stimulating hormone (FSH), luteinizing hormone (LH), and prolactin. These gonadotropic hormones regulate the menstrual cycle and secretion of male and female hormones. The relationship between the anterior pituitary and its target organs is seen in Figure 14–3.

adrenocorticotropic hormone
(ăd-rē″-nō-kŏr″-tĭ-kō-trŏp′-ĭk hŏr′-mōn)

gonadotropins
(gŏn″-ă-dō-tro′-pĭns)

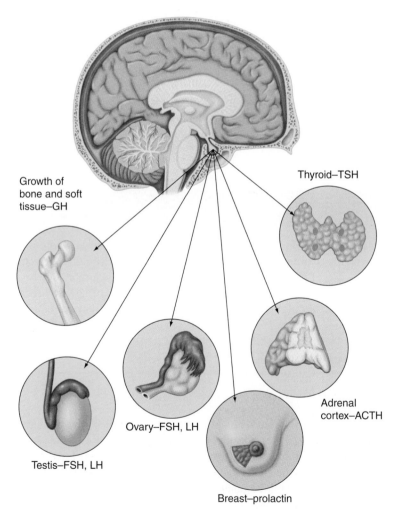

Growth of bone and soft tissue–GH

Thyroid–TSH

Ovary–FSH, LH

Testis–FSH, LH

Breast–prolactin

Adrenal cortex–ACTH

Figure 14–3
Anterior pituitary gland and its target organs.

➤ DISEASES OF THE ANTERIOR PITUITARY GLAND

Hyperpituitarism

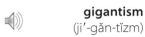

hyperpituitarism
(hī″-pĕr-pĭ-tū′-ĭ-tăr-ĭsm)

The most noticeable result of **hyperpituitarism** is the effect of excessive growth hormone. The condition produces a giant if the hypersecretion of growth hormone occurs before puberty. Normally, at puberty, the ends of the long bones seal with the shafts, and no further height is attained. Excessive growth hormone retards this normal closure of the bones. Sexual development is usually decreased, and mental development may be normal or retarded. **Gigantism** is usually the result of a tumor, an **adenoma,** of the anterior pituitary. Removal of the tumor or radiation treatment to reduce its size decreases the secretion of growth hormone.

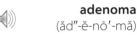

gigantism
(ji′-găn-tĭzm)

adenoma
(ăd″-ĕ-nō′-mă)

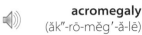

acromegaly
(ăk″-rō-mĕg′-ă-lē)

If the excessive production of growth hormone occurs after puberty, when full stature is attained, the result is different. This is the condition of **acromegaly;** the word element *megaly* means enlargement. The long bones can no longer grow in length, and bones of the hands, feet, and face enlarge. There is also excessive growth of soft tissues. The features of the face become coarsened; the nose and lips enlarge, and the lower jaw protrudes, producing an overbite that interferes with chewing. The skin and tongue thicken, the latter causing slurred speech. A curvature of the spine often develops, giving the person a bent appearance. The curvature is caused by an overgrowth of the vertebrae. This hyperactivity of the pituitary gland is generally due to a tumor. A patient with acromegaly is illustrated in Figure 14–4.

Treatment of acromegaly is complex. Surgery is used to remove or reduce the size of the tumor. Radiation and medication therapy is used to reduce overproduction of growth hormone. These treatments may not return growth hormone levels to normal for several years.

Disease by the Numbers x + ÷

Acromegaly occurs in 6 of 100,000 people. The name acromegaly comes from the Greek words for "extremities" and reflects one of its most common symptoms, the abnormal growth of bones in the arms, legs, and head. It is a rare, slowly progressive, chronic disorder that occurs in adults and is caused by increased secretion of growth hormone after normal growth has been completed. If left untreated, the risk of complications, such as arthritis and cardiovascular disease, increases. Patients with acromegaly have a mortality rate that is 2 to 4 times higher than the general population and a life expectancy that is 10 years shorter than for healthy individuals.

Hypopituitarism

Hypopituitarism can result from damage to the anterior lobe of the pituitary gland or from an inadequate secretion of hormones. A fracture at the base of the skull, a tumor, or ischemia (lack of blood flow) can cause pituitary destruction. Lack of blood flow causes an infarction, and the tissue becomes necrotic. Hypopituitarism can be mild or severe. If the entire anterior lobe of the pituitary is destroyed, the condition is called panhypopituitarism, *pan* meaning all. No pituitary hormones are secreted.

The abnormalities that result from the absence of tropic hormones are numerous. The thyroid gland, for example, is dependent on thyroid-stimulating hormone from the pituitary

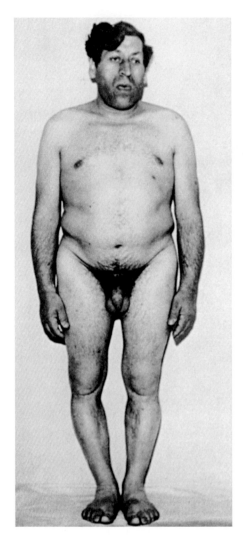
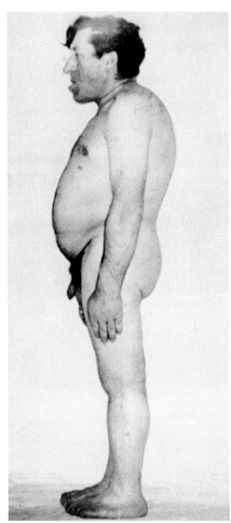

Figure 14–4
A 43-year-old patient with acromegaly. Note heavy, stocky build; broad chest; large head; and heavy hands and feet. Curvature of the spine causes the arms to appear excessively large. Thickening of the fingers interferes with manual dexterity.

for its functioning. Without that tropic hormone, the thyroid atrophies, and the functions of the thyroid cease. Mental dullness and **lethargy,** a condition of drowsiness, develop.

Lack of ACTH causes the adrenal cortex to atrophy. Inadequate cortical hormones result in a salt imbalance and improper metabolism of nutrients. The adrenal cortical hormones are essential to life.

Absence of the gonadotropic hormones depresses sexual functions. The gonads atrophy without stimulation of the tropic hormones. If the lack of hormones exists before puberty, sexual development is impaired. In an adult woman menstruation ceases; an adult male will lack sex drive or have **aspermia,** that is, no formation or emission of sperm. Figure 14–5 illustrates the glandular failure caused by severe hypopituitarism.

lethargy
(lĕth′-ăr-jē)

aspermia
(ă-spĕr′-mē-ă)

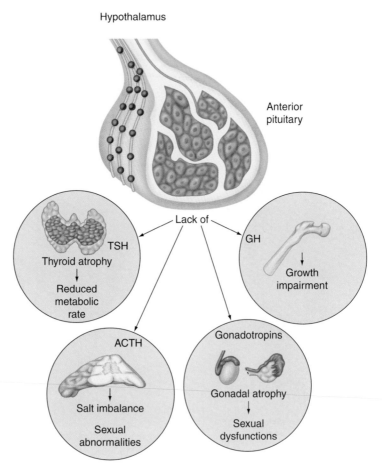

Figure 14–5
Effects of pituitary failure.

Hypopituitarism caused by a tumor may show additional symptoms. Pressure of the tumor may cause pain, a headache, or a peculiar form of blindness. Figure 14–6 shows the closeness of the pituitary gland to the optic nerves. As the tumor enlarges, it interferes with these nerves.

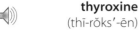

thyroxine
(thī-rŏks'-ēn)

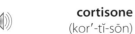

cortisone
(kor'-tĭ-sōn)

The patient suffering from hypopituitarism must be treated with hormonal supplements. Administration of **thyroxine, cortisone,** growth hormone, and sex hormones can compensate for the dysfunctional glands. It is significant that all these failures result from hypoactivity of the anterior pituitary. For this reason, the anterior pituitary is called the master gland.

A different form of hypopituitarism sometimes occurs in children. Inadequate growth hormone can cause a pituitary dwarf. This patient is mentally bright but small and underdeveloped sexually. All growth processes are retarded; teeth, for example, are late in erupting. A 28-year-old pituitary dwarf is shown in Figure 14–7. Replacement therapy with injections of growth hormone is currently used to treat children with pituitary dwarfism.

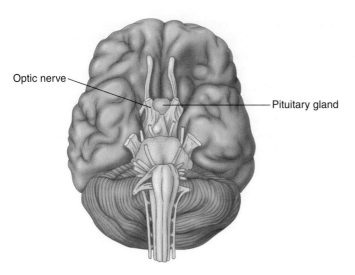

Optic nerve

Pituitary gland

Figure 14–6
Base of brain showing proximity of pituitary gland to optic nerves.

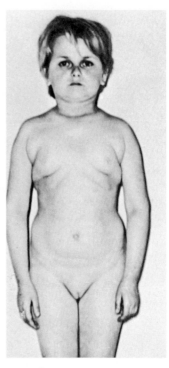

Figure 14–7
This 28-year-old pituitary dwarf is 45 inches tall, with the characteristic round face and fat deposits in breasts and abdomen. No sexual development is observed.

➤ FUNCTION OF THE POSTERIOR PITUITARY GLAND

The posterior pituitary, or neurohypophysis, secretes two hormones: **oxytocin** and **vasopressin,** also called **antidiuretic hormone** (ADH). Oxytocin causes smooth muscle, particularly that of the uterus, to contract and initiates milk secretion. It strengthens contractions during labor and helps prevent hemorrhage after delivery. Antidiuretic hormone prevents excessive water loss through the kidneys and makes the collecting ducts permeable to water. Water is then reabsorbed back into the bloodstream by the kidney tubules.

oxytocin
(ŏk″-sĭ-tō′-sĭn)

vasopressin
(văs″-ō-prĕs′-ĭn)

antidiuretic hormone
(ăn″-tĭ-dī-ū-rĕt′-ĭk
hŏr′-mōn)

➤ HYPOSECRETION OF THE POSTERIOR PITUITARY GLAND

Diabetes Insipidus

Diabetes insipidus is a disease that results from a deficiency of ADH. ADH is produced in the hypothalamus and is stored and released from the posterior pituitary gland. In the absence of ADH, water is not reabsorbed by the kidney and is lost in the urine. Extreme thirst or **polydipsia** and excessive production of dilute urine or **polyuria** results.

diabetes insipidus
(dī″-ă-bē′-tēz
ĭn-sĭp′-ĭ-dŭs)

polydipsia
(pŏlēdĭp′-sē-ă)

polyuria
(pŏl″-ē-ū′-rē-ă)

A condition of central diabetes insipidus can result from inadequate production of ADH by the hypothalamus or failure of the pituitary gland to release ADH into the bloodstream. Diabetes insipidus can also occur when ADH levels are normal. This condition, nephrogenic diabetes insipidus, involves a defect in the kidney. The kidney fails to concentrate urine in response to the instructions of ADH.

Excessive water loss can lead to dehydration quickly. Whenever possible, the underlying cause of diabetes insipidus must be corrected. Modified forms of ADH may be taken orally, by injection, or by nasal spray to maintain normal urine output. Figure 14–8 shows the normal action of ADH, and Figure 14–9 shows the effects of its absence.

➤ STRUCTURE AND FUNCTION OF THE THYROID GLAND

The activity of the thyroid gland affects the whole body. It regulates the metabolic rate, the rate at which calories are used. The thyroid gland, through its hormone, thyroxine, governs cellular oxygen consumption and, thus, energy and heat production. The more oxygen that is used, the more calories are metabolized ("burned up"). Thyroxine assures that enough body heat is produced to maintain normal temperature even in a cold environment.

Many people blame obesity on an underactive thyroid, a low rate of metabolism. Although there is a relationship between a person's body weight and metabolic rate, diet is still the critical factor in controlling obesity. A person with a low rate of metabolism requires fewer calories than someone who uses them at a faster rate.

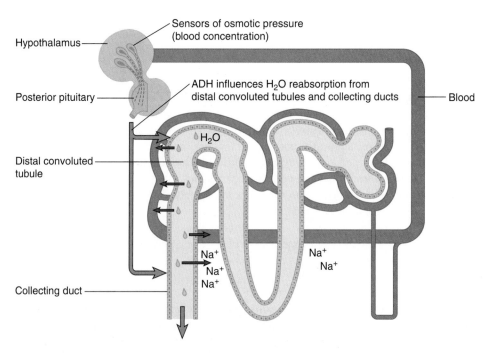

Figure 14–8
Normal action of antidiuretic hormone (ADH).

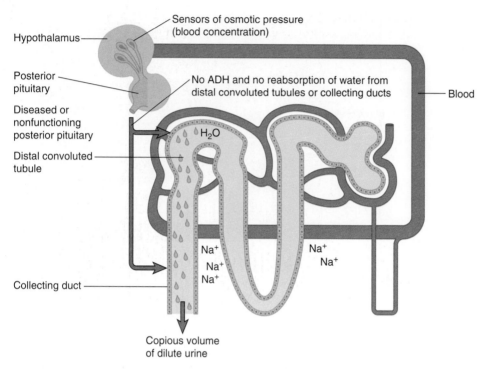

Figure 14-9
Effect of antidiuretic hormone (ADH) deficiency.

Structure of the Thyroid Gland

The thyroid gland is located in the neck region, one lobe on either side of the trachea. A connecting strip, or isthmus, anterior to the trachea, connects the two lobes. The thyroid gland lies just below the Adam's apple, the protrusion formed by part of the larynx. Figure 14–10 illustrates the thyroid gland. Internally, the thyroid gland consists of countless follicles, microscopic sacs. Within these protein-containing follicles, the thyroid hormones, thyroxine and **triiodothyronine,** are made. Thin-walled capillaries run between the follicles in a position ideal to receive the thyroid hormones.

triiodothyronine 🔊
(trī"-ī-ō"dō-thī'-rō-nēn)

Function of the Thyroid Gland

The thyroid gland synthesizes, stores, and releases thyroid hormones, which contain iodine. In fact, most of the iodide ions of the body are taken into the thyroid gland by a mechanism called the iodide trap. Iodine combines with an amino acid; two of these groups join, and the thyroid hormones are formed.

The hormones are stored until needed and then released into the blood capillaries. In the blood, the thyroid hormones combine with plasma proteins. Tests to determine the activity of the thyroid gland are based on this combination of tri-iodothyronine (T_3) and thyroxine (T_4) with plasma proteins. In the T_3 and T_4 tests, a sample of the patient's serum is incubated with radioactive thyroid hormones and resin. The resin absorbs the hormones that are not bound to the blood proteins. Radioactivity counts of the serum and resin are made, and the percentage of thyroid hormones absorbed by the resin is calculated. A low percentage of absorption indicates a poorly functioning thyroid gland. A high percentage of absorption indicates hyperactivity. In the latter case, the patient's own thyroid hormones had saturated the plasma proteins, and the radioactive hormones were absorbed by

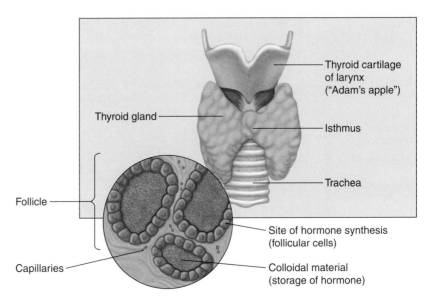

Figure 14–10
The thyroid gland.

the resin. This is a more accurate means of measuring thyroid activity than the test used for many years, the BMR, or basal metabolic rate. The term *basal metabolic rate,* however, is still used, and it refers to a person's oxygen consumption while at rest.

Effects of Thyroid Hormones

Although there is more than one thyroid hormone, for clarity the thyroid hormones are referred to here as thyroxine, the one that is secreted in the largest quantity. Thyroxine stimulates cellular metabolism by increasing the rate of oxygen use with subsequent energy and heat production.

Keeping in mind that thyroxine stimulates the rate of cellular metabolism, the effect of an increased thyroxine level on heart activity becomes clear. Think of it this way: Faster cellular metabolism increases the cell's demand for oxygen, so more oxygen must be circulated to the cells. Nutrients are converted to energy in the presence of oxygen and the waste products of metabolism, including carbon dioxide, are formed. These must be carried away from the cells. The circulatory system can meet these needs by increasing blood flow to the cells. Increased blood flow is obtained by greater cardiac output, more heart activity.

As cellular metabolism increases, respiration increases. The greater need for oxygen and a corresponding accumulation of carbon dioxide stimulate the respiratory center of the brain. Stimulation of the respiratory center results in a faster rate and greater depth of breathing.

Thyroxin increases body temperature. Heat is produced through cellular metabolism, and thyroxine stimulates this process. In a cold environment, thyroxine secretion increases to assure adequate body heat. If excessive body heat is produced, it is dissipated in two ways. Blood vessels of the skin dilate, increasing blood flow at the body surface, and giving the body a flushed appearance. As the blood flows through the skin blood vessels, excess heat escapes. The body is also cooled by the perspiration mechanism. Body temperature is controlled by a regulatory center in the brain.

Thyroxine also has a stimulatory effect on the gastrointestinal system. It increases the secretion of digestive juices and the movement of material through the digestive tract. Absorption of carbohydrates from the intestine is also increased under the influence of thyroxine, assuring adequate fuel for cellular metabolism. The effects of thyroxine are illustrated in Figure 14–11.

An understanding of these effects of thyroxine will make the diseases of the thyroid gland meaningful. Basically, the results of inadequate or excessive thyroxine secretion will be considered. The symptoms of each disease will be related to the function of thyroxine.

Control of Circulating Thyroxine Level

The anterior pituitary gland stimulates the thyroid by releasing thyroid-stimulating hormone, TSH. The thyroid, in turn, releases thyroxine, which circulates in the blood to all cells and tissues. When the level of circulating thyroxine is high, the anterior pituitary is inhibited and stops releasing TSH. This is an example of a negative feedback mechanism. An adequate level of thyroxine prevents further synthesis of the hormone. When the level of thyroxine falls, the anterior pituitary is released from the inhibition, and once again sends out TSH. This feedback mechanism is shown in Figure 14–12.

At times, this mechanism fails, constituting one basis for a thyroid disease. The thyroid gland may be perfectly healthy, but if the body's iodine supply is inadequate, the gland cannot produce thyroxine. It is possible for the thyroid gland to be overstimulated or understimulated by the anterior pituitary. The thyroid gland itself may be diseased, with a resultant hyperactivity or hypoactivity. These are some of the conditions that will be discussed.

➤ DISEASES OF THE THYROID GLAND

Goiter

Goiter is an enlargement of the thyroid gland. The enlargement may be caused by hypoactivity or hyperactivity of the thyroid or a deficiency in iodine needed to synthesize thyroid hormones.

goiter
(goy′tĕr)

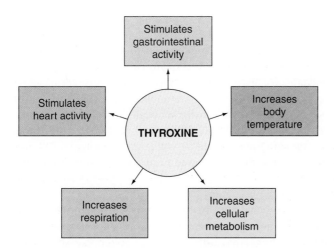

Figure 14–11
Effects of thyroxine.

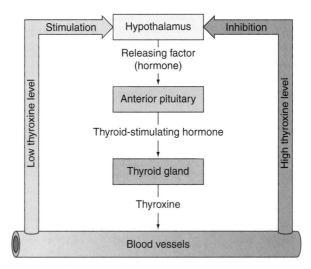

Figure 14–12
Control of thyroxine secretion (negative feedback mechanism).

The most common type of goiter is the diffuse colloidal goiter, or nontoxic goiter. The follicles of the thyroid gland normally contain colloid, a protein material. In this type of goiter, an excessive amount of colloid is secreted into the follicles, increasing the size of the gland. A diffuse colloidal goiter is also called an *endemic goiter* because it is common in a particular geographic region.

The usual cause of an endemic goiter is insufficient iodine in the diet. Inland areas, such as the Great Lakes region, and mountainous regions, like the Alps, have a very low iodine content in the soil and water. As a result, the inhabitants are unable to synthesize thyroxine adequately.

Normally, when the proper level of thyroxine is circulating, the anterior pituitary stops secreting thyroid-stimulating hormone. In the absence of thyroxine, there is nothing to inhibit the anterior pituitary. As a result, the continuous secretion of thyroid-stimulating hormone causes the thyroid gland to enlarge as a compensatory mechanism. The thyroid enlarges in an attempt to meet the demand of thyroid-stimulating hormone.

An enlargement of the neck is generally the only symptom (Figures 14–13 and 14–14). Usually enough thyroxine is produced to prevent the symptoms of hypothyroidism. The condition responds well to treatment with iodides, so the use of iodized salt prevents endemic goiter formation. If the goiter is very advanced, surgery may be necessary. A very large goiter puts pressure on the esophagus, causing difficulty in swallowing, or presses on the trachea, causing a cough or choking sensation.

Other factors can cause a simple diffuse colloidal goiter; for example, a defect in the thyroxine-synthesizing mechanism. A young girl entering adolescence may develop this type of goiter because of an increased need for thyroxine at this time.

Hyperthyroidism

Another type of goiter is the adenomatous or nodular goiter, named from adenoma, a glandular tumor. These nodules are secretory and produce an excessive amount of thyroxine, a condition of **hyperthyroidism.** Various goiters are shown in Figure 14–15.

The effects of thyroxine have been discussed, and an excessive amount of this hormone augments these effects. Hyperthyroidism causes nervousness and **tremors,** a shak-

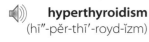
hyperthyroidism
(hī″-pĕr-thī′-royd-ĭzm)

tremors
(trĕm′-ŏrs)

side by side

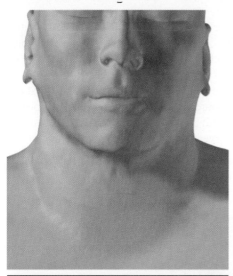

Figure 14–13

Normal anterior view of neck.

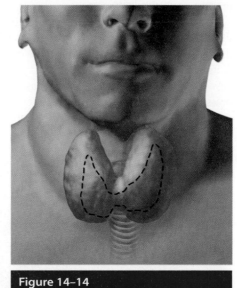

Figure 14–14

View of neck with goiter. Normal thyroid size is indicated by dashed line.

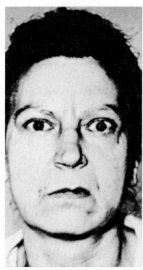

(a)

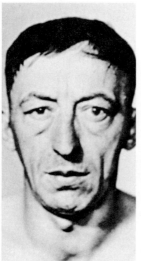

(b)

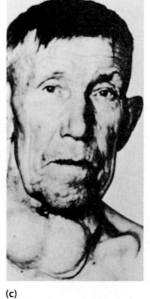

(c)

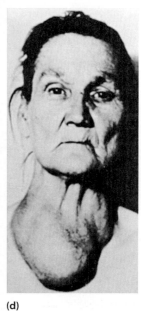

(d)

Figure 14–15
(a) A nontoxic, nodular goiter. (b) A 32-year-old man showing diffuse enlargement of the thyroid.
(c) An elderly man with a multinodular and cystic goiter. (d) A diffuse, multinodular colloid goiter.

iness, particularly in the hands. Metabolism increases, causing sweating and a rapid pulse. A nodule or adenoma may put pressure on the trachea or esophagus. Surgery is sometimes necessary to remove part of the thyroid gland, but medication is often effective in preventing further enlargement.

Graves' disease is another condition in which goiter develops. In this case, the entire gland hypertrophies, and there are no nodules. The person suffers from severe hyperthyroidism. Graves' disease is far more common in women than in men and usually affects young women.

A person with Graves' disease has a very characteristic appearance. The facial expression is strained and tense, and there is a stare in the eyes. The eyeballs protrude outward, a condition called **exophthalmos** (Figure 14–16). This is caused by edema in the tissue behind the eyes. The bulging of the eyes can be so severe that the eyelids do

exopthalmos
(ĕks″-ŏf-thăl′-mōs)

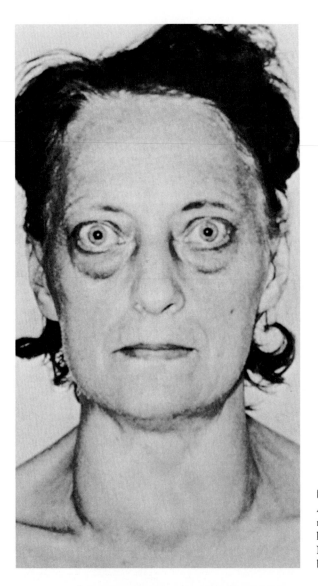

Figure 14–16
A Graves' disease patient with marked exophthalmos. The eyes have a fixed, staring expression. Note marked swelling of neck because of an enlarged thyroid.

not close, and the swelling sometimes damages the optic nerve. This symptom generally persists even when the hyperthyroidism is corrected.

The person has a tremendous appetite but loses weight to the point of appearing emaciated, as calories are burned up at a rapid rate. Thyroxine speeds the passage of food through the digestive tract. There is no time for the normal reabsorption of water from the large intestine, so diarrhea frequently accompanies the disease.

Tachycardia, rapid pulse rate, and palpitation are also among the symptoms. The person is extremely nervous, excitable, and is always tired but has difficulty sleeping because of the hyperactivity of the body. The high metabolic rate causes excessive heat production, which results in profuse perspiration. The skin is always moist, and an insatiable thirst follows the loss of water. The signs of Graves' disease are shown in Figure 14–17.

Graves' disease is an autoimmune condition in which antibodies to a thyroid antigen stimulate hyperactivity of the thyroid gland. This causes the thyroid to produce too much thyroxine.

Graves' disease can sometimes be treated with medication that inhibits the synthesis of thyroxine, or by administration of radioactive iodine, which destroys the thyroid gland. Removal of the thyroid gland, however, may be necessary. If the gland is removed, hormonal supplements must be given. Partial removal of the thyroid gland allows the remaining portion to secrete hormones.

Hypothyroidism

Myxedema is the condition of severe hypothyroidism, an inadequate level of thyroxine. The symptoms are just the opposite of those in Graves' disease. The person's face is bloated, the tongue is thick, and the eyelids are puffy. The skin is dry and scaly, and there is little perspiration. The person has no tolerance of a cold environment.

A person with myxedema experiences muscular weakness and somnolence, sleeping for 14 to 16 hours a day. The mental and physical processes are sluggish, the speech is slurred, and reflexes are slow. Heart rate is decreased, and the slowed circulation causes edema to develop. Lack of thyroxine increases the amount of circulating lipids, which leads to the development of atherosclerosis (Chapter 9). The digestive system works sluggishly, so the patient suffers from constipation. Weight gain also accompanies the disease.

myxedema
(mĭks″-ĕ-dē′-mă)

Exophthalmos

Profuse perspiration

Hand tremors

Enlarged thyroid

Severe weight loss

Nervousness and excitability

Rapid pulse

Insatiable thirst

Diarrhea

Rapid respiration

Insomnia

Figure 14–17
Signs of Graves' disease.

Myxedema affects women more than men, and usually affects women of middle age. It can result from radiation damage to the thyroid gland or develop after thyroid surgery if thyroxine is not administered. Myxedema can be a primary disease of the thyroid gland or secondary to pituitary disease. If the pituitary gland does not secrete thyroid-stimulating hormones, the thyroid gland ceases to function. Patients with myxedema are shown in Figure 14–18. Myxedema is treated by administering thyroxine. The condition generally responds well to treatment, and the symptoms disappear.

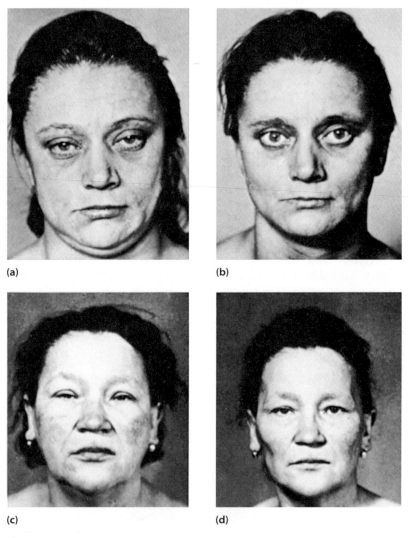

(a)　　　　　　　　　(b)

(c)　　　　　　　　　(d)

Figure 14–18
(a) A 29-year-old myxedema patient showing facial puffiness, muscle weakness, and drooping eyelids, which give a sleepy appearance. (b) The same patient after 2 months of thyroxine replacement. (c) A 62-year-old patient with myxedema exhibiting marked edema of the face and a somnolent look. The hair is stiff and without luster. (d) The same patient after 3 months of treatment with thyroxine.

Cretinism

Cretinism is a congenital thyroid deficiency in which thyroxine is not synthesized. Thyroxine is essential to both physical and mental development. Lack of this hormone in an infant or young child causes mental retardation and an abnormal, dwarfed stature. Cretinism can result from an error in fetal development if the thyroid gland fails to form or is nonfunctional. Cretinism sometimes occurs in areas of endemic goiter where the mother suffers from an inadequate iodine supply.

The cretin is a dwarf with a stocky stature and a characteristically protruding abdomen. The sexual organs do not develop, and the face of the cretin is typically misshapen: a broad, sunken nose, small eyes set far apart, puffy eyelids, and a short forehead. A thick tongue protrudes from a wide-open mouth, and the face is expressionless. Figure 14–19 shows an example of a cretin.

The earlier this condition is diagnosed and treated with thyroxine, the more optimistic is the prognosis. Lifelong hormonal therapy will be required. An untreated 14-year-old patient is shown in Figure 14–20.

Even less severe cases of hypothyroidism should be treated in infants. A baby may appear normal at first and only later give indications that the developmental processes are retarded. The baby may be slow in smiling, reaching, sitting, and standing. Newborns are routinely tested for hypothyroidism within two days of birth. Figure 14–21 shows the effectiveness of thyroxine replacement therapy.

cretinism
(krē′-tĭn-ĭzm)

➤ STRUCTURE AND FUNCTION OF THE ADRENAL GLANDS

The adrenal glands are located at the top of each kidney. Each of the glands consists of two distinct parts: an outer part (the cortex) and an inner section (the medulla). The cortex and the medulla secrete different hormones. The adrenal cortex is stimulated by ACTH, adrenocorticotropic hormone, from the anterior pituitary gland. The adrenal glands are shown in Figure 14–22.

The adrenal cortex secretes many steroid hormones, which can be classified into three groups. One group, the **mineralocorticoids,** regulates salt balance. The principal hormone of this group is **aldosterone.** Aldosterone causes sodium retention and potassium secretion by the kidneys. Another group, the **glucocorticoids,** helps regulate carbohydrate, lipid, and protein metabolism. The principal hormone of this group is **cortisol**

mineralocorticoids
(mĭn″-ĕr-ăl-ō-kŏr′-tĭ-koyds)

aldosterone
(ăl-dŏs′-tĕr-ōn)

glucocorticoids
(glū″-kō-kŏrt′-ĭ-koydz)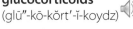

cortisol
(kŏr′-tĭ-sōl)

on the Practical Side

Muscle-Building Steroids

Anabolic steroids (muscle-building steroids) were used initially by athletes to increase strength and endurance during athletic competition. Anabolic steroids are closely related to the male hormone, testosterone, and did indeed build muscle. However, it was found that these steroids had serious side effects including kidney damage, increased risk of heart disease, and the development of liver cancer. Increased irritability and aggressive behavior developed, and in women, the growth of facial hair and deepening of the voice increased. Males were affected by diminished hormone secretion and sperm production. The use of anabolic steroids by athletes is now banned and, if they are found to be present, the athlete is severely punished.

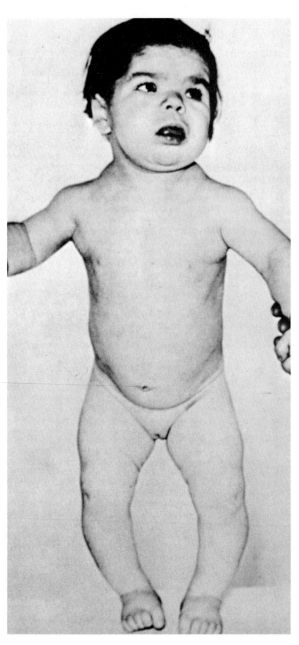

Figure 14–19
A 4-year-old child with congenital hypothyroidism. Note stunted growth (32 inches) and typical facial features: broad, flat nose; open mouth; and protruding tongue. The child cannot stand unsupported or speak.

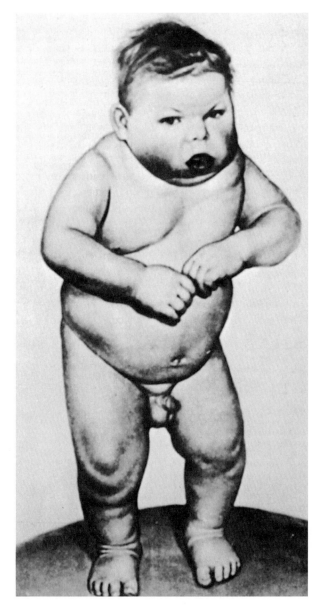

Figure 14–20
A 14-year-old untreated patient with severe, congenital hypothyroidism. The face is greatly swollen, the neck is obscured by fat, and the abdomen protrudes because of lack of muscle tone. The patient has difficulty in standing and walking.

androgens
(an'-drō-jĕns)

estrogen
(ĕs'-trō-jĕn)

epinephrine
(ĕp"-ĭ-nĕf'-rĭn)

or hydrocortisone. The third group of hormones are sex hormones: **androgens,** the male hormones, and **estrogen,** the female hormone.

The adrenal medulla secretes **epinephrine** and norepinephrine. These hormones are secreted in stress situations when additional energy and strength are needed. Epinephrine causes vasodilatation and increases heart rate, blood pressure, and respira-

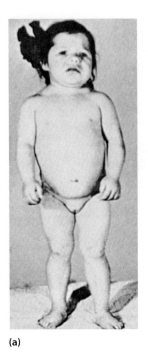
(a)

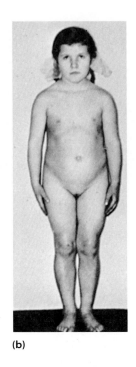
(b)

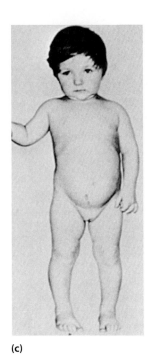
(c)

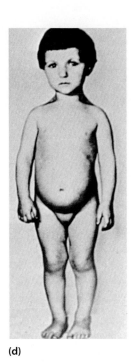
(d)

Figure 14–21
(a) A 6-year-old child with congenital hypothyroidism, exhibiting marked mental and physical retardation. (b) The same patient after 3 years of thyroxine therapy, which resulted in a spurt of growth and regression of pathological manifestations. Mental development is delayed. (c) A 5-year-old patient with congenital hypothyroidism. Mental and physical development are delayed. (d) The same patient after 3 months of thyroxine treatment. The child began to grow, lost weight, and became more alert.

tion. Norepinephrine brings about general vasoconstriction. Together epinephrine and norepinephrine help shunt blood to vital organs when required.

Hyperactivity of the adrenal cortex is usually caused by hyperplasia (enlargement of the glands), a tumor. Hyperactivity may also result from overstimulation by the anterior pituitary gland.

Hypoactivity of the adrenal cortex sometimes results from a destructive disease, such as tuberculosis. Some steroid hormones can cause the adrenal glands to atrophy by interfering with the normal control mechanism for corticosteroid release.

➤ DISEASES OF THE ADRENAL CORTEX

Hyperadrenalism

Overactivity of the adrenal cortex (hyperadrenalism) can take different forms depending on which group of hormones are secreted in excess. **Cushing's syndrome** develops from an excess of glucocorticoid hormones, the hormones that raise the blood sugar level. In excess, they cause **hyperglycemia.** Elevation of blood glucose caused by hypersecretion by the adrenal cortex is called adrenal diabetes. Glucocorticoids mobilize lipids, increasing their level in the blood. A characteristic obesity develops that is confined to the trunk of the body. A fat pad forms behind the shoulders and is referred to as a buffalo hump, but the arms and legs remain normal. The face is round and described as moon-shaped.

Cushing's syndrome
(koosh'-ĭngz sĭn'-drom)

hyperglycemia
(hī"-pĕr-glī-sē'-me-ă)

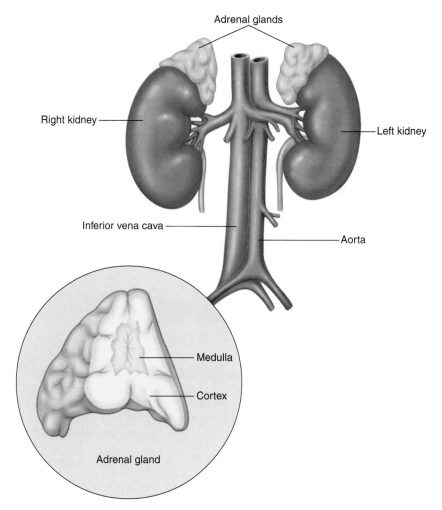

Figure 14–22
The adrenal glands.

The person with Cushing's syndrome retains salt and water, resulting in hypertension, and atherosclerosis develops as a result of excess circulating lipid. Muscular weakness and fatigue accompany the disease, and the person finds it difficult even to climb stairs. The skin is thin and tends to bruise easily. Red striae (stretch marks) develop on the abdomen, buttocks, and breasts as a result of a loss of elastic tissue and fat accumulation. Figure 14–23 shows a patient with Cushing's syndrome. Wounds heal poorly, and the patient is very susceptible to infection. Bones, particularly the vertebrae and ribs, are likely to fracture. These symptoms result from a decrease in protein synthesis. Surgical removal of the enlarged glands or tumor can correct the condition. Hormonal therapy is then required to replace the hormones normally secreted by the adrenal cortex.

Conn's syndrome is another form of hyperadrenalism. In this disease, aldosterone is secreted in excess. This causes retention of sodium and water, and abnormal loss of potassium in the urine. Hypertension develops as a result of the salt imbalance and water retention. Muscles become weak to the point of paralysis. The person has an excessive thirst (polydipsia) caused by the salt retention, and polyuria follows the great intake

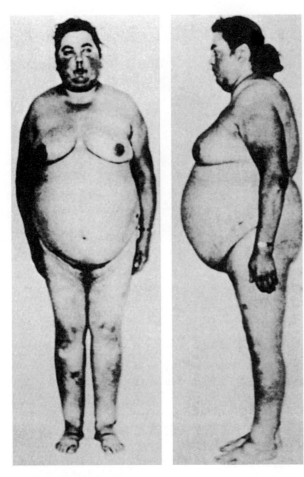

Figure 14–23
Cushing's syndrome patient showing round, red face; stocky
neck; and marked obesity of the trunk with protruding
abdomen. Note bruises on trunk and legs and also stretch
marks. Note fat pads above the collarbone and on the back of
the neck, which produce the "buffalo hump."

of water. Conn's syndrome is usually caused by a tumor that can be removed surgically,
and the prognosis is usually good.

Adrenogenital syndrome is another form of hyperadrenalism, also called *adrenal
virilism*. In this case, androgens, male hormones, are secreted in excess. If this occurs
in children, it stimulates premature sexual development. Sex organs of a male child
greatly enlarge. In a girl, the clitoris enlarges, a male distribution of hair develops, and
the voice deepens. This condition is seen in Figure 14–24.

This excessive production of androgens is usually caused by a block in the synthesis of cortisol from cholesterol or from other corticosteroids. Cortisone is generally
inactive until it is converted to cortisol. Cortisone is prepared synthetically from animal
and plant tissue. Inasmuch as steroids cannot be converted to cortisol, because of the
blockage in the pathway, they are converted to androgens. Cortisol treatment can prevent this overproduction.

Excessive androgen secretion in a woman causes masculinization (adrenal virilism).
Hair develops on the face, a condition called **hirsutism,** and the hairline recedes. The

**androgenital
syndrome**
(ăn″-drō-jĕn′-ĭ-tăl
sĭn′-drōm)

hirsutism
(hŭr′-sūt-ĭzm)

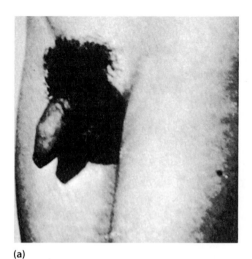
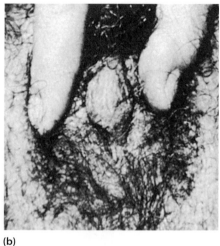

(a)   (b)

Figure 14–24
(a) Genitalia of a 6-year-old boy with adrenogenital syndrome, showing precocious sexual development. The penis is enlarged, but the testes remain small. **(b)** Genitals of an 18-year-old woman with adrenogenital syndrome. The enlarged clitoris resembles a penis, and growth of pubic hair is excessive.

breasts diminish in size, the clitoris enlarges, and ovulation and menstruation cease. In an adult, the cause is usually an androgen-secreting tumor of the glands. Adrenal virilism is shown in Figure 14–25.

➤ DISEASES OF THE ADRENAL MEDULLA

Pheochromocytoma
Pheochromocytoma is a rare tumor of the adrenal medulla that causes overproduction of epinephrine and norepinephrine. This condition is rare and occurs equally in men and women, most commonly between the ages of 30 and 60. Symptoms of palpitations, increased blood pressure, rapid heart rate, chest pain, and weight loss may appear suddenly and sporadically. The best treatment is to remove the tumor. Medications are also used before surgery to control symptoms caused by excessive epinephrine and norepinephrine.

Hypoadrenalism
Addison's disease results when the adrenal glands fail to produce corticosteroids—aldosterone and cortisol. The adrenal glands may be destroyed by cancer, infections, or inhibited by chronic use of steroid hormones, such as *prednisone*. Many cases are called idiopathic, where Addison's disease results from unknown causes.

Aldosterone deficiency renders the patient unable to retain salt and water. The kidneys are unable to concentrate urine and, eventually, dehydration ensues. Severe dehydration can ultimately lead to shock. Cortisol deficiency leads to low blood sugar, impaired protein and carbohydrate metabolism, and generalized weakness.

The pituitary gland produces more corticotropin in response to a deficiency of corticosteroids. Corticotrophin normally stimulates the adrenal gland and production of a skin-darkening pigment called melanin. Persons with Addison's disease develop a peculiar yellow-brown discoloration. Normally pigmented areas such as the areola surrounding the nipples and parts of the genitals become even darker. Areas of the body such as the palms and elbows also darken, and pigment develops in scars.

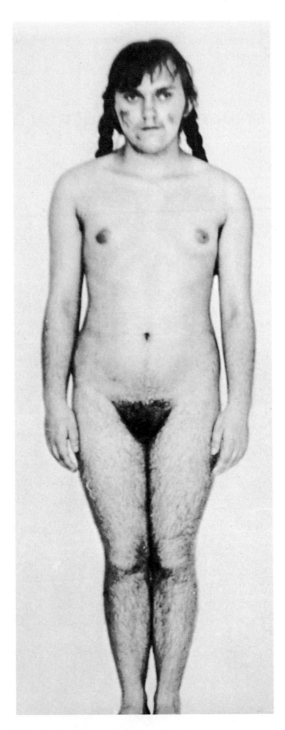

Figure 14–25
A 15-year-old girl with congenital adrenogenital
syndrome. Note typical masculine build of broad
shoulders and narrow hips. Breast development is poor,
and excessive hair has developed on the face, abdomen,
and legs.

Addison's disease can be life-threatening and must be treated with corticosteroid replacement. Injectable cortisol treatment is used initially to treat severe cases. Oral cortisol treatment is required for life. Medication to restore normal excretion of salt and water is also administered.

➤ STRUCTURE AND FUNCTION OF THE PARATHYROIDS

Structure of the Parathyroids

The parathyroids are four tiny glands located on the posterior side of the thyroid gland (Figure 14–26). Before the function of the parathyroid glands was understood, they were sometimes removed with a thyroidectomy. The hormone secreted by the parathyroids is **parathormone,** also called parathyroid hormone.

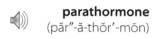

parathormone
(păr″-ă-thŏr′-mōn)

Function of the Parathyroids

The parathyroid glands are extremely important in regulating the level of circulating calcium and phosphate. Ninety-nine percent of the body's calcium is in bone, but the remaining 1 percent has many important functions. Calcium is essential to the blood-clotting mechanism. It increases the tone of heart muscle and plays a significant role in muscle contraction.

Bone is not inert, but rather there is a constant exchange of calcium and phosphate between bone and the blood. Two kinds of cells are at work within bone: **osteoblasts** (which form bone tissue) and **osteoclasts** (which resorb salts out of bone, dissolving it). These salts are then released into the blood. The balance between these two processes, osteoblastic and osteoclastic, is governed by the parathyroid hormone.

osteoblasts
(ŏs′-tē-ō-blăsts)

osteoclasts
(ŏs′-tē-ō-klăsts)

When the calcium level falls, parathormone is secreted. The hormone acts at three distinct sites to raise the level of calcium to normal. Parathormone increases the amount of calcium that is absorbed out of the digestive tract by interaction with ingested vitamin D. It prevents a loss of calcium through the kidneys and releases calcium from bones by stimulating osteoclastic activity. When the proper level of circulating calcium is restored, parathormone is no longer released. An excess or a deficiency of calcium can

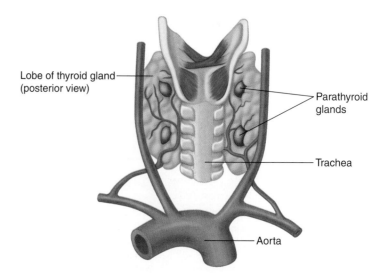

Lobe of thyroid gland (posterior view)

Parathyroid glands

Trachea

Aorta

Figure 14–26
Parathyroid glands.

have disastrous results. These conditions are usually the result of hyperactivity or hypoactivity of the parathyroid glands.

➤ DISEASES OF THE PARATHYROID GLAND

Hyperparathyroidism

An overactive parathyroid gland secretes too much parathormone (**hyperparathyroidism**). Excessive parathormone raises the level of circulating calcium above normal, the condition called **hypercalcemia.** Much of the calcium comes from bone resorption mediated by parathormone. As the calcium level rises, the phosphate level falls.

With the loss of calcium, the bones are weakened. They tend to bend, become deformed, and fracture spontaneously. Giant cell tumors and cysts of the bone sometimes develop. Excessive calcium causes formation of kidney stones because calcium forms insoluble compounds. Calcium deposited within the walls of the blood vessels makes them hard. It may also be found in the stomach and lungs. Effects of hyperparathyroidism are illustrated in Figure 14–27.

Hyperparathyroidism, with its concurrent excess of calcium, causes generalized symptoms. There may be pain in the bones that is sometimes confused with arthritis. The nervous system is depressed, and muscles lose their tone and weaken. Heart muscle is affected and the pulse slows. Gastrointestinal disturbances, abdominal pain, vomiting, and constipation develop. These symptoms result from deposits of calcium in the mucosa of the gastrointestinal tract. Deposits of calcium sometimes form in the eye, causing irritation and excessive tearing. Hyperparathyoidism usually results from a tumor. If the tumor is removed, parathormone secretion returns to normal, and the level of circulating calcium is again properly controlled.

Hyperparathyroidism can develop from other conditions that reduce the level of circulating calcium. Any decrease in calcium stimulates the parathyroid glands to hypertrophy and to increase their rate of secretion. During pregnancy and lactation, the mother's supply of calcium is reduced. This reduction will stimulate the parathyroid glands to secrete parathormone.

Hypoparathyroidism

The principal manifestation of hypoparathyroidism is **tetany,** a sustained muscular contraction. In hypoparathyroidism, the muscles of the hands and feet contract in a characteristic fashion. The typical tetanic contraction of the hand is seen in Figure 14–28.

hyperparathyroidism
(hī″-pĕr-păr″-ă-thī′-roy-dĭzm)

hypercalcemia
(hī″-pĕr-kăl-sē′-mē-ă)

tetany
(tĕt′-ă-nē)

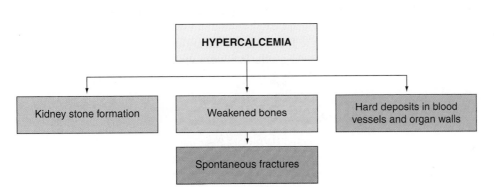

Figure 14-27
Complications of hyperparathyroidism—hypercalcemia.

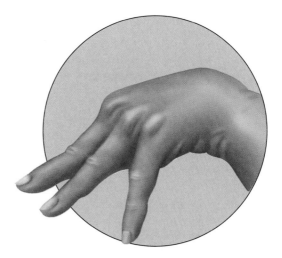

Figure 14–28
Tetany of the hand in hypoparathyroidism.

Laryngeal muscles are very susceptible to these spasms, which can obstruct the respiratory tract, and death may follow.

The low level of calcium in the blood, hypocalcemia, makes the nervous system hyperexcitable. As the nerves discharge spontaneously, the skeletal muscles are overstimulated. Administration of calcium and vitamin D, which assists in the absorption of calcium from the gastrointestinal tract, will correct the condition.

➤ ENDOCRINE FUNCTION OF THE PANCREAS

The structure of the pancreas and its role as an exocrine gland were described in Chapter 12. The pancreas has another critical function: the control of glucose level in the blood. This is accomplished through the secretion of two hormones, insulin and glucagon.

Insulin is secreted by certain cells of the pancreas called beta cells, located in patches of tissue named the islands of Langerhans or pancreatic islets. Glucagon is secreted by the alpha cells of the islets. This arrangement is illustrated in Figure 14–29. These hormones work antagonistically to each other. Insulin lowers the level of blood glucose and glucagon elevates it. The combined effect of these hormones maintains the normal level of blood glucose.

Insulin is secreted when the blood glucose level rises. Through a complex mechanism, not completely understood, insulin facilitates the entry of glucose into the cells

 PREVENTION *PLUS!*

Nearly three-fourths of adults with diabetes lack basic information about their disease—information that can help control their disease. Studies have shown that better control of diabetes improves overall diabetes management and helps prevent complications that may develop over time.

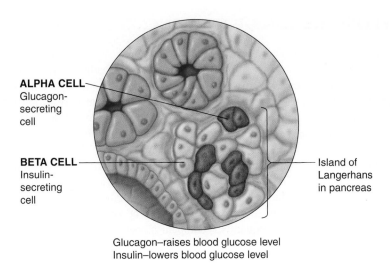

Figure 14–29
Islands of Langerhans.

where it is primarily stored as glycogen and metabolized for energy. Glucose enters primarily skeletal muscle cells and fat cells.

As glucose enters cells and is converted to glycogen by the liver, the level of blood glucose falls. The normal level of glucose in the blood is about 90 mg/100 ml (or 90 mg/dl) of blood. This is also expressed as 90 mg percent.

When the level of blood glucose falls below normal, glucagon is released. Glucagon circulates to the liver and stimulates the release of glucose from its stored form, glycogen. This raises the level of blood glucose to normal. The control of glucose is illustrated in Figure 14–30.

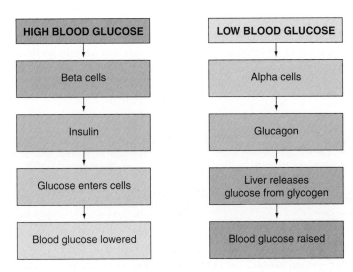

Figure 14–30
Control of blood glucose level.

➤ HYPOSECRETION OF THE PANCREAS

Diabetes Mellitus (Hyperglycemia)

diabetes mellitus
(dī″-ă-bē′-tēz
mě-lī′-tŭs)

Diabetes mellitus is an endocrine disease in which the beta cells fail to secrete insulin or target cells fail to respond to insulin. In the absence of insulin, glucose cannot enter the cells. The glucose level in the blood increases greatly, resulting in hyperglycemia. A diabetic's sugar level can range from 300 to 1200 mg/dl of blood and even higher. The cells are deprived of their principal nutrient, glucose, for the production of energy.

Insulin dependent diabetes mellitus (IDDM) or Type I diabetes most commonly occurs before the age of 30. This is the most serious form where the patient requires multiple injections of insulin daily. Non-insulin dependent diabetes mellitus (NIDDM) or Type II diabetes usually occurs after the age of 45 and becomes more common with advancing age. Type II diabetes frequently accompanies obesity and can often be controlled by weight loss, diet, and exercise.

Development of Type I and Type II diabetes may have a genetic basis. Other less common causes of diabetes are abnormally high levels of corticosteroids, pregnancy or gestational diabetes, and drugs that interfere with production or utilization of insulin.

Symptoms of Diabetes Mellitus One of the principal symptoms of diabetes mellitus is excessive urination, or polyuria (Table 14-1). This is caused by the great amount of glucose that filters into the kidney tubule and the volume of water required to carry it away. The glucose acts as a diuretic. Normally, glucose that enters the kidney tubules is reabsorbed and does not appear in the urine. In diabetes, however, the amount of glucose that the kidney tubules can reabsorb, the tubular maximum, is surpassed. The excess glucose is excreted in the urine, a condition called **glycosuria.** Glycosuria is a major sign of diabetes mellitus.

glycosuria
(glī″-kō-sū′-rē-ă)

The great loss of water with the glucose could result in dehydration, but the diabetic has an excessive thirst, polydipsia. By drinking large amounts of water, the diabetic compensates for the fluid loss. An unusual thirst is also one of the symptoms of diabetes.

Cells prefer to metabolize glucose, but in its absence, cells metabolize fats first and proteins last. This is known as the "protein-sparing effect." Because glucose cannot enter the cells without the action of insulin, the diabetic metabolizes a large amount of fat. Fat metabolism produces a large number of fatty acids and **ketone bodies,** acetone, and related substances. The presence of ketone bodies in the urine is another sign of diabetes mellitus.

ketone bodies
(kē′-tōn bŏd′-ēz)

TABLE 14–1. WARNING SIGNS OF DIABETES

TYPE I OR INSULIN-DEPENDENT DIABETES MELLITUS	TYPE II OR NON-INSULIN DEPENDENT DIABETES MELLITUS
• Frequent urination • Excessive thirst • Extreme hunger • Weight loss • Fatigue • Irritability	• Any of the Type I symptoms • Frequent infections • Recurring skin, gum, or bladder infections • Blurred vision • Cuts and bruises that heal slowly • Numbness or tingling sensations in the hands or feet

From the American Diabetes Association.

The production of acids lowers the body's pH, and the condition of **acidosis** results. This is one of the most serious consequences of diabetes. The normal pH range is 7.35 to 7.45. If the pH drops below 6.9 to 7.0, the person goes into a coma and will die if not treated.

Another sign of diabetes mellitus is weight loss, although the diabetic's appetite is good. The patient tires easily and lacks energy. In the absence of glucose to metabolize, the diabetic uses the body's tissue fat and protein, as well as that in the diet, which explains the loss of weight. There is an increased breakdown of tissue protein and a decrease in protein synthesis that results in poor wound healing. Susceptibility to infection also accompanies diabetes.

Complications of Diabetes Mellitus   Lipid is mobilized from fat tissue, and the level of blood lipid, particularly cholesterol, increases. Much of this lipid is deposited within the walls of the blood vessels, causing atherosclerosis. This is one of the greatest dangers in long-term uncontrolled diabetes because blood vessels tend to become occluded. Blockage of a coronary artery causes a myocardial infarction, as explained in Chapter 8. Thromboembolic strokes are also frequent complications of untreated diabetes. Occlusion of a leg artery can result in gangrene. Atherosclerosis generally causes poor circulation, which is another reason for poor wound healing.

Another complication of diabetes is diabetic retinopathy, a vascular disorder of the retina that can result in blindness. The minute retinal blood vessels become sclerotic and rupture. The nervous system is affected by poor circulation, as manifested by pain, tingling sensations, loss of feeling, and paralysis. The kidneys are usually affected by long-standing diabetes, and kidney failure is frequently the cause of death in the diabetic. The complications of diabetes are summarized in Figure 14–31.

Treatment of Diabetes Mellitus   Important factors in treating diabetes are weight loss, diet, and exercise. The insulin dosage prescribed accompanies a carefully regulated diet. The diet cannot be altered without creating an insulin excess or deficiency. A person who exercises actively requires less insulin than one who does not. A diabetic's exercise pattern is a factor in prescribing insulin.

Regulation of the proper insulin dosage takes time. Certain factors—illness or emotional stress—can temporarily alter a patient's needs. There are different types of insulin (fast-, intermediate-, and slow-acting), which are effective over various time periods. These are often prescribed in combination. Monitoring blood sugar levels is an essential part of diabetes care. Self-monitoring of blood glucose enables the diabetic to determine his or her blood glucose and adjust insulin dosage according to a measured reading. The test involves taking a small sample of blood from a finger prick and checking it with a portable glucose-monitoring device.

Insulin must be given by injection because it is a protein and would be digested in the gastrointestinal tract. There are oral compounds that can be used for some Type II diabetes, but they are not insulin. These are oral hypoglycemic agents, which stimulate secretion of insulin from beta cells that still have some capacity or make cells more responsive to insulin. These are oral hypoglycemic agents, which stimulate secretion of insulin from the beta cells and make cells in the body more sensitive to insulin. There are several choices of injectors and needle sizes that are easy to use. The automatic insulin pump administers a measured dose of insulin into the body via a tube with its tip embedded under the skin.

Diabetic Coma and Insulin Shock   Diabetic coma develops when a person with severe diabetes fails to take enough insulin or deviates markedly from a prescribed diet.

acidosis
(ăs″-ĭ-do′-sĭs)

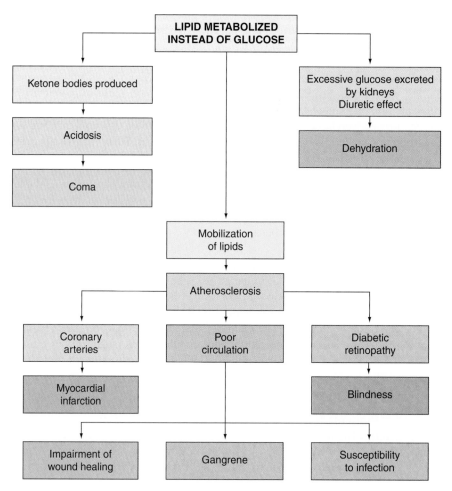

Figure 14–31
Complications of diabetes mellitus.

Acidosis and dehydration result, and death can follow if proper treatment is not given immediately. One symptom of diabetic coma is deep, labored breathing, which results from the effect of the acidosis on the respiratory center of the brain. The person's breath has a fruity, acetone smell. The skin is flushed and dry, and the tongue is dry because of the dehydration. A diabetic coma may have a gradual onset, during which time the patient is drowsy and lethargic. If urine and blood samples are taken, a high level of sugar is found.

Treatment of diabetic coma (diabetic ketoacidosis) requires urgent replacement of fluids intravenously to correct the dehydration. Insulin, usually given intravenously, is necessary as well. Because diabetic coma adversely affects sodium and potassium, the serum electrolytes must be checked frequently as therapy proceeds.

Insulin shock, also called hypoglycemic shock, results from too much insulin, not enough food, or excessive exercise. The person feels light-headed and faint, trembles, and begins to perspire. Taking sugar in some form, candy or orange juice for example, may be adequate treatment at this stage. If the glucose level is not raised, the condition becomes more serious. The person's speech becomes thick and walking becomes unsteady because the low level of glucose affects the brain. Double vision may be experienced, and loss of consciousness may follow.

If the person becomes comatose, it is difficult for the untrained to determine if the cause is a diabetic coma or insulin shock. A significant difference is that the deep, rapid breathing and acetone breath characteristic of diabetic coma are not present in insulin shock. The person in insulin shock breathes shallowly. Intravenous injections of glucose must be given immediately for insulin shock. The administration of epinephrine also raises the blood sugar level. Figure 14–32 illustrates the differences between diabetic coma and insulin shock.

Tests for Diabetes Mellitus   A simple urine test can show the presence or absence of glucose or ketones in the urine. Urine tests are helpful for initial screening and for those who are prone to ketoacidosis. Fasting blood sugar level, glucose tolerance testing, and glycosylated hemoglobin tests are used to monitor and diagnose diabetes. The fasting blood sugar level helps diagnose and monitor diabetes. A sample of blood is taken after the person has fasted for eight hours. The glucose tolerance test challenges the body's ability to secrete and use insulin. The test is performed after a 10-hour fast. The patient drinks a standard glucose solution, and blood and urine samples are taken and analyzed for the next three hours. No glucose should appear in the urine, and the blood glucose level should not exceed 170 mg/dl of blood if insulin is being produced and utilized. Glycosylated hemoglobin determination is a simple blood test that is used to monitor long-term control of diabetes. It generally indicates the average blood sugar over the past 90 days. Normal values should be below 6, and ideal levels for diabetics should be less than 7.

Education of the Diabetic Patient   The American Diabetes Association, physicians, nurses, and dieticians have made a great effort to assist the diabetic patient in leading a normal life. The diabetic who understands the disease knows the importance of weight control, diet, exercise, and either insulin or oral agents for leading a normal life. A safety precaution advised by the American Diabetes Association is that anyone who takes insulin should carry an identification card explaining the emergency treatment required if an insulin reaction occurs.

➤ ABNORMALITIES IN SECRETION OF SEX HORMONES

The gonads (ovaries and testes) are endocrine glands as well as the source of the ova and sperm (Chapter 15). They secrete the hormones estrogen and testosterone directly into the blood.

DIABETIC COMA	INSULIN SHOCK
Deep, labored breathing due to acidosis	Shallow breathing
Skin and tongue dry due to dehydration	Patient perspires
Fruity, acetone smell to breath	Odor of breath normal
Patient drowsy and lethargic before onset	Patient feels light-headed and faint before onset
Comatose	Comatose
Requires large dose of insulin	Requires glucose intravenously
Fluid and salts needed	

Figure 14–32
Differences between diabetic coma and insulin shock.

Hypergonadism (Hypersecretion)

Abnormally increased functional activity of the gonads before puberty produces precocious sexual development in both sexes. In a male child, excessive production of testosterone may be caused by a tumor in the testes. This causes rapid growth of musculature and bones but premature uniting of the epiphyses and shaft of long bones. Normal height, therefore, is not attained. Hypersecretion of ovarian hormones in the female is rare because of the negative feedback mechanism with gonadotropic hormones.

Hypogonadism in the Male   Several factors can cause hypogonadism, that is, the decreased functional activity of the gonads. A person may be born without functional testes, the testes may fail to descend and thus atrophy, or the testes may be lost through castration. Testes fail to develop because of a lack of gonadotropic hormones.

Loss of the male gonads before puberty causes the condition of eunuchism, in which sexual characteristics do not develop. Development of male traits depends on testosterone secretion by the testes. Castration after puberty causes some regression of secondary sexual characteristics, but masculinity is retained. Hormonal therapy, the administration of testosterone, can be effective.

Hypogonadism in the Female   Hyposecretion of hormones by the ovaries may be caused by poorly formed or missing ovaries. When ovaries are absent or fail to develop, female eunuchism results. Secondary sexual characteristics do not develop. A characteristic of this condition is excessive growth of long bones because the epiphyses do not seal with the shaft of the bone as normally occurs at adolescence.

➤ DIAGNOSTIC PROCEDURES FOR ENDOCRINE DISEASES

Indications of pituitary hyperactivity or hypoactivity can be confirmed by serum assays (tests). Growth hormone (GH) level can detect hyperpituitarism (gigantism and/or acromegaly) and hypopituitarism (dwarfism). Thyroid-stimulating hormone (TSH) assay is useful in confirming primary hypothyroidism or hyperthyroidism. Activity of the posterior pituitary can be evaluated by the water deprivation and vasopressin injection test. A urine specimen is taken after controlled water deprivation, and a blood sample is drawn. Dilute urine and high osmotic pressure in the blood indicates that water is not being absorbed by the kidney tubules. If vasopressin injection corrects the massive polyuria, diabetes insipidus is confirmed.

Diseases of the thyroid gland are diagnosed on the basis of the T_3 and T_4 tests previously described, and by the serum level of thyroid-stimulating hormone. An elevated TSH indicates low T_4 function. A low TSH indicates an excess of T_4, which may be caused by a functioning adenoma or carcinoma. A thyroid scan provides visualization of the thyroid gland after administration of radioactive iodine. It is usually recommended after discovery of a mass, an enlarged gland, or an asymmetric goiter. Thyroid ultrasonography evaluates characteristics of thyroid nodules and distinguishes between solid or cystic masses in the gland.

Diagnostic tests for parathyroid gland activity measure parathyroid hormone and calcium levels in the blood and can detect hyperparathyroidism.

Adrenal gland activity can be evaluated by the level of plasma cortisol from the adrenal cortex. Abnormal levels indicate hyperfunction (Cushing's syndrome) or hypofunction (Addison's disease). Urine tests measure steroid level and detect hyperactivity of the gland.

A fasting blood glucose test helps detect diabetes mellitus and evaluate the clinical status of diabetic patients. An oral glucose tolerance test, previously described, challenges the ability of the pancreas to secrete insulin in response to large doses of glucose.

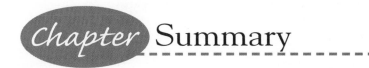

Chapter Summary

The endocrine system provides a means of chemical communication between body parts. The tiny anterior pituitary gland controls activities of the thyroid, adrenals, and sex glands. It also stimulates growth, development, and tissue repair. The pituitary is called the "master gland" for these reasons. Pituitary activity is governed by the hypothalamus of the brain.

Hyperpituitarism causes an excess of growth hormone. This condition, if present before puberty results in gigantism. In an adult, excessive production of growth hormone leads to abnormal enlargement of facial bones, bones of hands and feet, and soft tissue. This growth in an adult is called acromegaly.

Severe hypopituitarism impedes growth and development in a child, causing the child to be dwarfed in stature. Glands dependent on stimulation by the anterior pituitary—the thyroid, adrenals, and sex glands—cease functioning in hypopituitarism at any age. The posterior pituitary gland secretes vasopressin, also called antidiuretic hormone, and oxytocin. Hypoactivity of this gland causes diabetes insipidus.

The rate of metabolism is controlled by the thyroid gland. An enlargement of this gland is a goiter. Hyperthyroidism, an excess of thyroxine, accelerates heart and respiratory activity, increases metabolic rate, and raises body temperature. Graves' disease is an example of severe hyperthyroidism. A congenital lack of thyroxine results in cretinism, a condition of mental and physical retardation. Myxedema is a disease of severe hypothyroidism in an adult.

Hormones of the adrenal cortex are essential to life. Aldosterone regulates salt balance and cortisol affects the metabolism of nutrients. The sex hormones estrogen and androgen are also produced by this gland. Hypoactivity of the adrenal cortex is called Addison's disease.

Hyperactivity of the adrenal cortex causes different diseases, depending on which hormones are in excess. Cushing's syndrome results from an excess of cortisol, and Conn's syndrome results from excessive aldosterone. Precocious puberty and adrenal virilism develop from too much androgen secretion.

The parathyroid hormone, parathormone, regulates the level of circulating calcium and phosphate. Hyperactivity of the parathyroids causes hypercalcemia. The high level of calcium is primarily from bone resorption that weakens the bones. Hypoparathyroidism reduces the level of calcium in the blood. This causes the nervous system to become hyperexcitable, skeletal muscles are overstimulated, and tetany results. Hormones of the pancreas, insulin and glucagon, control blood sugar level. Lack of insulin causes an increase in blood glucose, the condition of diabetes mellitus.

Hypoglycemia, abnormally low blood glucose, results from insulin excess. This condition can develop in the diabetic from an overdosage of insulin. A tumor of the insulin-producing cells of the pancreas can also cause hypoglycemia. The absence of glucocorticoids in an Addison's disease patient results in low blood glucose.

Categories	* Disease ❑ Condition	Signs and Symptoms
Pituitary disease	* Hyperpituitarism, GH excess in child	Gigantism as bone length increases rapidly, slow sexual development
	* Acromegaly, GH excess in adult	Enlargement of hands, feet, face as bones grow in diameter, soft tissue growth; nose, lips, lower jaw protrude, tongue and skin thicken
	* GH lack in child	Pituitary dwarf; normal mentality, slow growth, sexual development lacking
	* Panhypopituitarism	Lack of TSH, ACTH, FSH, LH leads to lack of gland activity; mental dullness, lethargy, salt imbalance, abnormal nutrient metabolism, lack of sexual function
	* Diabetes insipidus	Polyuria, polydipsia
Parathyroid glands	* Hyperparathyroidism	Weakened bones, deform and fracture easily, kidney stones form, pain in bones, depressed nervous system, weak muscles, slow heart rate, abdominal pain, vomiting, constipation
	* Hypoparathyroidism	Muscular and nervous systems overexcitable, typical pattern of tetanic contractions in hands, laryngeal spasm
Thyroid disease	❑ Goiter	Enlargement of thyroid gland; accompanies overactivity, underactivity, or normal activity
	* Endemic goiter, nontoxic goiter, diffuse colloidal goiter	Enlargement of neck, may cause difficulty swallowing, cough, choking sensation, lower level thyroxine production
	* Hyperthyroidism, adenomatous or nodular goiter and Grave's disease	Exophthalmos, increased nervous activity, tremor, high metabolic rate, sweating and thirst, rapid pulse, increased appetite and weight loss, diarrhea, difficulty sleeping
	* Hypothyroidism in adult, myxedema	Edema, weight gain, dry skin, little sweat, low body temperature, muscular weakness, somnolence, slow heart rate, atherosclerosis, constipation
	❑ Hypothyroidism in infants, congenital cretinism	Mental retardation, dwarf growth, weak muscles, protruding abdomen, no sexual development, characteristic face—protruding tongue, broad nose, short forehead, small wide-set eyes, expressionless

Affected Organ/Body Region	Diagnostic Procedure	Treatment
Bones	Serum assay for GH	None
Bones, skin connective tissues, muscle	Serum assay for GH	None
Bones	Serum assay for GH	GH injections
Thyroids, adrenals, ovaries, testes	Serum assay for GH, TSH, thyroxine, cortisol	Thyroid hormone, cortisol, GH, sex hormones
Kidneys	Urinalysis in water deprivation/vasopressin injection test	Administer ADH
Bones, calcium level in blood, muscles, nerves	High serum calcium, patient history, kidney stones	Surgery, medication to lower calcium
Calcium level in blood, muscles, nerves	Low serum calcium, patient history	Administer calcium and vitamin D
Thyroid gland	Ultrasound thyroid scan, serum assay for thyroxine	Varies with cause, surgery
Metabolic rate, all cells	Ultrasound, thyroid scan, serum assay for thyroxine	Add iodine to diet
Metabolic rate, all cells, nervous system	Ultrasound, thyroid scan, serum assay for thyroxine	Radioactive iodine, medication, surgery
Metabolic rate, all cells, nervous system	Ultrasound, serum assay for thyroxine	Administer thyroid hormone
Metabolic rate, all cells, nervous system	Serum assay for thyroxine	Administer thyroid hormone

Endocrine System (continued)

Categories	* Disease ❏ Condition ➢ Complications of a Disease	Signs and Symptoms
Adrenal glands	* Hyperadrenalism, Cushing's syndrome	Hyperglycemia, adrenal diabetes, obesity of trunk, buffalo hump, moon face, hypertension, atherosclerosis, muscle weakness and fatigue, thin skin, easily bruised, stretch marks, increased susceptibility to infection, wounds heal poorly, weak bones
	* Hyperadrenalism, Conn's syndrome	Weak muscles due to loss of potassium; polydipsia, polyuria, hypertension due to salt and water retention
	* Hyperadrenalism, Adrenogenital syndrome	Premature sexual development in children; masculinization in adult women
	* Hypoadrenalism, Addison's disease	Dehydration, loss of salt and water with low BP, muscle weakness, weight loss, fatigue, GI disturbances, dark skin pigmentation increases
Pancreas, Beta cells of islands	* Hyposecretion, Insulin Dependent Diabetes Mellitus (IDDM), Type I Diabetes, Juvenile Diabetes	Polyuria, polydipsia, increased appetite (polyphagia) with weight loss, glycosuria, hyperglycemia, ketone bodies in urine, acidosis, poor wound healing, increased susceptibility to infection
	* Hyposecretion, Non-Insulin Dependent Diabetes Mellitus (NIDDM), Type II Diabetes, Maturity-onset Diabetes	May or may not have polyuria, polydipsia, polyphagia, weight loss; individual often obese, onset of disease gradual, may have nonspecific symptoms such as itching, recurrent infections, visual changes, abnormal sensations
	➢ Diabetic coma	Ketosis, acidosis and dehydration; deep labored breathing, fruity, acetone smell of breath, skin flushed and dry, tongue dry, gradual onset involving drowsiness and lethargy
	➢ Insulin shock, hypoglycemic shock	Light-headed feeling, faintness, trembling, perspiration, double vision, speech thick, unsteady walk, loss of consciousness, shallow breathing, breath odor normal
Gonads, Ovaries, Testes	* Hypergonadism (hypersecretion)	Before puberty, produces precocious sexual development
	* Hypogonadism (hyposecretion)	Before puberty, loss of sexual development, eunuchism

Affected Organ/Body Region	Diagnostic Procedure	Treatment
Metabolic regulation of foods, fat tissue, bones, skin, heart and vessels	Serum cortisol level, urinalysis, physical exam	Surgery and hormone replacement
Kidneys, muscles	Serum aldosterone level, urinalysis	Surgical
Primary and secondary sex characteristics	Serum androgen and cortisol levels	Surgical, and cortisol
Kidneys, muscles	Serum cortisol and aldosterone levels	Administer cortisol, aldosterone
Cells have lowered ability to absorb glucose (except for nerve cells)	Urinalysis, fasting blood sugar levels, oral glucose tolerance test, physical exam, patient history	Diet, insulin injections, exercise
Cells have lowered ability to absorb glucose (except for nerve cells)	Urinalysis, fasting blood sugar levels, oral glucose tolerance test, physical exam, patient history	Diet, oral hypoglycemic medications, exercise
Characteristic crisis for Type I diabetic Failure to take insulin, deviation from diet	High level glucose in blood and urine samples	Insulin, fluids, sodium chloride, sodium bicarbonate, electrolyte balance
Characteristic crisis for Type I diabetic Excess insulin taken, failure to eat, excessive exercise	Low blood sugar	Sugar (candy or orange juice); if unconscious IV glucose, epinephrine
Reproductive organs, secondary sex characteristics	Serum level of sex hormones	Administration of sex hormones
Reproductive organs, secondary sex characteristics	Serum level of sex hormones	Administration of sex hormones

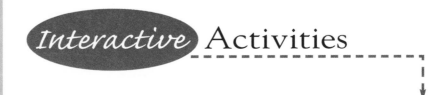

Interactive Activities

CASES FOR CRITICAL THINKING

1. Mom brings her 5-year-old son to the pediatrician with complaints that her son has been "wetting the bed" consistently. The child has a good appetite, and drinks a lot of water and a "high metabolism" according to the mother. On examination, the doctor notes that the child has lost 10 pounds since his last physical six months ago. What diseases should be ruled out?

2. A 59-year-old woman reports to the doctor's office with a chief complaint of "terrible headaches" especially between her eyes. Her blood pressure, blood sugar, and cholesterol level is high. The doctor also notes a terrible bruise on her leg that was there since her last examination 2 months ago. What diseases should be ruled out?

3. A 45-year-old man reports to the emergency room with terrible dehydration. He has a yellowish appearance and can hardly stand without assistance. His blood level of potassium is extremely high and his legs feel "tingly." His heartbeat is very rapid, and his breathing is shallow. What diseases does this man possibly have?

MULTIMEDIA EXTENSION ACTIVITIES

www.prenhall.com/mulvihill
Use the above address to access the free, interactive companion Website created for this textbook. Included in the features of this site are chapter specific activities, internet links, and an audio-glossary.

Audio Glossary
Use the CD-ROM disk enclosed with your textbook to hear the pronunciation of the key terms in this chapter.

Diseases at a Glance: Endocrine System

Use the chart on page(s) 298–301 to answer the following:

1. List 5 types of diseases or conditions that affect the endocrine system.

2. What are the major signs and symptoms of the diseases or conditions you named?

Quick Self Study

MULTIPLE CHOICE

1. Acromegaly results from the anterior pituitary _____.
   a. hypoactivity   b. hyperactivity

2. Glucose should be administered in _____.
   a. diabetic coma   b. insulin shock

3. Hypoglycemia is a sign in _____.
   a. Cushing's disease   b. Addison's disease
   c. Diabetes   d. Graves' disease

4. The trunk is obese in _____.
   a. Graves' disease   b. Cushing's disease
   c. Addison's disease

TRUE OR FALSE

_____ 1. Kidney stones are likely to form in hypoparathyroidism.

_____ 2. Hypercalcemia causes tetany.

_____ 3. Glucagon prevents hyperglycemia.

_____ 4. Steroids that suppress the inflammatory response, as in arthritis, are produced by the thyroid.

_____ 5. Hypertension accompanies Addison's disease.

_____ 6. Cretinism results from a congenital thyroid deficiency.

_____ 7. A person with Graves' disease is very sensitive to cold.

_____ 8. Dehydration can develop in diabetes mellitus.

FILL-INS

1. Overproduction of growth hormone before puberty is called
   _____, whereas an overproduction of growth hormone after
   puberty is called _____.

2. The posterior pituitary secretes _____ and
   _____.

3. Chronic hypoadrenalism, accompanied by weight loss and muscle weakness, is known
   as _____.

4. A tumor of the adrenal medulla, or _____, causes overproduction of epinephrine and norepinephrine.

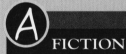

FICTION

In persons with nephrogenic diabetes insipidus, the kidney forms an inability to respond to normal amounts of antidiuretic hormone. These patients develop severe dehydration because of excessive urinary water loss. Nephrogenic diabetes insipidus is difficult to control and is ironically treated with diuretic medication.

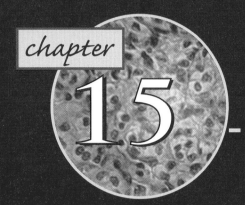

chapter

15

Diseases of the Reproductive Systems and Sexually Transmitted Infections

New life is created through the reproductive system. The female body produces ova, nurtures the developing fetus in the uterus, and nourishes the baby at the breast. The male body produces sperm and transmits it to the female. The fertilization that ensues combines characteristics of each parent, and an embryo begins to develop.

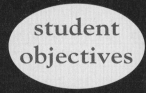

student objectives

After studying this chapter, students should be able to

- ➤ Describe the normal functions of the reproductive organs
- ➤ Describe the key characteristics of major diseases of the female reproductive system
- ➤ Describe the key characteristics of major diseases of the male reproductive system
- ➤ Name the causes of diseases of the reproductive system
- ➤ Name the diagnostic procedures for diseases of the reproductive system
- ➤ Describe the treatment options for diseases of the reproductive system

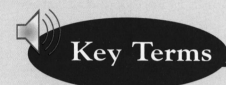

Key Terms

Amenorrhea
Aseptic
Bulbourethral gland
Carcinoma in situ
Cervix
Chancre
Chorionic gonadotropin
Clitoris
Corpus luteum
Cryptorchidism
Curettage
Dermoid cyst
Diethylstilbestrol
Dilatation
Dysmenorrhea
Dyspareunia
Eclampsia
Ectopic pregnancy
Ejaculatory duct
Endometriosis
Epididymis
Fallopian tubes
Fibrocystic disease
Fimbriae
Graafian follicles
Hydatiform mole
Hydrosalpinx
Hymen
Hyperplasia
Laparoscopy
Leiomyoma
Leukorrhea
Lumpectomy
Mammography
Mastectomy

Menarche
Menopause
Menorrhagia
Metrorrhagia
Mons pubis
Nocturia
Orchitis
Ovaries
Paget's disease
Paresis
Placenta
Preeclampsia
Premenstrual syndrome
Prepuce
Primary follicle
Prostate
Prostatitis
Puerperal sepsis
Puerperium
Pyosalpinx
Salpingitis
Scrotum
Seminal vesicle
Seminiferous tubules
Seminoma
Septicemia
Syphilis
Teratoma
Toxic shock syndrome
Trichomonas
Uterus
Vagina
Vaginitis
Vas deferens
Vulva

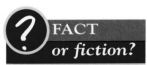

vagina
(vă-jī′-nă)

uterus
(ū′-těr-ŭs)

fallopian tubes
(făl-ō′-pē-ăn tūbz)

ovaries
(ō′-vă-rēs)

cervix
(sĕr′-vĭks)

fimbriae
(fĭm′-bri-ā)

primary follicle
(prī′-mă-rē fŏl′-lĭ-kŭl)

vulva
(vŭl′-vă)

mons pubis
(mons pū′-bĭs)

clitoris
(klĭ′-tō-rĭs)

➤ ANATOMY OF THE FEMALE REPRODUCTIVE SYSTEM

The female reproductive system consists of the **vagina,** the **uterus,** the **fallopian tubes,** and the **ovaries.** The vagina is a tubular structure extending backward and upward to the **cervix,** the lowest part of the uterus. The expanded, upper portion of the uterus tapers down to form the narrow cervix, giving the organ a pear-shaped appearance. The uterine wall is very strong, comprised of smooth muscle and lined with a mucosal membrane, the endometrium. It is responsive to hormonal changes. Figure 15–1 shows the female reproductive system.

The fallopian tubes extend laterally from each side of the uterus. The outer ends of the tubes are open to receive a released ovum. Fringelike projections at the outer ends, the **fimbriae,** propel the ova into the tube.

The ovaries, small, oval-shaped glands, are anchored near the open end of the fallopian tubes by ligaments. The ovaries contain hundreds of thousands of ova, which are present at birth. Each ovum is surrounded by a single layer of cells comprising a **primary follicle.** The relationship between the ovaries and the fallopian tubes is shown in Figure 15–2.

The external genitalia, the **vulva,** consists of the **mons pubis,** the labia majora and labia minora, the **clitoris,** and the vaginal opening. The urinary meatus is between the clitoris and the vaginal opening. The mons pubis, a pad of fat tissue over the pubic symphysis, becomes covered with hair at puberty. Extending back from the mons pubis to the anus are two pairs of folds, the labia majora and the labia minora. The clitoris, a tuft of erectile tissue, similar to that of the penis, is located at the anterior junction of the

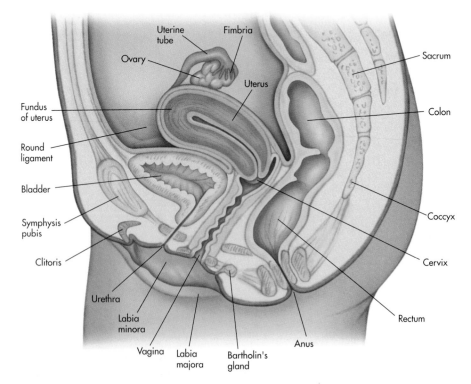

Figure 15–1
Sagittal section of the female pelvis, showing organs of the reproductive system.

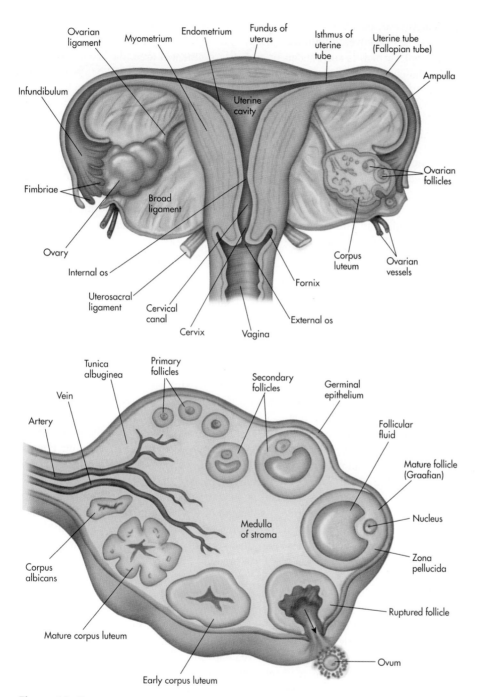

Figure 15–2
The uterus, ovaries, and associated structures.

minor lips. A membranous fold, the **hymen,** partly or completely closes the vaginal opening. Occasionally this membrane is imperforate or abnormally closed and requires a minor surgical procedure to open it. A pair of mucus-secreting glands, Bartholin's glands, are situated at the vaginal entrance. These glands produce a lubricating secretion during sexual intercourse.

hymen
(hī-mĕn)

The breasts, accessory organs of reproduction, consist of milk glands supported by connective tissue covered with fatty tissue and skin. Ducts of the milk glands converge at the nipple, which is surrounded by a darkly pigmented area, the areola. The breasts overlie the pectoral muscles of the chest.

➤ PHYSIOLOGY OF THE FEMALE REPRODUCTIVE SYSTEM

The cyclic hormonal changes in the life of a woman prepare the uterus monthly for a possible pregnancy. The secretion of female hormones, estrogen and progesterone, is governed by the gonadotropic hormones of the anterior pituitary gland, which is controlled by the hypothalamus of the brain. Failure of the ovary to secrete sex hormones or to ovulate may result from pituitary disease or disturbances in the central nervous system.

menarche
(měn-ăr′-kē)

menopause
(měn′-ō-pawz)

Graafian follicles
(grăf′-ē-ăn
fŏl′-lĭ-kŭlz)

A woman's reproductive life begins with the onset of menstruation, the **menarche,** occurring generally between ages 10 and 15. The reproductive years terminate with the cessation of menstrual periods, **menopause,** which usually begins in the late 40s or early 50s. At the beginning of each monthly cycle, a pituitary gonadotropic hormone stimulates ovarian follicles to develop. The particular follicles that are stimulated begin to grow and develop into **Graafian follicles.** One of these matures first and is released at the midpoint of the cycle, which is the process of ovulation. Ovulation is also controlled by a gonadotropic hormone.

As the follicles are growing, during the first half of the cycle, the ovary secretes estrogen, which is carried by the blood to the uterus. Estrogen stimulates the endometrium of the uterus to thicken and become more vascular. This is in preparation for pregnancy and is called the proliferative phase.

corpus luteum
(kor′-pŭs lā-tĕ-ŭm)

Once the ovum has been released from the ovary, the empty follicle is converted into the **corpus luteum,** which begins to secrete progesterone. Progesterone continues the stimulation of endometrial growth and promotes the storage of nutrients for nourishing a fertilized ovum. This is the secretory phase of the uterus.

placenta
(plă-sen′-tă)

If no fertilization occurs, the corpus luteum ceases to secrete hormones approximately 8 to 12 days after ovulation. At the end of the monthly cycle, the level of estrogen and progesterone drops, and menstruation, the sloughing of the endometrial lining, occurs. If pregnancy occurs, the corpus luteum greatly enlarges and continues to secrete high levels of progesterone. The **placenta** gradually assumes the role of the corpus luteum in secreting these hormones.

The placenta is formed from both maternal and embryonic tissue. Near the site of implantation in the uterus, the endometrium greatly thickens, becomes highly vascular, and develops large blood sinuses. An embryonic membrane, the chorion, develops fingerlike projections called villi, which dip into the maternal blood sinuses. This interdigitation of embryonic and maternal tissue constitutes the placenta.

The umbilical arteries extend into the chorionic villi, where the exchange of carbon dioxide for oxygen and waste material for nutrients occurs. Maternal and fetal blood do not mix; the exchange of these substances is by diffusion across the blood vessel walls. Oxygen and nutrients return to the fetus through the umbilical vein.

➤ DISEASES OF THE FEMALE REPRODUCTIVE SYSTEM

Infections, tumors, and cysts develop in the reproductive organs and in the breasts. Abnormalities of the menstrual cycle and of pregnancy also occur.

Pelvic Inflammatory Disease (PID)

The pelvic reproductive organs become inflamed as a result of bacterial, viral, fungal, or parasitic invasion. The subsequent infection can ascend to the cervix, the endometrium, the fallopian tubes, and even to the ovaries. Gonorrhea is one of the most common causes of pelvic inflammatory disease. Chlamydia and other sexually transmitted infections also cause PID. Streptococcal and staphylococcal organisms can enter the female reproductive tract after an abortion or delivery in which sterile procedures were not carefully followed. The symptoms of pelvic inflammatory disease are lower abdominal pain, fever resulting from the infection, and a vaginal discharge of pus. If the infection is not treated, abscesses form. PID may also result in infertility if untreated. Antibiotics, aspirin, bed rest, and fluids are the usual treatments.

Salpingitis

Salpingitis is an inflammation of the fallopian tubes; the term *salpinx* refers to a tube. Untreated sexually transmitted diseases can cause this inflammation, as can a streptococcal or staphylococcal invasion. These pyogenic organisms cause a purulent, pus-producing infection.

    The fallopian tubes become red and swollen, and if the outer ends remain open, the infection spreads out into the pelvic cavity to cause pelvic peritonitis. The outer ends of the tubes usually close and the tubes fill with pus, which is then called a **pyosalpinx.** When the inflammation subsides after treatment with antibiotics, the tube is filled with a watery fluid and is referred to as a **hydrosalpinx.** Both tubes are usually affected as the inflammation ascends through the uterus. Sterility results from salpingitis if the ends of both tubes close. Adhesions may form that affect the tubes and cause sterility. Menstrual disturbances generally accompany salpingitis, as do ectopic pregnancies.

Vaginitis

Vaginitis, inflammation of the vagina, is a common disease caused by several organisms. A parasite, **trichomonas,** that can be transmitted by sexual intercourse is one causative agent. Trichomonas is sometimes admitted from fecal material. *Candida albicans,* a fungus, is another cause of vaginitis, a yeast infection. An overgrowth of fungus can develop from antibiotic treatment that destroys the normal flora. The normal flora consists of nonpathogenic microorganisms that are generally present and help keep down the number of harmful microbes. If the normal flora is wiped out by antibiotics, fungi, and viruses, antibiotic-resistant organisms thrive. A foul-smelling vaginal discharge is the principal sign of vaginitis. The discharge causes itching, burning, and soreness of the surrounding tissues. Any vaginal discharge other than blood is referred to as **leukorrhea.** Atrophic vaginitis can be a postmenopausal condition. The vaginal lining changes with the loss of estrogen secretion when the ovaries atrophy, and the mucosa becomes more susceptible to infection. Hormonal therapy, antibiotic ointments, or steroid creams may be prescribed.

Inflammation of Bartholin's Glands

Bartholin's glands are susceptible to infections caused by gonococcal, streptococcal, and staphylococcal organisms. If the duct of the gland becomes occluded from the inflammation, pus collects in the gland and abscesses form. Such abscesses require surgical lancing to allow drainage of the pus.

Puerperal Sepsis

Puerperal sepsis is an infection of the endometrium after childbirth or an abortion. The **puerperium** is the period after childbirth, when the endometrium is open and particu-

salpingitis
(săl″-pĭn-jī′-tĭs)

pyosalpinx
(pī″-ō-săl′-pĭnks)
hydrosalpinx
(hī-drō-săl′-pĭngks)

vaginitis
(văj″-ĭn-ī′-tĭs)
trichomonas
(trĭk″-ō-′-mō′-năs)

leukorrhea
(loo″-kō-rē′-ă)

puerperal sepsis
(pū-ēr′-pĕr-ăl
sĕp-sĭs)
puerperium
(pū″-ĕr-pē′-rē-ŭm)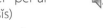

larly susceptible to infection. The trauma and blood loss encountered during delivery provide a portal of entry for invading microorganisms through the birth canal. The lesions of the endometrium favor bacterial growth. Streptococci are the principal causative organisms, but staphylococci and *E. coli* enter the uterus through a lack of **aseptic** technique. Necrosis of the endometrium develops from the infection.

Infected blood clots can break loose and travel as septic emboli. A systemic infection of the blood, **septicemia,** is often the result. The deep veins of the leg are frequently affected, resulting in thrombophlebitis, a condition previously described in Chapter 9. The symptoms of puerperal sepsis are fever, chills, and profuse bleeding. A foul-smelling vaginal discharge indicates infection. Pain is experienced in the lower abdomen and pelvis. Puerperal sepsis responds well to antibiotic treatment.

aseptic
(ā-sĕp′-tĭk)

septicemia
(sĕpt-ĭ-sē′-mē-a)

Neoplasms of the Female Organs

Early detection, diagnosis, and treatment of any abnormal mass or lump is extremely important in preventing the growth and spread of cancer. Many tumors and cysts are harmless, but tests are required to differentiate between malignant and benign growths.

Carcinoma of the Cervix Carcinoma of the cervix is one of the cancers most easily diagnosed in the early stages. Incidence of this malignancy has decreased significantly since the development of the Pap smear. The Pap smear, explained in Chapter 4, enables physicians to obtain cell samples from the cervix. These scrapings are examined microscopically. Biopsies of suspected lesions are taken if cell abnormalities indicate precursors of cancer. **Carcinoma in situ,** a premalignant lesion, is the earliest stage of cancer; the underlying tissue has not yet been invaded. Progression from a carcinoma in situ to an invasive malignancy may be slow. Ulceration then occurs, causing vaginal discharge and bleeding. The cancer spreads to surrounding organs: the vagina, bladder, rectum, and pelvic wall. Widespread cancer becomes inoperable, and radiation therapy is the usual treatment. Carcinoma of the cervix is strongly associated with infection by human papillomavirus. Early sexual activity and promiscuity are also related to the incidence of this cancer.

carcinoma in situ
(kăr-sĭ-nō′-ma
ĭn sī′-too)

Carcinoma of the Endometrium Carcinoma of the endometrium, the lining of the uterus, occurs most often in postmenopausal women who have had no children. The malignant tumor may grow into the cavity of the uterus or invade the wall itself. Ulcerations develop, and erosion of blood vessels causes vaginal bleeding. Surgery and radiation are the usual treatments.

Fibroid Tumors Benign tumors of the smooth muscle of the uterus, **leiomyomas** or fibroid tumors, are the most common tumors in females and frequently cause no symptoms. Fibroids are often multiple and vary greatly in size. Fibroid tumors, some of which are stalked or pedunculated, are shown in Figure 15–3. Fibroid tumor growth is stimulated by estrogen because the tumors develop only during the reproductive years. Large tumors putting pressure on surrounding organs and nerve endings cause pelvic pain. Fibroid tumors can also interfere during delivery. Abnormal bleeding between periods or excessively heavy menstrual flow is a common symptom of fibroid tumors. A hysterectomy is generally required if bleeding continues.

leiomyoma
(lī″-ō-mī-ō′-ma)

Ovarian Neoplasms The most common ovarian neoplasm is the cyst, a fluid-filled sac. Many cysts cause no symptoms but are discovered during a pelvic examination. Large cysts that can interfere with blood flow are removed surgically.

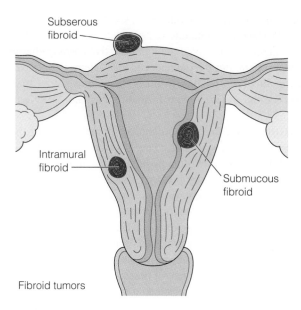

Subserous fibroid

Intramural fibroid

Submucous fibroid

Fibroid tumors

Figure 15–3
Types of uterine fibroid tumors.

Primary malignant tumors of the ovary are relatively rare. Primary tumors tend to cause few symptoms and, therefore, are discovered only when the disease is advanced. A malignant tumor can be removed surgically before metastases or treated with chemotherapy once it has spread.

A peculiar benign tumor of the ovary is the **dermoid cyst,** or **teratoma,** described in Chapter 4. The dermoid cyst may contain many kinds of tissues: skin with its oil glands and hair follicles, teeth, and bone. The cyst is filled with oily material from the glands, and hair grows into the cavity. The tumor is harmless unless its size or other symptoms necessitate surgery.

dermoid cyst
(dĕr′-moyd sĭst)

teratoma
(tĕr-ă-tō′-mă)

Hydatidiform Mole The **hydatidiform mole** is a benign tumor of the placenta. It can develop after a pregnancy or in association with an abnormal one. The tumor consists of multiple cysts and resembles a bunch of grapes. The tumor secretes **chorionic gonadotropic** hormone (CGH), the hormone that indicates a positive pregnancy test. The uterus enlarges greatly, although no fetus develops. Bleeding usually occurs, and the mole is expelled. Scraping of the uterus, the procedure of **dilatation** of the cervix and **curettage** (D&C), removes any fragments of the tumor or placenta.

hydatiform mole
(hĭ″-dă-tĭd′-ĭ-form mōl)

chorionic gonadotropin
(kō-rē-ŏn′-ĭk gō-năd-ō-trō′-pĭn)

dilatation
(dī-lă-tā′-shŭn)

curettage
(kū″-rĕ-tăzh′)

Choriocarcinoma Choriocarcinoma is a highly malignant tumor of the placenta. A part of the placenta is formed by the embryonic membrane called the chorion. This tumor may develop after a hydatidiform mole, a normal delivery, or an abortion. A choriocarcinoma, like the hydatidiform mole, secretes large amounts of chorionic gonadotropic hormone. Presence of this hormone in the urine in the absence of pregnancy is significant diagnostically. The tumor is highly invasive and metastasizes rapidly. Chemotherapy rather than surgery is the usual treatment.

Adenocarcinoma of the Vagina Adenocarcinoma of the vagina has been linked to the synthetic hormone **diethylstilbestrol (DES),** which was used to prevent spontaneous

diethylstilbestrol
(dī-ĕth″-ĭ-stĭl″-bĕs′-trŏl)

abortion. This rather rare cancer has developed in some young girls whose mothers were given diethylstilbestrol during pregnancy.

Daughters of women who received diethylstilbestrol therapy should be checked for possible cancer development, but the incidence is low. Diethylstilbestrol appears to have only slight effects in sons born to these women. Testes have been found to be smaller than normal in some cases, and some cyst formation has been found in the epididymis.

Malignant Neoplasms of the Breast Adenocarcinoma, cancer of the breast ducts, is the most common breast malignancy. Breast cancer is the second leading cause of cancer death in U.S. women. It occurs more often in single women, in women who have had no children, and in women with a family history of breast cancer. Adenocarcinoma of the breast usually develops around the time of the menopause, and development of this cancer seems to be related to estrogen activity. Women are strongly urged to examine their breasts monthly for a possible lump. The American Cancer Society and the National Cancer Institute have done a great deal to encourage this practice, and they provide valuable information on the procedure. A genetic screen for breast cancer is also available. The BRC gene increases the risk for the development of breast cancer. Results should be interpreted cautiously because having BRC does not mean a woman will definitely develop cancer.

The signs that indicate a malignant tumor are presented by an advanced cancer. A hard, fixed lump in the upper, outer quadrant is one such sign. Benign tumors, because they are encapsulated (Chapter 4), are not fixed to underlying structures. The nipple often retracts and the skin dimples due to contraction of dense fibrous connective tissue that extends to the chest muscles and skin. (Figures 15–4 and 15–5).

The lymph nodes of the axillary region may be swollen. Carcinoma spreads principally through the lymph system. Metastases are frequent to the lungs, liver, brain, and bone. **Mammography** can detect small, early cancers and should be performed on the recommended schedule according to age. A biopsy of the suspected malignancy confirms the diagnosis or shows the tumor to be benign (Figure 15–4 and Figure 15–5.)

Treatment of breast cancer varies. In a simple mastectomy, only the breast is removed. The breast, chest muscles, and axillary lymph nodes are removed in a radical **mastectomy.** Some studies indicate that prognosis after a radical mastectomy is not necessarily better than that after a less mutilating procedure. Less mutilating procedures involve removal of the tumor only, a **lumpectomy,** and radiation therapy. The ovaries are often removed to prevent the stimulating effect of estrogen on tumor growth when disease is metastatic.

Paget's disease of the nipple is a rare cancer involving inflammatory changes that affect the nipple and the areola. The nipple becomes granular and crusted with lesions resembling eczema. In advanced Paget's disease, ulceration develops and there is a discharge from the nipple. The breast becomes edematous and is characterized as having a "pigskin" appearance. Treatment depends on the extent of the disease. A significant feature in Paget's disease is that it is accompanied by an underlying infiltrating duct cancer.

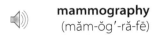
mammography
(măm-ŏg′-ră-fē)

mastectomy
(măs-těk′-tŏ-mē)

lumpectomy
(lŭm-pěk′-tŏ-mē)

Paget's disease
(păj′-ěts dĭ-zēz′)

PREVENTION *PLUS!*

Self-screening for Cancer

Early detection of cancer is key to favorable outcomes. Tissue changes associated with testicular cancer and breast cancer may be detected at home through regular self-screening. Suspicious changes detected at home can be reported to a physician, who can determine the nature of the tissue changes and begin treatment if necessary.

side by side

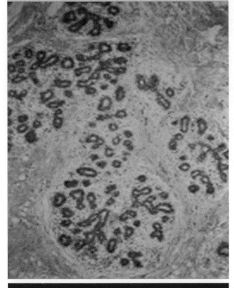

Figure 15–4

Normal microscopic view of breast tissue and ducts.

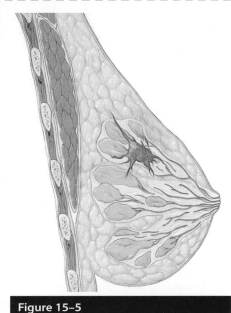

Figure 15–5

Carcinoma of breast tissue and ducts.

Benign Tumors of the Breast   The most common benign tumor of the breast is a fibroadenoma. It is a firm, movable mass easily removed by surgery. The fibroadenoma does not become malignant.

Cystic **hyperplasia** or **fibrocystic disease** (Figure 15–6) is very common and not serious. Development occurs at any age with the formation of numerous lumps in the breast. The lumps are fluid-filled cysts, not tumors. They tend to be painful at the time of the menstrual period as the breasts themselves respond to hormonal changes, enlarging and regressing. These cysts are often aspirated: A needle is inserted to remove fluid. The withdrawal of fluid confirms that the lump is a cyst and not a solid tumor. There may be a higher incidence of breast cancer development in women who have cystic hyperplasia. These women should be examined regularly to prevent mistaking a tumor for a cyst.

hyperplasia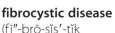
(hī″-pĕr-plā′-zē-ă)

fibrocystic disease
(fī″-brō-sĭs′-tĭk
dĭ-zēz′)

Menstrual Abnormalities

Amenorrhea is the absence of menstrual periods and is known as primary amenorrhea if menstruation fails to begin. Lack of gonadotropic hormones from the pituitary gland or a diseased ovary can cause the abnormality, and administration of hormones may be effective treatment. The cessation of menstrual periods for more than a year is termed secondary amenorrhea. This can result from an ovarian or uterine disease, as well as hormonal imbalance; pituitary failure and thyroid disease can cause amenorrhea. The absence of menstruation is a sign of a disease that must be diagnosed and treated.

amenorrhea
(ă-mĕn″-ō-rē′-ă)

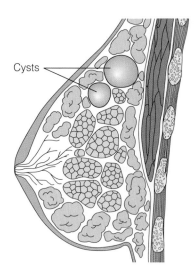

Cysts

Figure 15–6
Cystic hyperplasia of the breast.

Certain psychological states—extreme depression, worry, and continuous stress—can cause cessation of menstruation. Certain eating disorders and/or excessive exercise, both of which deplete body fat, can cause amenorrhea. The hypothalamus of the brain governs the release of pituitary hormones, including the gonadotropins. The condition of amenorrhea may correct itself if the stressful conditions can be eliminated.

menorrhagia
(měn″-ō-rē′-ă)

Menorrhagia is excessive or prolonged bleeding during menstruation. It can result from tumors of the uterus, pelvic inflammatory disease, or endocrine imbalance. Failure to ovulate can also cause menorrhagia. If a corpus luteum is not formed, progesterone is not secreted and estrogen continues to stimulate endometrial thickening. Treatment varies according to the cause of the disease. Tumors should be removed surgically, pelvic inflammatory disease should be treated with antibiotics, and hormonal therapy should be administered for endocrine insufficiency.

metrorrhagia
(mě″-trō-rē′-ă)

Metrorrhagia is bleeding between menstrual periods or extreme irregularity of the cycle. It results from an abnormal buildup and sloughing of endometrial tissue. Hormonal imbalance may be the cause of metrorrhagia, or the endometrial response to the hormones may be incorrect. A D&C is often performed and the endometrium returns to normal.

Toxic Shock Syndrome

toxic shock syndrome
(tŏk-sĭk shŏc sĭn′-drōm)

Toxic shock syndrome (TSS) is caused by an infection of *Staphylococcus aureus*. The signs include high fever, rash, skin peeling, and decreased blood pressure. Other systemic involvements may include gastrointestinal complaints, elevated liver enzymes, and neuromuscular disturbances. Treatment includes fluid replacement to counteract shock and administration of selected antibiotics.

The relationship between particular tampons and development of toxic shock syndrome is thought to be an increase in staphylococcal toxin production in the environment of certain synthetic fibers. These fibers were found to be the ones used in "super" tampons to increase absorbency. The fibers apparently remove magnesium from the vagina, and this produces an environment that encourages growth of the bacteria that make toxins. These fibers are no longer used. It was found that some surgical dressings also contained the same fibers, a finding that may explain some cases of toxic shock syndrome in nontampon users.

Recommendations for women who use tampons include avoidance of the superabsorptive type, daytime use only, and frequent changes of tampons.

Premenstrual Syndrome

Most women experience some mild premenstrual symptoms during their reproductive years but when symptoms become temporarily disabling, disrupt family, business, and social relationships, **premenstrual syndrome** (PMS) is indicated.

PMS consists of a group of severe symptoms, emotional, physical, and behavioral, that are associated with the menstrual cycle. They usually begin at the mid-point of the cycle and worsen until the onset of bleeding.

Physical symptoms include lower abdominal bloating, breast swelling and soreness, headache, and constipation. Episodes of depression, anxiety, irritability, and hostility are characteristics of emotional changes. Typical behavioral symptoms include crying, binge eating, and clumsiness. No tests or physical examinations confirm the presence of PMS. A daily diary that shows the relationship of the monthly cycle and the symptoms can assist in the diagnosis.

The cause of PMS is unknown but researchers suspect that the production of cyclic ovarian hormones affect the production of other hormones and chemicals, specifically neurotransmitters. These chemicals may cause the symptoms, but it is not understood why some women are affected and others are not. Whereas in the past it was thought that PMS was emotional in origin or caused by stress, it is now known to have a physical cause (Figure 15–7).

Treatment has to be individually prescribed as women respond differently to various suggestions. For some women, dietary changes during the week before the onset of menstruation are helpful. These changes might include the avoidance of salt, sugar, caffeine, and alcohol. Aerobic exercise, brisk walking, or swimming is helpful for others. Support groups and stress management techniques can be positive means of coping with the condition.

Endometriosis

Endometriosis is a disease condition in which endometrial tissue from the uterus becomes embedded elsewhere. The tissue may have been pushed backward through the fallopian tubes during menstruation or carried by blood or lymph. It then takes hold on some structure in the peritoneal cavity, such as the ovary. The endometrial tissue by nature responds to hormonal changes even when outside the uterus. This tissue goes through a proliferative and secretory phase, along with the sloughing-off phase with subsequent bleeding. Endometriosis causes pelvic pain, abnormal bleeding, and painful menstruation (**dysmenorrhea**). Sterility and pain during sexual intercourse (**dyspareunia**) can result. Treatment

premenstrual syndrome (prĕ-mĕn′-stroo-ăl sĭn′-drōm)

endometriosis (ĕn″-dō-mē″-trē-ō′-sĭs)

dysmenorrhea (dĭs-mĕn-ō-rē′-ă)

dyspareunia (dĭs″-pă-rū′-nē-ă)

on the Practical Side

Hot Flashes

One of the most common complaints of menopausal women is the discomfort of hot flashes. The range in severity is broad but generally involves vasodilation, redness, heat, and sweating. The extensive dilatation of superficial blood vessels and increased blood flow accounts for the rapid temperature fluctuations. The cause of hot flashes is attributed to decreased levels of estrogen and progesterone in response to gonadotropic hormone stimulation from the anterior pituitary gland.

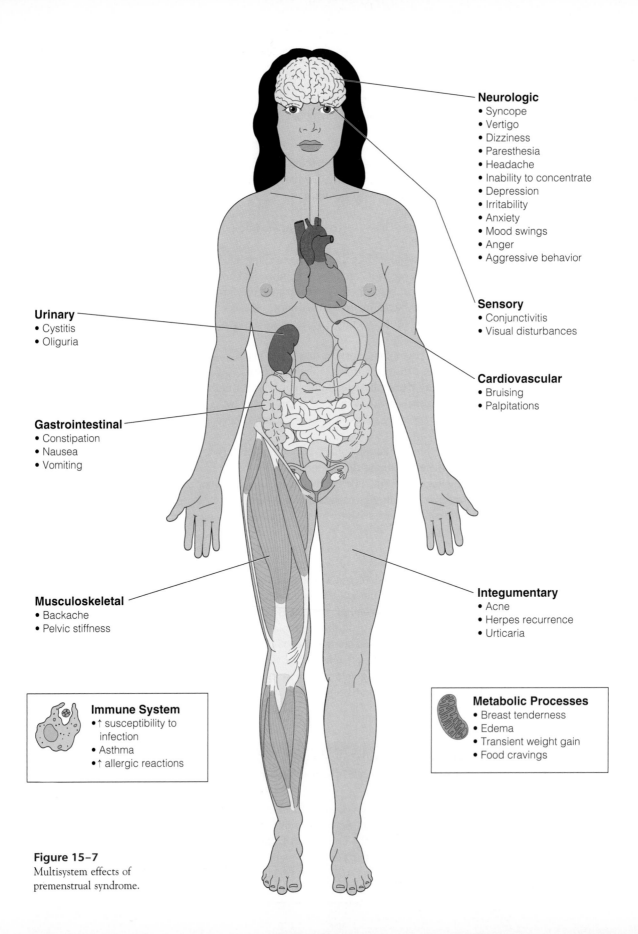

Neurologic
- Syncope
- Vertigo
- Dizziness
- Paresthesia
- Headache
- Inability to concentrate
- Depression
- Irritability
- Anxiety
- Mood swings
- Anger
- Aggressive behavior

Sensory
- Conjunctivitis
- Visual disturbances

Cardiovascular
- Bruising
- Palpitations

Integumentary
- Acne
- Herpes recurrence
- Urticaria

Metabolic Processes
- Breast tenderness
- Edema
- Transient weight gain
- Food cravings

Immune System
- ↑ susceptibility to infection
- Asthma
- ↑ allergic reactions

Musculoskeletal
- Backache
- Pelvic stiffness

Gastrointestinal
- Constipation
- Nausea
- Vomiting

Urinary
- Cystitis
- Oliguria

Figure 15–7
Multisystem effects of premenstrual syndrome.

of endometriosis varies according to the extent of the abnormal growth and the age of the patient. The only certain means of diagnosing endometriosis is by seeing it. Direct visualization is possible through **laparoscopy** in which an illuminated tube is inserted through a small abdominal incision. A tissue biopsy can be taken and examined. Hormonal therapy is generally used for the young patient. Pregnancy, with the absence of menstruation, tends to hold the condition in check. Extensive proliferation of endometrial tissue requires surgery, and cysts filled with blood are usually found at this time.

laparoscopy
(lăp-ăr-ŏs′-kō-pē)

➤ ABNORMALITIES OF PREGNANCY

A most important factor during pregnancy is good prenatal care. The pregnant woman should be checked regularly for weight gain, blood pressure, and urine abnormalities. She should be instructed on the importance of proper diet and exercise. Most pregnancies progress normally, but occasionally some problems do arise.

Ectopic Pregnancy

An **ectopic pregnancy** is a pregnancy in which the fertilized ovum implants in a tissue other than the uterus. The most common site of an ectopic pregnancy is in the fallopian tubes. The fertilized ovum becomes trapped because of a stricture or obstruction such as a tumor. Salpingitis is a predisposing condition for a tubal pregnancy due to the inflammatory effect on the mucosal lining. Embryonic development proceeds for about 2 months, at which time the pregnancy terminates. The tube often ruptures, causing severe internal hemorrhage into the abdominal cavity. Intense pain and bleeding from the uterus result, and the embryo is usually destroyed by the trauma. Once the diagnosis has been made, the ruptured tube and embryo have to be removed surgically.

ectopic pregnancy
(ĕk-tŏp′-ĭk prĕg′-năn-sē)

Spontaneous Abortion

A spontaneous abortion, commonly called a *miscarriage,* usually results from a genetic abnormality. The fetus is expelled before it is able to live outside of the uterus, and this usually occurs in the second or third month of pregnancy. The first sign is vaginal bleeding with cramping. The woman who has aborted should receive medical attention at once to reduce the hazards of hemorrhage and infection. A D&C is usually performed to remove any tissue that remains in the uterus.

A woman who has repeated spontaneous abortions should be examined comprehensively to determine the cause. Hormonal imbalances are sometimes responsible and can be corrected by replacement hormones. Emotional and psychological factors may be involved, and professional counseling is advised.

Toxemia of Pregnancy

Toxemia of pregnancy sometimes develops during the last trimester. The condition is poorly named because no toxin appears to cause the disease and the cause is not known. The principal signs are hypertension, albuminuria, edema (particularly in the face and arms), and a significant weight gain. These signs are presented in Figure 15–8. In the first phase of toxemia, pregnancy-induced hypertension (PIH), symptoms include headache, visual disturbances, abdominal pain, and vomiting. A spasm of blood vessels apparently causes the headache and visual disturbances. If this condition is not treated, **eclampsia** develops and convulsions and coma occur.

Preventive treatment for toxemia consists of early prenatal care, in which blood pressure is regularly checked, urine is analyzed for albumin, and weight gain is con-

eclampsia
(ĕ-klămp′-sē-ă)

SIGNS	SYMPTOMS
Hypertension	Headache
Albuminuria	Visual disturbances
Edema of face and extremities	Abdominal pain
Significant weight gain	Vomiting

Figure 15–8
Pregnancy-induced hypertension.

preeclampsia
(prē-ĕ-klămp′-sē-ă)

trolled. **Preeclampsia,** diagnosed early and treated, responds well. Restriction of salt (which tends to increase blood pressure), a nutritious low-calorie diet, and diuretics may be prescribed. This must be done with great care to prevent injury to the fetus. Anticonvulsant medications can be prescribed for eclampsia.

➤ ANATOMY OF THE MALE REPRODUCTIVE SYSTEM

The male reproductive system consists of a pair of testes in which the sperm develop and hormones are produced, a system of tubules that convey sperm to the outside, and the penis, which transmits the sperm into the female tract. Accessory glands contribute to the formation of semen.

scrotum
(skrō′-tŭm)

The testes are suspended in the **scrotum,** a saclike structure outside the body wall. The testes contain highly coiled tubules called the **seminiferous tubules,** which are the site of sperm development. When the sperm reach a certain maturity they enter the **epididymis,** a coiled tube that lies along the outer wall of the testis. The epididymis leads into another duct, the **vas deferens,** that passes through the inguinal canal into the abdominal cavity.

seminiferous tubules
(sĕ-mĭ-nĭf′-ĕr-ŭs tūb′-ūlz)

epididymis
(ĕp″-ĭ-dĭd′-ĭ-mĭs)

vas deferens
(văs-dĕf′-ĕr-ĕnz)

Near the base of the urinary bladder the vas deferens joins a duct of the **seminal vesicle,** an accessory gland, to form the **ejaculatory duct.** The ejaculatory ducts from each side penetrate the **prostate** gland to enter the urethra. Ducts of the prostate open into the first part of the male urethra. Another pair of glands, the **bulbourethral glands,** secrete into the urethra as it enters the penis. The male reproductive system is illustrated in Figure 15–9.

seminal vesicle
(sĕm′-ĭn-ăl vĕs′-ĭ-kŭl)

ejaculatory duct
(ē-jăk′-ū-lā-tor-ē dŭkt)

The penis consists of three cylindrical bodies of cavernous tissue also known as erectile tissue. This tissue is filled with spaces, or sinuses, that become engorged with blood. The urethra passes through one of these cylindrical bodies as it extends to the outside and connective tissue supports the erectile structures. The distal, expanded end of the penis is the glans penis. A flap of loosely attached skin covering the glans, the **prepuce** or foreskin, is often removed shortly after birth, which is the procedure called circumcision.

prostate
(prŏs′-tāt)

bulbourethral gland
(bŭl″-bō-ū-rē′-thrăl glăndz)

➤ PHYSIOLOGY OF THE MALE REPRODUCTIVE SYSTEM

prepuce
(prē′-pūs)

Spermatogenesis, the formation of sperm, begins in the male at puberty and continues through life. The development of sperm and the secretion of the male hormone, testosterone, are processes stimulated by gonadotropic hormones of the anterior pituitary gland. Maturation of sperm continues in the epididymis, where they acquire motility. Sperm are stored in both the epididymis and vas deferens and can live for several weeks in the male genital ducts. Once they are ejaculated, they live for only 24 to 72 hours in the female reproductive tract.

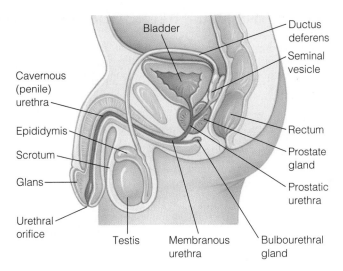

Figure 15–9
The male reproductive system.

The accessory glands contribute to the nourishment and protection of the sperm, and mucoid secretions from these glands form the semen. The seminal vesicles provide fructose, other nutrients, and prostaglandin, which increases uterine contractions. This helps to propel the sperm toward the fallopian tubes. The seminal vesicles release their secretions into the ejaculatory ducts at the same time the vas deferens empty the sperm. The muscular prostate gland, which surrounds the first part of the urethra, contracts during ejaculation, releasing its secretions. The secretion is alkaline, which buffers the highly acidic vaginal secretions that can inhibit sperm motility.

Sexual stimulation of the male transmits impulses into the central nervous system, which initiates the male response. Erection of the penis is the first effect. Nerve impulses cause the dilation of penile arteries, allowing blood to flow under high pressure into the erectile tissue. The high pressure temporarily impedes the emptying of the penile veins and causes the penis to become hard, elongated, and erect.

Intense sexual stimulation causes peristaltic contractions in the walls of the epididymis and vas deferens, propelling sperm into the urethra. The seminal vesicles and prostate gland simultaneously release their secretions, which mix with the mucous secretion of the bulbourethral glands forming the semen, the process of emission. Ejaculation of the semen—the culmination of the sexual act—occurs when contraction of this musculature increases pressure on the erectile tissue, and the semen is expressed through the urethral opening.

on the Practical Side

Semen Analysis in Evaluating Sterility
Several factors are analyzed in evaluating possible sterility. Sperm counts below 20 million/ml of semen and/or a high percentage of abnormally shaped sperm are indicators of sterility. Motility of the sperm is essential and a factor that is analyzed. The semen and sugar content, specifically fructose, are also evaluated to determine possible obstruction or absence of accessory glands and ducts.

➤ DISEASES OF THE MALE REPRODUCTIVE SYSTEM

The most common diseases of the male reproductive system are those affecting the prostate gland. This gland can become inflamed or enlarged as a result of bacterial invasion and cause urinary problems (Figure 15-10). Cancer sometimes develops in the prostate as well as in the testes.

Diseases of the Prostate Gland

Inflammation of the prostate can result from urinary tract infections or sexually transmitted diseases. Conversely, an enlarged prostate can cause urinary tract infections by obstructing the outflow of urine from the bladder.

prostatitis
(prŏs″-tă-tī′-tĭs)

Prostatitis   The cause of **prostatitis,** inflammation of the prostate, is not always known. Infection frequently develops from gonococci in a male with gonorrhea or from *E. coli* that has caused a urinary tract infection. Prostatitis causes pain and a burning sensation during urination. The prostate may be tender, and pus from the tip of the penis is sometimes noted. Penicillin is the usual treatment unless hypersensitivity to the drug necessitates the use of other antibiotics.

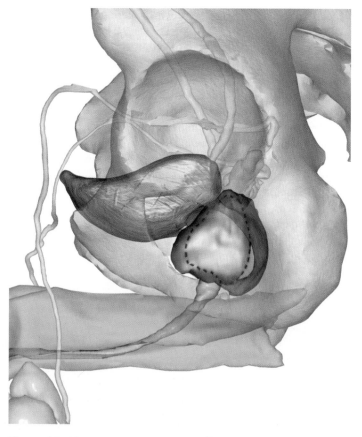

Figure 15–10
Enlarged prostate gland. Dashed line indicates the normal size.

Benign Prostatic Hyperplasia Enlargement of the prostate gland, benign prostatic hyperplasia, is a common occurrence in men over 50. The incidence increases with age, and the enlargement can be felt through rectal examination.

The symptoms resemble urinary tract disturbances (see Chapter 10) as the enlarged prostate partially blocks the flow of urine from the bladder. If the bladder cannot be fully emptied, residual urine provides a medium for bacterial infection and cystitis develops.

The blockage of urine outflow places back pressure on the ureters, which causes them to become congested with urine, a condition called *hydroureters*. This back pressure can extend to the kidneys; they swell with fluid, and hydronephrosis results. An imbalance of sex hormones frequently causes prostatic enlargement. The level of testosterone generally decreases with age, but estrogen from the adrenal cortex continues to be secreted, changing the ratio of the two. Treatment for benign prostatic hyperplasia, which is highly symptomatic, is surgical removal.

Carcinoma of the Prostate Gland Carcinoma of the prostate is common in old age, but the tumor may be small and asymptomatic. Rectal examination may reveal an enlarged prostate that is very hard, harder than a benign enlargement. Men over 40 should have annual rectal exams. Prostate-specific antigen (PSA) levels rise and can help predict the risk of having prostate cancer. Signs of prostatic cancer are urinary tract obstruction, urinary infections, the need to urinate during the night, or **nocturia,** and at times urinary incontinence.

nocturia
(nŏk-tŭ′-rē-ă)

Prognosis for this carcinoma is poor, as the malignancy spreads rapidly to nearby organs like the bladder and rectum. The cancer invades the lymph and blood vessels and metastasizes to the bone and other organs. Early diagnosis is key to a favorable outcome (Figure 15–11 for a classification of clinical manifestations of prostate cancer).

CLINICAL MANIFESTATIONS OF PROSTATE CANCER

GENITOURINARY	
Dysuria	Hematuria
Frequency of urination	Abnormal prostate on
Reduction in urinary stream	digital rectal examination
Nocturia	
MUSCULOSKELETAL	
Bone or joint pain	Back pain
Migratory bone pain	
NEUROLOGIC	
Nerve pain	Bowel or bladder dysfunction
Bilateral lower	Muscle spasms
extremity weakness	
SYSTEMIC	
Weight loss	Fatigue

Figure 15–11
Some manifestations of prostate cancer.

Treatment depends on the extent of the cancer, which may be inoperable, and hormonal therapy is generally prescribed. Because testosterone stimulates growth of the tumor, removal of the testes—the source of the hormone—may reduce its size. Estrogen, which has an inhibitory effect on the tumor's growth, is administered.

Diseases of the Testes and Epididymis

The testes and epididymis can become inflamed from injury, infection, or some rare tumors that develop in the testes.

Epididymitis   Inflammation of the epididymis (epididymitis) is frequently caused by gonococci, but a urinary tract infection or prostatitis can also be the source of epididymitis. Abscesses sometimes form, and scar tissue develops that can cause sterility if both sides are affected. Symptoms include severe pain in the testes, swelling, and tenderness in the scrotum. Antibiotic treatment is effective when combined with rest and the avoidance of irritants such as alcohol and spicy food.

orchitis
(or-kī'-tĭs)

Orchitis   **Orchitis,** inflammation of the testes, can follow an injury or viral infection such as mumps, with the development of inflammatory edema and pain. The most common cause of orchitis is mumps in an adult man. Swelling of the testes and severe pain usually develop about a week after mumps, an inflammation of the parotid salivary glands. In severe cases, atrophy of the testes can occur, and if both sides are affected, sterility results.

seminoma
(sĕm"-ĭ-nō'-mă)

Testicular Tumors   Tumors of the testes are rare, but when they occur it is usually in young men, and these tumors are highly malignant. One such tumor is the **seminoma,** a cancer of the seminiferous tubules. The seminoma is quite radiosensitive, so the prescribed treatment is irradiation.

teratoma
(tĕr-ă-tō'-mă)

Another tumor of the testes is the **teratoma,** similar in form to the dermoid cyst of the ovary described previously. The teratoma evidently arises from a primitive germ cell, and the tumor contains a variety of tissues. Whereas the dermoid cyst in the ovary is benign, the teratoma of the testes is highly malignant and spreads through the lymphatics and blood vessels. Chemotherapy and radiotherapy are the usual means of treatment.

Impotence   Impotence, the inability of the male to achieve and maintain an erection sufficient for sexual intercourse, is often caused by emotional disturbances. Stress decreases the output of gonadotropic hormones, and, consequently, testosterone production and spermatogenesis are diminished. The dilation of penile arteries that leads to engorgement of the erectile tissue of the penis and then erection is under the control of the autonomic nervous system. Anxiety, fear, and worry are emotions that affect the nervous system. The onset of impotence may be due to fatigue, a form of stress, or distraction.

Impotence may also be physiologic in nature. Arteriosclerosis, inadequate blood flow, diabetes mellitus, surgical complications, urologic disorders, and premature ejaculation are all possible causes. The onset of impotence may be caused by certain medications, drug abuse, or alcoholism; changes in these areas may correct the impotence.

Impotence is said to be primary if the man has never been able to complete intercourse successfully. The inability to maintain an adequate erection may stem from worry about satisfactory sexual performance or from psychological concerns about events in adolescence. Impotence is secondary if intercourse has been achieved successfully at least once.

Whether the cause is psychological or physiological in nature, treatment should be directed toward the source of the problem, which requires openness on the part of the patient with the physician or therapist. The man must be helped to overcome his personal insecurity and frustration, and his partner should also be supported and instructed about the problem. With correct treatment, impotence can usually be overcome. Recently, Viagra has been shown to improve sexual function for some men. Those with heart conditions or other cardiovascular disease should discuss this with their physicians, because of potentially dangerous side effects.

Cryptorchidism   **Cryptorchidism** is not a disease but a failure of the testes to descend from the abdominal cavity, where they develop during fetal life, to the scrotum. This condition should be corrected through surgery or hormonal therapy. Sterility results if this condition is not rectified. Maturation of the sperm cannot occur in the abdominal cavity, where the temperature is slightly higher than that of the scrotum. If the testes are not brought down into the scrotum, they should be removed. Undescended testes atrophy and may become the potential site of cancer.

cryptorchidism
(krĭpt-or′-kĭd-ĭsm)

➤ SEXUALLY TRANSMITTED INFECTIONS (STIs)

The incidence of sexually transmitted infections has increased dramatically in recent years, especially among women and teenagers. If untreated, serious conditions may develop that can gravely affect a person's life. An estimated 1 million women contract pelvic infections each year as a result of undetected STIs. Infected individuals are often asymptomatic and spread the diseases to other sexual partners. Infected women may spread STIs to their offspring during pregnancy and childbirth. Sterility and life-threatening ectopic pregnancies are common complications of sexually transmitted infections.

HIV/Aids

HIV is not only transmitted sexually but can also be acquired as a blood-borne infection. Because the immune system is destroyed by HIV, the disease is discussed in Chapter 2 with Immunity.

Gonorrhea

Gonorrhea is one of the most common and widespread of sexually transmitted infections. It is caused by the bacterium *Neiserria gonorrhoeae,* the gonococcus, and is transmitted through sexual intercourse. Gonococci do not live outside the body, and the organisms are acquired by direct sexual contact with an infected person.

The initial site of infection is the genitals or urethra. Symptoms usually occur within 2 to 8 days of infection. The vaginal glands in the female are frequently affected and fill with pus; the organisms may spread to the cervix. Symptoms of urethritis or cervicitis may be ignored in the female or she may be asymptomatic. The female can be a reservoir for organisms and not be aware that she is infected. Acute urethritis develops in the male, causing difficulty and pain during urination. A copious discharge of pus ensues, and prostatitis frequently develops with abscess formation.

Gonorrhea usually responds rapidly to penicillin but early detection and treatment are extremely important. Diagnosis of gonorrhea is made by examining pus from the urethra or vaginal discharge for the presence of gonococci.

If untreated, a chronic condition develops, and the infection spreads from the initial site of infection. The inflammation causes fibrosis, which can produce a stricture in the male urethra or in the vas deferens. If both vas deferens become stenotic, sterility results.

The fallopian tubes in the female are frequently affected by untreated gonorrhea, and salpingitis results. The pus-filled tubes can empty into the peritoneal cavity, causing peritonitis.

One of the most common causes of pelvic inflammatory disease (PID) is untreated gonorrhea. Chills, fever, and weakness develop with intestinal upset. Chronic pelvic inflammatory disease causes abscesses to develop in the fallopian tubes, with fibrous scarring and sterility resulting. Ectopic pregnancies may also result.

The baby of an infected mother can be born with acute purulent conjunctivitis, inflammation of the conjunctiva. The gonococcal organisms enter the eye during delivery, and if the cornea becomes ulcerated, blindness results. To prevent this infection from developing, a drop of erythromycin is routinely placed in the eyes of newborn babies.

Although penicillin can control gonorrhea, resistant gonococci have evolved. Thus, prevention is key to controlling the spread of gonorrhea. Measures such as condom use or abstinence are effective.

Syphilis

syphilis
(sĭf-ĭ-lĭs)

chancre
(shăng′-kĕr)

Syphilis, commonly called "lues," is a serious STI. The causative bacterium is a spirochete. ***Treponema pallidum,*** transmitted by sexual intercourse or intimate contact with an infectious lesion. The baby of an infected mother may be born syphilitic.

A **chancre,** or ulceration, develops on the genitals in the primary stage of infection. This lesion, which may vary from a small erosion to a deep ulcer, appears within a few days to a few weeks after sexual contact. The chancre usually develops on the vulva of the female and on the penis of the male as shown in Figure 15–12. The chancre may develop elsewhere: on the lips, the tongue, or anus. Anal chancres are common in male homosexuals.

The lesion, which sometimes goes unnoticed, heals after a few weeks. If untreated with penicillin, the secondary phase of the disease occurs in a matter of weeks. The principal sign of the secondary phase is a nonitching rash that affects any part of the body: the trunk, soles of the feet, palms, mouth, vulva, or rectum. The person is still infectious at this stage, but he or she can be treated with penicillin.

An untreated case of syphilis may be dormant for many years, but the organisms remain in the bloodstream and cause a systemic infection known as tertiary syphilis. The

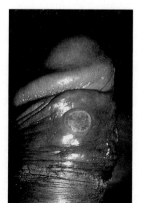

Figure 15–12
Chancre of primary syphilis on the penis.

appearance of symptoms, years after the primary infection, marks the tertiary and most serious phase of syphilis.

The cardiovascular system is severely damaged at this stage of infection. The inflammatory response to the spirochetes in the blood causes fibrosis, scarring, and obstruction of blood vessels, particularly of the aorta. Lesions develop on the cerebral cortex, causing mental disorders, deafness, and blindness. Loss of sensation in the legs and feet due to spinal cord damage cause a characteristic gait to develop. **Paresis,** a general paralysis associated with organic loss of brain function, results in death if untreated. The tertiary lesions of the syphilitic infection are irreversible.

Congenital defects are numerous in an infant born to an infectious mother; mental retardation, physical deformities, deafness, and blindness are common. The syphilitic infection can cause death of the fetus and spontaneous abortion.

The severe consequences of syphilis point out the urgent need for early detection and treatment. Diagnostic procedures include screening tests—the VDRL test perfected by the Venereal Disease Research Laboratory of the United States Public Health Service, and the rapid plasma reagin (RPR) test. The most sensitive and specific test for syphilis is the *Treponema pallidum* immobilization test (TPI), which detects specific antibodies against the spirochete. Treatment with penicillin is successful except in reversing tertiary lesions. Development of resistant strains is a serious threat. As for gonorrhea, the most effective methods for controlling syphilis include the use of a condom or abstention.

paresis
(păr′-ĕ-sĭs)

Genital Herpes

Genital herpes is an extremely painful, viral disease that tends to recur periodically and for which there is no cure. Herpes virus is transmitted by intimate contact between mucous membrane surfaces, the site of herpes virus affinity. There are two types of herpes simplex virus—type I, causing "fever blisters" or "cold sores," and type II, involving the mucous membranes of the genital tracts.

Symptoms generally appear within 3 weeks after exposure to the virus. The symptoms intensify from a burning, itching sensation to severe pain. Multiple blisters appear on the genitalia and at times on the buttocks or thigh. As the blisters rupture, they become secondarily infected and ulcerate. Painful urination and vaginal discharge are common (Figure 15–13).

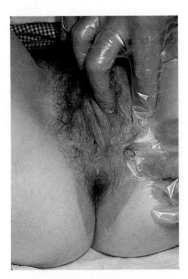

Figure 15–13
Genital herpes blisters as they appear on the labia.

The active phase subsides as the lesions heal, but the virus remains dormant in ganglia until reactivated, perhaps at a time of stress or low resistance. Then, the painful lesions recur.

The disease is transmitted by contact with an active sore that is releasing (shedding) the infectious virus. The virus can be spread from a cold sore on the lips to the genitals; the reverse is also true. Great caution should be used to avoid self-infection of the mucous membrane of the eye.

Use of condoms provides partial protection from transmitting the virus during intercourse, but abstention from sexual contact during the active phase is essential.

Diagnosis is most accurate based on a positive viral culture on living tissue. The Tzanck smear test, which involves examination of lesion fluid, is also available.

There is no cure for a herpes infection, but secondary infections can be prevented and healing promoted. The lesions must be kept clean and dry, and ice-cold compresses may be used to relieve the pain. Prescription medications can control the activation of dormant infections. Examples include acyclovir or AZT.

Active herpes genitalis has very serious consequences during pregnancy, not only causing spontaneous abortion or premature delivery, but also increasing the risk of transmitting the infection to the newborn.

Genital Warts

Genital or venereal warts can develop in both men and women and are caused by a virus in the group called HPV (human papilloma virus), which also causes other types of warts. The warts may appear within weeks after sexual relations—vaginal, anal, or oral—with an infected partner, or they might not develop for several months. In men, the warts occur on the penis or scrotum. In women, the most common site is the peritoneum, but they may occur on the vulva, vaginal opening, or skin of the thighs. The warts may even develop within the vagina and on the cervix.

Genital warts may cause symptoms such as itching or bleeding, although often they are first detected during a physical exam. An abnormal Pap smear might be an indication of human papilloma virus infection. The types of human papilloma virus that cause genital warts are considered as risk factors for cervical cancer when combined with other factors such as multiple sex partners, first intercourse at an early age, and other sexually transmitted infections. Treatment of genital warts depends on their size and number. Some are treated with medication applied by a healthcare provider, but the procedure is very painful. Electrocautery (burning), cryosurgery (freezing), and laser surgery are alternative treatments. Some prescription drugs are now available for home use.

Chlamydial Infections

Chlamydial infections are now the most prevalent STI in the United States. *Chlamydia trachomatis* is the bacterium responsible for sexually transmitted genitourinary infections in both men and women, as well as in newborns of infected mothers. The disease is a leading cause of pelvic inflammatory disease (PID) in women, with resultant infertility, and severe urethritis in both sexes. Women are often asymptomatic carriers of the infection and continue to infect partners and offspring. Improved tests for the diagnosis of chlamydial infection have recently been developed. The disease responds to certain antibiotics but not to penicillin. The infection often coexists with gonorrhea. Again, abstention or condom use are the best methods for controlling Chlamydia.

Disease by the Numbers x + ÷

EPIDEMIOLOGY—HOW COMMON ARE STIs?

According to the Centers for Disease Control and Prevention, which tracks reportable infectious diseases, Chlamydia cases now outnumber gonorrhea. Moreover, Chlamydia is the first among *all* reportable infectious diseases. Second and third among *all* reportable infectious diseases are gonorrhea and HIV. In fact, STIs account for 87% of the top 10 reported diseases.

Chapter Summary

Disease can affect the reproductive system in many ways. In the female, tumors and cysts develop in the ovary, uterus, and breast. Infections invade the vagina and vaginal glands, the fallopian tubes, and the endometrium. Menstrual abnormalities result from a diseased organ or from a hormonal imbalance. A pregnancy can develop in the fallopian tubes, a fetus can be spontaneously aborted, and toxemia can occur in pregnancy.

Diseases of the male affect the prostate gland by infection, enlargement, or tumor formation, causing urinary complications. Infections of the testes and epididymis can result in sterility. Inadequate testosterone secretion affects the male secondary characteristics.

Sexually transmitted infections were discussed. HIV/AIDS, the most devastating disease in today's society, a sexually transmitted but also a blood-borne infection, was discussed in Chapter 2 as a failure of the immune system. Gonorrhea and syphilis have far-reaching consequences if untreated. Early detection of these diseases and administration of penicillin prevent numerous complications providing that a superinfection does not develop. Chlamydial infections, among the most prevalent venereal diseases, responds to certain antibiotics but not to penicillin.

There is no cure for genital herpes, which tends to recur periodically. Types of the human papilloma virus (HPV) that causes genital warts are considered as risk factors for cervical cancer.

Diseases at a Glance:
Unique to Female Reproductive System

Categories	* Disease ❏ Condition ● Disorder	Signs and Symptoms
Malignancies	* Breast cancer	Lump in breast, swollen axillary lymph nodes, breast skin dimpling, nipple retraction
	* Ovarian cancer	Asymptomatic or pelvic pain
	* Cervical cancer	Cellular abnormalities in Pap smear
	* Choriocarcinoma	Enlargement of uterus, often follows hydatiform mole
Infections	* PID (pelvic inflammatory disease)	Fever and pelvic/back pain
	* Salpingitis	Menstrual disturbances, pain, fever
	* Vaginitis	Itching, burning, vaginal discharge
	* Puerperal sepsis	Fever, chills, profuse uterine bleeding, pain in lower abdomen and pelvis
	* Toxic shock syndrome	High fever, rash, skin peeling, reduced blood pressure
Other abnormal structure/function	* Leiomyomas (fibroids)	Abnormal bleeding between periods or excessive bleeding during menstruation
	* Fibrocystic disease	Fluid-filled sacs change in size during menstrual period, may be painful
	❏ Premenstrual syndrome	Abdominal bloating, breast pain, swelling, headache, emotional changes (anxiety, depression)
	* Endometriosis	Pelvic pain, abnormal bleeding, painful menstruation
	* Hydatiform mole	Enlargement of uterus, no fetus present, bleeding
	❏ Amenorrhea	Lack of menstruation
	❏ Menorrhagia	Excessive bleeding in menstruation

Affected Organ/Body Region	Diagnostic Procedures	Treatment
Breast	Mammography, needle biopsy	Lumpectomy, mastectomy, chemotherapy, radiation
Ovaries	Ultrasonography, laparoscopy, biopsy	Surgery, radiation, chemotherapy
Cervix of uterus	Pap smear	Hysterectomy, chemotherapy, radiation
Placental tissue in uterus	CGH in absence of pregnancy	Surgical
Female reproductive system	Microbiological analysis of discharge	Antibiotics, aspirin, bed rest, fluids
Fallopian tubes	Microbiological analysis of discharge	Antibiotics
Vagina	Microbiological analysis of vaginal smears	Varies with cause (protozoal, fungal, bacterial infection)
Uterus	Recent childbirth, microbiological analysis of discharge	Antibiotics
Systemic disease	Physical exam, microbiological analysis	Antibiotics, fluids for shock
Uterus	Ultrasound, laparoscopy	Hysterectomy
Breast	Physical exam, needle aspiration, ultrasound	Dietary changes, regular exams
Systemic	Patient history	Diet changes, stress relief, exercise & counseling
Pelvis, abdomen	Laparoscopy, biopsy	Hormones, surgery
Placenta tissue in uterus	Ultrasound, hormone analysis for CGH	D&C
Ovaries, uterus, pituitary gland	Physical exam, hormone levels	Hormone replacement, dietary change, counseling
Uterus	Patient history, hormone analysis, ultrasound, microbiological analysis	Varies by cause; hormones, tumor removal, antibiotics

Unique to Female Reproductive System (continued)

Categories	* Disease ❑ Condition ● Disorder	Signs and Symptoms
	❑ Metrorrhagia	Bleeding between periods
	❑ Ectopic pregnancy	Intense pain and bleeding upon rupture of fallopian tube
	❑ Spontaneous abortion	Vaginal bleeding, cramping, loss of fetus
	* Toxemia of pregnancy	Headaches, visual disturbances, abdominal pain, vomiting; with progression, hypertension, albuminuria, edema of face and arms, significant weight gain; with eclampsia, convulsions and coma

Unique to Male Reproductive System

Categories	* Disease ❑ Condition ● Disorder	Signs and Symptoms
Malignancies	* Prostate cancer	Enlarged prostate, urinary tract obstruction and infection, pelvic pain later as bone is involved
	* Seminoma (malignant)	Abnormal lump upon palpation
	* Teratoma (malignant)	Abnormal lump upon palpation
Infections	* Prostatitis	Pain and burning upon urination
	* Epididymitis	Severe pain in testes, swelling, tenderness in scrotum
Inflammations	❑ Benign prostatic hyperplasia	Difficulty starting and maintaining urine stream, frequency, nocturia, urinary infection more common
	* Orchitis	Swelling and severe pain in testes after mumps
Other abnormal structure/function	● * Impotence	Inability to achieve and maintain erection
	❑ Cryptorchidism	Failure of testes to descend normally from abdominal cavity into scrotum

Affected Organ/Body Region	Diagnostic Procedures	Treatment
Uterus	Patient history, hormone analysis, microbiological analysis	D&C
Fallopain tubes	Patient history; ultrasound if suspected before crisis	Surgery
Uterus	Physical exam	D&C, hormones in habitual miscarriage
Systemic disease	Prenatal care physical examinations	Early intervention; low-salt diet, low-calorie diet, diuretics

Affected Organ/Body Region	Diagnostic Procedures	Treatment
Prostate	Rectal exam, biopsy	Hormone therapy, removal of testes, surgery
Seminiferous tubules of testicles	Palpation, biopsy	Radiation
Testicles	Palpation, biopsy	Chemotherapy and radiation
Prostate	Microbiological analysis of discharges	Penicillin, other antibiotics
Epididymis	Microbiological analysis of discharges	Antibiotics, rest
Prostate	Rectal examination, ultrasound	Surgery, drug treatment
Testicles	History of infection	Anti-inflammatory drugs
Penis	Patient history	Altered medications, counseling, Viagra
Testes, inguinal canal	Palpation of scrotum	Surgical correction

STIs Affecting Both Male & Female

Categories	* Disease ❑ Condition ● Disorder	Signs and Symptoms
Infections	* Gonorrhea	Male: acute urethritis, painful urination, urethral discharge Female: urethritis, cervicitis, or asymptomatic
	* Syphilis	Primary: painless chancres at infection site, chancres heal Secondary: non-itching rash on trunk, palms, soles Tertiary: Gumma formation, destruction of brain blood vessels, other organs
	* Genital herpes	Painful blister at infection site, painful urination, secondary infections common
	* Genital warts	Painful growths on skin or mucous membranes, itching and bleeding, secondary infections
	* Chlamydia	No or few symptoms, or urethritis with painful urination and urethral discharge
Other abnormal structure/function	❑ Sterility	Male: failure to produce sperm Female: failure to ovulate

Affected Organ/Body Region	Diagnostic Procedures	Treatment
Reproductive system	Microbiological analysis of pus or vaginal discharge	Penicillin (except for antibiotic-resistant strains)
Starts in reproductive system, develops into systemic disease	VDRL test, RPR test, TPI test	Penicillin
External genitalia, mouth	Positive viral culture in live tissue; Tzanck smear test	Acyclovir, AZT, not curable
External genitalia, perineum, anus, mouth	Physical exam; HPV detected by abnormal Pap smear	Medication, electrocautery, cryosurgery, laser surgery
Reproductive system	Tissue culture, antigen detection	Antibiotics (penicillin not effective)
Male: testes Female: ovaries	Male: Semen analysis Female: Basal body temperature, cervical mucus exam, endometrial biopsy	Male: none Female: hormones

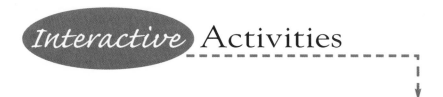

Interactive Activities

CASE FOR CRITICAL THINKING

A young woman reports severe pain and cramping in her lower abdomen. Laparoscopic examination found ectopic endometrial tissue on the uterine wall and ovaries. Name this disease. What is meant by ectopic endometrial tissue? She was prescribed oral contraceptives. Why would these be useful?

MULTIMEDIA EXTENSION ACTIVITIES

www.prenhall.com/mulvihill
Use the above address to access the free, interactive companion Website created for this textbook. Included in the features of this site are chapter specific activities, internet links, and an audio-glossary.

Audio Glossary
Use the CD-ROM disk enclosed with your textbook to hear the pronunciation of the key terms in this chapter.

Diseases at a Glance:
Reproductive Systems

Use the chart on page(s) 328–333 to answer the following questions.

1. List 5 types of diseases or conditions that affect the reproductive systems.

2. What are the major signs and symptoms of the diseases or conditions you named?

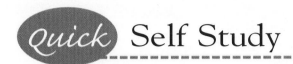 Self Study

MULTIPLE CHOICE

1. Which is the most common tumor among females?
   a. ovarian cysts
   b. breast cancer
   c. uterine leiomyomas
   d. cervical cancer

2. Diseases are matched to descriptions. Which match is *INCORRECT?*
   a. recurrent painful sores on genitals: genital herpes
   b. watery discharge from urethra: Chlamydia infection
   c. transmission to newborns can cause blindness: gonorrhea
   d. caused by *Treponema pallidum:* genital warts

3. Which is *FALSE* about syphilis?
   a. sores of primary syphilis may disappear and heal with no scars
   b. a fetus can be affected and born with major physical and mental abnormalities
   c. mental confusion may be part of tertiary syphilis
   d. secondary syphilis is characterized by gummas that form in several organs

4. Which disease can lead to pelvic inflammatory disease and sterility?
   a. gonorrhea
   b. cystitis
   c. prostatitis
   d. herpes

TRUE/FALSE

_____T____ 1. Pelvic inflammatory disease can lead to infertility

_____F____ 2. The Pap smear detects endometriosis.

_____F____ 3. Family history is not a risk factor for breast cancer.

_____F____ 4. Herpes simplex virus causes syphilis.

FILL-INS

1. Fluid-filled sacs in breast tissue are signs of _____ disease.

2. After mumps, some males experience _____, a painful swelling of the testes.

3. The most prevalent reportable sexually transmitted infection is ___gon_____.

4. Human papilloma virus infection is strongly associated with __uterian_____ cancer.

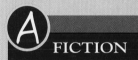 **FICTION**

STIs are serious diseases and some, such as gonorrhea, are difficult to treat because the bacteria have acquired antibiotic resistance.

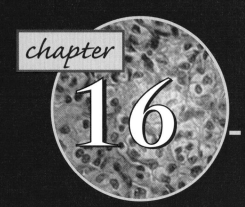

16

Diseases of the Nervous System

The body is constantly subjected to changes in its internal and external environment. The body's response is to react appropriately to these changing conditions. How is this response accomplished unconsciously?

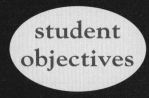

student objectives

After studying this chapter, students should be able to

➤ Recognize the normal structures and functions of the nervous system, including the meninges and the blood-brain barrier

➤ List and describe demyelination diseases of the nervous system

➤ Recognize and describe infectious diseases of the nervous system, listing their causes, symptoms, and effects

➤ List and describe degenerative diseases of the nervous system

➤ Identify and describe inherited and congenital diseases of the nervous system

➤ Describe a seizure, and recognize diseases involving seizures

➤ List and describe the effects of trauma in the nervous system

➤ Identify the causes and effects of CVA (strokes)

➤ List and describe prevention, diagnosis, and treatment of diseases of the nervous system

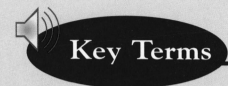

Key Terms

Amyotrophic

Anaerobic

Aneurysms

Antitoxin

Aphasia

Astrocytoma

Aura

Basal ganglia

Bradykinesia

Cerebrospinal

Concussion

Contusion

Dementia

Dopamine

Electroencephalogram

Electromyogram

Encephalitis

Endarterectomy

Epidural

Epilepsy

Extradural

Glioblastomas

Gliomas

Hemiplegia

Huntington's chorea

Hydrocephalus

Lumbar puncture

Meninges

Meningitis

Meningocele

Meningomyelocele

Myelin

Myelocele

Nystagmus

Palsy

Pathologic aspiration

Petit mal

Poliomyelitis

Rabies

Reye's syndrome

Seizures

Shingles

Spina bifida

Strabismus

Stroke

Subarachnoid

Subdural

Tetanus toxoid

myelin
(mī′-ĕ-lĭn)

➤ STRUCTURAL ORGANIZATION OF THE NERVOUS SYSTEM

The basic organization of a very complex nervous system includes two major sections: the central nervous system (CNS) and the peripheral nervous system (PNS). The CNS is composed of the brain and spinal cord. The PNS comprises all those nerves outside the CNS, beginning with the 12 pairs of cranial nerves and the 31 pairs of spinal nerves that connect the spinal cord to other innervated parts of the body.

The basic unit of the nervous system is the neuron or nerve cell. The neuron consists of a cell body and long filamentous extensions or fibers and a single axon leading from the cell body. A neuron is shown in Figure 16–1. Some neurons are sensory nerve cells, capable of detecting environmental changes and transmitting messages to the brain or spinal cord. Other neurons, the motor neurons, convey messages from the central nervous system to muscles causing contraction, or to glands, triggering secretion. The fibers of sensory and motor neurons are insulated by a lipid covering called the **myelin** sheath, which facilitates the rate of transmission of an impulse. Deterioration of this sheath is characteristic of multiple sclerosis, a disease to be described.

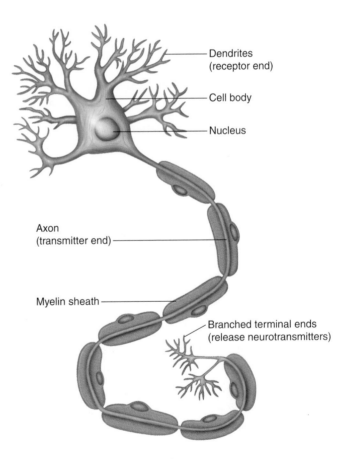

Figure 16–1
Typical neuron.

The Brain

The largest portion of the brain is the cerebrum, or cerebral hemispheres. The surface is highly convoluted with many elevations and depressions. The outer surface of the brain, the cortex, consists of gray matter, where nerve cell bodies are concentrated. The inner area consists of white matter, the nerve fiber tracts. Deep within the white matter are concentrations of nerve cell bodies known as **basal ganglia,** which help control position and automatic movements. It is the basal ganglia (also gray matter) that are affected in Parkinson's disease.

Within the brain are four spaces called ventricles where cerebrospinal fluid is formed, which are continuous with the central canal of the spinal cord. This fluid, derived from plasma, flows out of the ventricles through small openings and is channeled to circulate over the brain and spinal cord. It flows under the arachnoid covering, acting as a watery, protective cushion. Cerebrospinal fluid is reabsorbed into the venous sinuses of the dura mater, and new fluid is formed. Obstruction of cerebrospinal fluid circulation results in hydrocephalus, which will be described.

basal ganglia
(bā'-săl
găng'-glē-ă)

The Spinal Cord

The spinal cord is housed within the vertebral column and is continuous with the brain stem (Figure 16–2). Numerous tracts of nerve fibers within the cord ascend to and descend from the brain, carrying messages destined for muscles and glands. Three coverings, the **meninges,** protect the delicate nerve tissue. The innermost covering is the pia mater, the middle layer is the arachnoid, and the toughest, outermost covering is the dura mater. Meningitis is an inflammation of these coverings that also surround the brain.

meninges
(měn-ĭn'-jēz)

The Autonomic Nervous System

Another component of the nervous system is the autonomic nervous system. This system controls internal functioning of the body. The autonomic nervous system contains the sympathetic and the parasympathetic nervous systems, which often work antagonistically to each other. The hypothalamus, located within the brain, controls activity for a large portion of the autonomic nervous system, but it is also affected by other parts of the central nervous system.

The autonomic nervous system controls arterial blood pressure, heart rate, gastrointestinal functions, sweating, temperature regulation, and many other involuntary actions. Whereas the peripheral nerves affect skeletal or voluntary muscle, the autonomic nervous system acts on smooth or involuntary muscle and cardiac muscle. Diseases of the digestive system such as stress—ulcers, regional enteritis, and ulcerative colitis (Chapter 11) are influenced by the autonomic nervous system.

The Sensory Nervous System

Sensations detected by sensory neurons in the skin, muscles, tendons, or internal organs are transmitted to the spinal cord, where they may trigger a simple reflex response. A synapse is made with a motor neuron that will bring about an action. More complex responses require that the impulse be sent to various parts of the brain. Impulses reaching the brain stem and cerebellum bring about many unconscious automatic actions, but sensory information involving thought processes must reach the highest area of the brain, the cerebral cortex.

The cerebral cortex has specialized areas to receive sensory information from all parts of the body, such as the feet, the hands, or the abdomen. These areas are just pos-

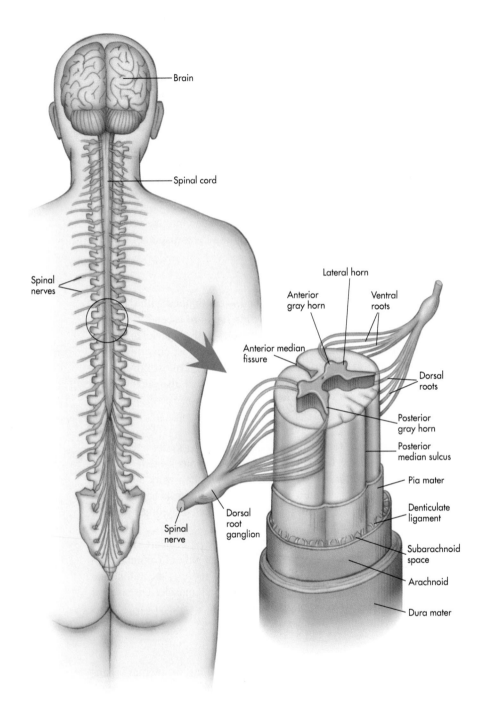

Figure 16–2
The brain, spinal cord, and spinal nerves. An expanded view of the spinal cord is shown.

terior to the central sulcus. Visual impulses are transmitted to the posterior part of the brain, whereas olfactory and auditory impulses are received in the lateral parts. Association areas of the brain interpret deeper meaning of the sensations, and all the sensory messages are integrated in the "knowing area" where they may be stored as memory. Creative thought becomes possible through use of all sensory input.

The Motor Nervous System

Just as the cerebral cortex has areas specialized for the reception of sensory information, there are areas that govern motor activity. The primary motor cortex, anterior to the central sulcus, controls discrete movements of skeletal muscles. Because the nerve fibers cross over in the medulla and/or spinal cord, stimulation on one side of the cerebral cortex affects particular muscles on the opposite side of the body.

Anterior to the primary motor cortex is the premotor cortex, which controls coordinated movements of muscles. This process is accomplished by stimulating groups of muscles that work together. Also the speech area is located here and is usually on the left side in right-handed people. Specialized areas of the brain are shown in Figure 16–3.

Damage to any part of the brain from trauma, hemorrhage, blood clot formation with subsequent ischemia, or infection will have varying effects on motor responses depending on the degree of injury and the location of the lesion.

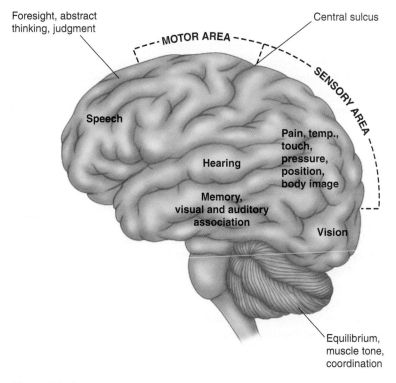

Figure 16–3
Specialized areas of the brain.

➤ DISEASES OF THE NERVOUS SYSTEM

The nervous system is affected by disease in numerous ways. For example, bacteria and viruses can invade the system and cause infection. Degeneration of nerve tissue can lead to disease. Seizures result from abnormal transmission of neuronal impulses in the brain. Errors in fetal development are responsible for other neural disorders. The brain may be damaged by trauma, cerebral hemorrhages, blood clot formation, and tumors. Many diseases of the nervous system manifest themselves in abnormal muscular activity.

---

on the Practical Side

Drugs and the Nervous System: "Uppers" and "Downers"

Amphetamines, known as "uppers," "pep pills," and "speed," are stimulants to the central nervous system. They are subject to abuse as they produce wakefulness and euphoria, but they also produce a dangerous dependency. Amphetamines are sometimes used in "diet pills" to suppress appetite, but they are ineffective for weight reduction. Appetite returns when the pills are discontinued, lost weight is regained, and it is difficult to get off the pills. Abuse of amphetamines can lead to compulsive behavior, paranoia, hallucinations, and suicidal tendencies.

Barbiturates, or "downers," are sedatives or hypnotics and depress the central nervous system. Blood pressure and body temperature are depressed, and the drugs become addictive.

Infectious Diseases of the Nervous System

Many diseases are neurotropic in that the causative agent, a virus or bacterium, has an affinity for the nervous system. Most viruses in this class affect the nerve tissue directly, whereas the toxin produced by bacteria is the offending agent in another neural disease.

Infectious neural diseases have numerous causes, such as a systemic infection, a contaminated puncture wound from a dog, or insect bite, or exposure to chicken pox.

meningitis
(měn"-ĭn-jī'-tĭs)

Meningitis **Meningitis** is an acute inflammation of the first two meninges that cover the brain and spinal cord, the pia mater and the arachnoid. It is a disease usually affecting children and young adults and may have serious complications if not diagnosed and treated early. There are many forms of meningitis, some being more contagious than others. The most common causative organism is the *Neisseria meningitidis,* but other bacteria, as well as viruses, may cause meningitis.

The infecting organisms can reach the meninges from the middle ear, upper respiratory tract, or frontal sinuses; or they can be carried in the blood from the lungs or other infected sites. Healthy children may be carriers of the bacteria and spread the organisms by sneezing or coughing. Viral meningitis may be caused by mumps, polio viruses, and occasionally by herpes simplex.

The *symptoms* of meningitis are high fever, chills, and a severe headache caused by increased intracranial pressure. The person has a very stiff neck and holds the head rigidly. Any movement of neck muscles stretches the meninges and increases the pain. Nausea, vomiting, and a rash may also be symptomatic. The high fever often causes delirium and convulsions in children, and they may lapse into a coma.

lumbar puncture
(lŭm'-băr
pŭnk'-chŭr)

Diagnosis of meningitis is made by performing a **lumbar puncture** (Figure 16–4) or spinal tap, in which a hollow needle is inserted into the spinal canal between verte-

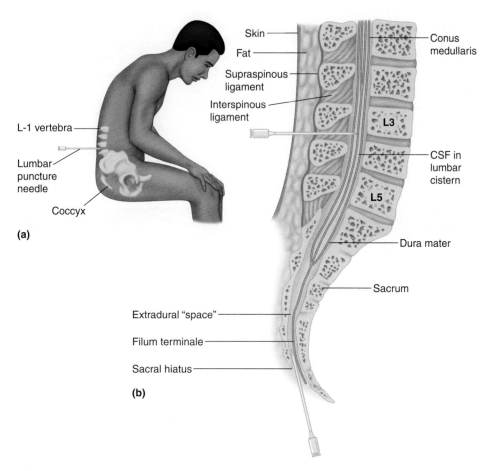

Skin
Fat
Supraspinous ligament
Interspinous ligament
L-1 vertebra
Lumbar puncture needle
Coccyx
(a)
Conus medullaris
L3
CSF in lumbar cistern
L5
Dura mater
Sacrum
Extradural "space"
Filum terminale
Sacral hiatus
(b)

Figure 16–4
(a) Shows lumbar puncture, also known as spinal tap. (b) Section of the vertebral column showing the spinal cord and membranes. A lumbar puncture needle is shown at L3-4 and in the sacral hiatus.

brae near L-4 in the lumbar region. This procedure is possible because the spinal cord terminates at or near the first lumbar vertebra although a sac containing cerebrospinal fluid extends down to the sacrum. Increased pressure of the cerebrospinal fluid with an elevated protein level, numerous polymorphs, and infecting organisms confirms the diagnosis of meningitis. The level of glucose in the cerebrospinal fluid is below normal because the bacteria use the sugar for their own growth.

The *prognosis* depends on the cause of meningitis and prompt treatment. Treatment with antibiotics is very effective if the meningitis is bacterial. If not treated, permanent brain damage usually results, manifesting itself by sight or hearing loss, paralysis, mental retardation or death. The opening in the roof of the fourth ventricle may become blocked by the pyogenic infection. This blockage results in the accumulation of cerebrospinal fluid in the brain causing a form of **hydrocephalus** (Figure 16–5 and 16–6).

Encephalitis **Encephalitis,** an inflammation of the brain and meninges, is caused by a viral infection. The virus may be harbored by wild birds and transmitted to man by mosquitoes. There are many forms of the disease, and they may occur in epidemics. Lethargic encephalitis, or "sleeping sickness," is one type of encephalitis in which

hydrocephalus
(hī″-drō-sĕf′-ă-lŭs)

encephalitis
(ĕn-sĕf″-ă-lī′-tĭs)

side by side

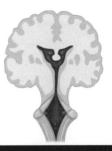

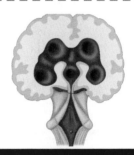

Figure 6–5	Figure 6–6
Normal ventricles.	Enlarged ventricles.

persistent drowsiness, delirium, and sometimes result in coma. Symptoms of encephalitis range from mild to severe and may include headache, fever, cerebral dysfunction, disordered thought patterns, and, often, seizures. Secondary encephalitis may develop from viral childhood diseases, such as chicken pox, measles, and mumps.

Diagnosis of encephalitis is made by lumbar puncture. Treatment is essentially aimed at the symptoms, control of the high fever, maintenance of fluid and electrolyte balance, and careful monitoring of respiratory and kidney function.

In serious cases involving extensive brain damage, convalescence is slow and requires prolonged physical rehabilitation. Nerve damage may cause paralysis. Personality changes occur as well as emotional disturbances requiring therapy. Amphetamines may be used to challenge lethargy and drowsiness.

poliomyelitis
(pōl″-ĭ-ō-mī″-ĕl-ī′-tĭs)

Poliomyelitis **Poliomyelitis,** once a crippling and killing disease that primarily struck children, has nearly been eradicated through the development of the Salk and Sabin vaccines. Immunization programs were designed to assure that all children were protected.

Polio is an infectious disease of the brain and spinal cord caused by a virus. Motor neurons of the medulla oblongata and of the spinal cord are primarily affected, and without motor nerve stimulations, muscles become paralyzed. If the respiratory muscles are affected, artificial means of respiration are required.

Symptoms of poliomyelitis are stiff neck, fever, headache, sore throat, and gastrointestinal disturbances. When diagnosed and treated early, severe damage to the nervous system is prevented.

The tremendous value of Dr. Jonas Salk's vaccine to prevent poliomyelitis cannot be measured. Salk used inactivated polio virus, injected intramuscularly, which stimulated production of antibodies against polio. The decrease in the number of polio cases with the institution of immunization programs was immediate. Dr. Albert Sabin developed an oral vaccine against polio that is more convenient to administer, particularly to large groups, and is extremely effective. The Sabin vaccine, because it is taken orally, stimulates the production of antibodies within the digestive system, where the viruses first reside. Destruction of the viruses in the digestive system prevents their transmission and eliminates carriers, which the Salk vaccine does not do. Many researchers believe, however, that the Salk vaccine is the better choice because the use of killed virus ensures a zero contraction rate for polio. The Centers for Disease Control and Prevention has recommended a combination of Sabin/Salk vaccine. It may be worthwhile to consult a physician about treatment options.

Polio has essentially been eliminated in the U.S., although worldwide the problem of polio still exists. Consequently, it is important to immunize people to prevent them from contracting and spreading this dreaded disease. Between 1988 and 1998, however, polio declined 85% worldwide. Those who survive paralytic polio may show excessive fatigue, muscular weakness, pain, and other difficulty some 20 to 30 years after the onset of the disease. This condition, known as post polio syndrome (PPS), has recently led to major disruptions in careers and lifestyle. Currently, rest seems to be the only relief for this debilitating disease.

Rabies **Rabies** is primarily a disease of warm-blooded animals such as dogs, cats, raccoons, skunks, wolves, foxes, and bats; but it can be transmitted to humans through bites or scratches from a rabid animal. Rabies is an infectious disease of the brain and spinal cord caused by a virus that is transmitted by the secretions (saliva) of an infected animal.

The virus passes from the wound along nerves to the spinal cord and brain where it causes acute encephalomyelitis. The incubation period is long, 40 to 60 days or more, depending on the severity of the wound and the distance of the wound from the brain. Bites on the face, neck, and hands are most serious. The mode of tetanus and rabies transmission to the central nervous system is illustrated in Figure 16–7.

rabies
(rā′-bēz)

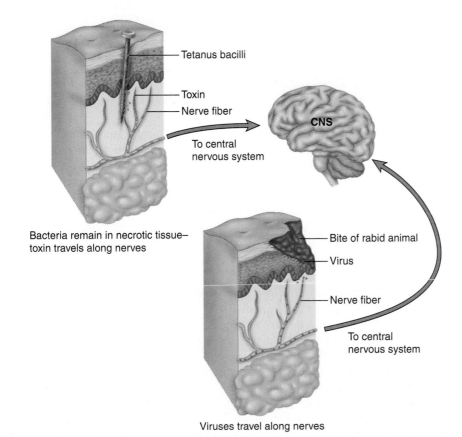

Figure 16–7
Nerve involvement in tetanus and rabies.

Symptoms of rabies include fever, pain, mental derangement, rage, convulsions, and paralysis. The muscles of the throat go into spasm at the sight of water, and the person is unable to drink. Hydrophobia is an aversion to water related to rabies. Because of the inability to swallow, a profuse, sticky saliva that is secreted.

The disease is fatal in humans once it reaches the central nervous system and the symptoms described have developed. A series of antirabies injections must be administered before the virus reaches the brain.

In the case of an animal bite, it is extremely important to know if the animal is rabid; thus, investigation of the animal must be made whenever possible. If rabies is suspected, immunization injections are started on the infected person. The person receives repeated injections of an altered virus to stimulate antibody production and an immune serum to provide passive immunity.

The severity of rabies explains the critical need for the vaccination of dogs and cats against the disease. Certain signs indicate that an animal is rabid. The animal goes through several stages, the first of which is an anxiety stage manifested by a change of temperament. As an example, wild animals may act friendly. A furious stage follows in which the animal bites at everything. When paralysis of the throat occurs, the animal cannot swallow, and it foams at the mouth. The last stage of rabies is called the dumb stage. The animal appears to have something caught in the throat but makes no attempt to remove it, and death then follows.

shingles
(shĭng'-lz)

Shingles *(Herpes Zoster)*   **Shingles** is an acute inflammation of nerve cells caused by the chicken pox virus, herpes zoster. It is manifested by pain and a rash characterized by small water blisters surrounded by a red area. The lesions follow a sensory nerve, forming a zone toward the midline of the torso. The rash is generally confined to one side of the body and does not cross the midline. The optic nerve can be affected, causing severe conjunctivitis. If not properly treated, ulcerations can form on the cornea and results in scarring. The lesions dry up and become encrusted. The lesions cause severe itching, pain, and scarring.

Shingles can develop from exposure to a person with shingles in the infectious stage. It may also develop from exposure to chicken pox with an incubation period of about 2 weeks. It sometimes accompanies other diseases, such as pneumonia or tuberculosis. Shingles may also result from trauma or reaction to certain drug injections. If there has been no known exposure to the virus, it is theorized that the chicken pox virus may be dormant in the body for a time and then reactivated.

Treatment of shingles is directed toward alleviating the symptoms to relieve the pain and itchiness. Lotions such as calamine are often prescribed. Glucocorticoids may also be prescribed to suppress the inflammatory reaction.

Reye's syndrome
(rīz sĭn'-drōm)

Reye's Syndrome   **Reye's syndrome** is a potentially devastating neurologic illness that sometimes develops in young children after a viral infection. Viruses associated with Reye's syndrome include Epstein-Barr, influenza B, and varicella, which causes chicken pox. There is a negative link between these viral infections and the use of aspirin. Tylenol is preferred in these cases. The actual cause of the disease is unknown.

Manifestations of Reye's syndrome include persistent vomiting, often a rash, and lethargy about 1 week after a viral infection. Neurologic dysfunction can progress from confusion to seizures and coma. The encephalopathy includes cerebral swelling with elevated intracranial pressure.

Management is geared toward lowering intracranial pressure. Meticulous monitoring of all vital functions is essential with correction of any imbalances. Blood gases and blood pH also must be analyzed.

The outcome is very satisfactory when diagnosed early and proper therapy is given. The recovery rate is about 85% to 90%.

Tetanus Most people are familiar with the need for a tetanus shot after a puncture wound or an animal bite. Why are these wounds particularly dangerous?

Tetanus, commonly called "lockjaw," is an infection of nerve tissue caused by the rod-like tetanus bacillus that lives in the intestines of animals and human beings. The organisms are excreted in fecal material and persist as spores indefinitely in the soil. The bacilli are prevalent in rural areas and in garden soil fertilized with manure. Fecal remains (manure) especially from horse farms or race tracks (urban) are major locations for potential tetanus.

The organism that enters the wound with dirt remains in the wound. This organism flourishes in the necrotic tissue of a pus infection and in the absence of oxygen. Deep wounds with ragged, lacerated tissue contaminated with fecal material are the most dangerous type. The bacillus produces a powerful toxin that migrates to the nerves (Figure 16–7). The toxin becomes anchored to motor nerve cells and stimulates them, which in turn stimulate muscles.

Muscles become rigid, and painful spasms and convulsions develop. The jaw muscles are often the first to be affected, hence the name lockjaw. These muscles cannot relax, and the mouth is tightly closed. The neck is stiff, and swallowing becomes difficult. If the muscles of respiration are affected, asphyxiation occurs. Death can result from even a minor wound if the condition is not treated.

Tetanus has an incubation period ranging from 1 week to a few weeks. The toxin travels slowly, so the distance from the wound to the spinal cord is significant. Treatment includes a thorough cleansing of the wound, removal of dead tissue and any foreign substance. Immediate immunization to inactivate the toxin before it reaches the spinal cord is crucial.

The type of immunization administered depends on the patient's history. If the patient has had no previous immunization, tetanus **antitoxin** is given. If 5 years have elapsed since the previous tetanus injection, the person receives a booster injection of **tetanus toxoid** to increase the antitoxin level.

Additional treatment includes the administration of antibiotics to prevent secondary infections and the use of sedatives to decrease the frequency of convulsions. Oxygen under high pressure is also used as the bacillus is **anaerobic,** that is, it thrives in the absence of oxygen.

Tetanus may be prevented by adequate immunization. Tetanus toxoid, which stimulates antibody formation, should be given to infants and small children at prescribed times. This inoculation may be done in combination with diphtheria toxoid and pertussis vaccine, which prevents whooping cough.

Abscess of the Brain Pyogenic organisms such as streptococci, staphylococci, and *E. coli* can travel to the brain from other infected areas and cause a brain abscess. Infections of the middle ear, skull bones, or sinuses, as well as pneumonia and endocarditis are potential sources for brain abscess. Figure 16–8 shows abscesses of the brain.

The symptoms of brain abscess may be misleading. The individual has a fever and headache caused by increased intracranial pressure, which can suggest a tumor. Analysis of the cerebrospinal fluid shows increased pressure and the presence of neutrophils and lymphocytes, indicating infection.

Once the diagnosis of a brain abscess has been made, the abscess must be opened surgically and drained, and the patient must be treated with antibiotics. Brain abscesses are not as common today because the spread of most infections is checked by antibiotics.

antitoxin
(ăn″-tĭ-tŏk′sĭn)

tetanus toxoid
(tĕt′-ă-nŭs
tŏks′-oyd)

anaerobic
(ăn″-ĕr-ō′bĭk)

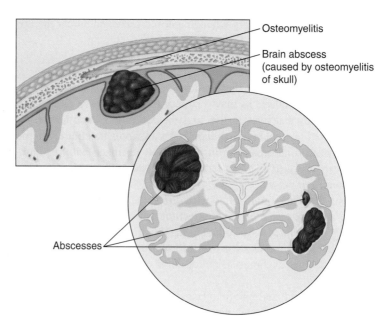

Figure 16–8
Abscesses of the brain.

Degenerative Neural Diseases

Some diseases of the nervous system involve the degeneration of nerves and brain tissue. Abnormalities in muscle function result from neural degeneration.

Multiple Sclerosis   Multiple sclerosis (MS) is a major disorder of the central nervous system. It is a chronic, progressive disease of unknown origin. Possible causes that have been studied are viruses or immunologic reaction to a virus, bacteria, trauma, autoimmunity, and heredity, but the findings of this research have remained inconclusive.

At first, the disease manifests itself by muscle impairment. The person experiences a loss of balance and poor coordination. Tingling and numbing sensations progress to a shaking tremor and muscular weakness. The person has difficulty in speaking clearly, and bladder dysfunction frequently develops.

Vision may suddenly be impaired, and double vision frequently occurs. Lesions on the optic nerve can lead to blindness. The person may have **nystagmus,** an involuntary, rapid movement of the eyeball. Emotional changes may also accompany the disease.

 nystagmus
(nĭs-tăg′-mŭs)

Multiple sclerosis usually affects young adults between the ages of 20 and 40. The disease is difficult to diagnose in the early stages, as many disorders of the nervous system have similar symptoms. It is characterized by periods of remissions and exacerbations and progresses at very different rates.

The degeneration of nerve tissue in MS involves a breaking up of the neuronal myelin sheath due to chronic inflammation. Therefore, patchy areas of demyelination appear and become sclerotic. Because the myelin sheath protects the neuron and acts as an insulator to promote the velocity of nerve impulse transmission, the degeneration of myelin impairs nerve conduction. MRI (magnetic resonance imaging) demonstrates plaques of demyelination of nerve fibers.

To date, there is no effective treatment for MS. Physical therapy enables the person to use the muscles that are operable. Muscle relaxants help reduce spasticity, and steroids are often helpful. Psychological counseling is advantageous in dealing with the emotional changes brought about by the disease.

Another degenerative disorder that attacks the myelin sheath of nerves is Tay-Sachs disease. This inheritable disease involves a metabolic breakdown whereby particular chemicals known as gangliosides, which are necessary for proper neuron membrane integrity, are not handled properly. This error of lipid metabolism causes an accumulation of materials (sphingolipids) that result in the deterioration of the neurons. The specific cellular organelle involved is the lysosome. The corrupted lysosomes lack a particular enzyme (hexosaminidase A). This enzyme is necessary to metabolize a special binding lipid found in relatively high concentrations in the nervous system. Tay-Sachs disease tends to afflict the Ashkenazi Jewish population of Eastern Europe descent and is fatal by about the age of 4.

With MS there is an erosion of the myelin membrane or demyelination, but in Tay-Sachs disease there is an accumulation of unwanted material that causes a lack of nervous control/function. In both cases, the myelin membrane is involved, and the impulse capability of the nerve is impaired.

Amyotrophic Lateral Sclerosis (ALS)   **Amyotrophic** lateral sclerosis, also known as Lou Gehrig's disease, is a chronic, terminal neurologic disease in which there is a progressive loss of motor neurons. Cause of the disease is not known. ALS is characterized by disturbances in motility and atrophy of muscles of the hands, forearms, and legs because of degeneration of neurons in the ventral horns of the spinal cord. Also affected are certain cranial nerves, particularly the hypoglossal, trigeminal, and facial nerves, which impair muscles of the mouth and throat. Swallowing and tongue movements are affected, and speech becomes difficult or impossible. ALS occurs later in life, most commonly in the 50s and 60s, and is slightly more common in men than in women.

ALS is diagnosed by an **electromyogram** (EMG), which shows reduction in the number of motor units active with muscle contraction. Also observed are fasciculations; the spontaneous, uncontrolled discharges of motor neurons seen as irregular twitchings.

ALS requires early education of the patient and the patient's family so that a proper management system may be provided to anticipate and prevent certain hazards. Specifically, the prevention of upper airway obstruction and **pathologic aspiration,** drawing of vomitus or mucus into the respiratory tract. Aspiration can occur from weakened respiratory musculature and an ineffective cough. Death usually occurs within 3 to 4 years after onset of symptoms and generally results from pulmonary failure. However, as the renowned British scientist Stephen Hawkings attests, survivorship of ALS does vary.

Parkinson's Disease (PD)   Parkinson's Disease, also known as shaking **palsy,** is a disease of brain degeneration that appears gradually and progresses slowly. It is a chronic disabling disease that usually develops late in life. Early symptoms include mild tremors of the hands and a nodding movement of the head. Because postural reflexes are lost, the person is likely to fall frequently.

As the disease progresses, muscular movements become slower and more difficult. The stiffness of the muscles affects the facial expressions, making them rigid and masklike. A characteristic tremor develops in the fingers, referred to as a pill-rolling tremor. This tremor disappears with voluntary movement of the hands. The posture is stooped. The forward-leaning position causes a peculiar shuffling gait to maintain balance.

Three obvious signs of Parkinson's disease are **bradykinesia** (slowness of movement), tremor, and rigidity. Actions that were once automatic become deliberate. Experts recommend frequent brief rests, moving slowly, and learning how to manage difficult

amyotrophic
(ă-mī″-ō-trŏf′-ĭk)

electromyogram
(ē-lĕk″-trō-mī′-ō-grăm)

**pathologic
aspiration**
(păth-ō-lŏj′-ĭk
ăs-pĭ-rā′-shŭn)

palsy
(pawl′-zē)

bradykinesia
(brăd″-ē-kĭ-nē′-sē-ă)

movements, such as descending stairs. The most important factor is prescribed exercise to maintain flexibility, motility, and mental well-being. Relaxation is particularly important for PD patients because stressful situations worsen the condition. Figure 16–9 summarizes possible effects of PD.

dopamine
(dō'-pă-mēn)

The degeneration of nerve cells occurs in the basal ganglia, the nerve centers responsible for regulation of certain involuntary body movements. It has been discovered that a neuronal transmitter substance, **dopamine,** is inadequately produced. Treatment includes the administration of L-dopa, a substance that is converted to dopamine in the brain. Although the drug therapy does not stop the neuronal degeneration, the symptoms are improved. The drug is not recommended for individuals with a history of mental disorders or cardiovascular disease. Alcohol consumption should be limited because alcohol acts antagonistically to L-dopa.

Physical therapy, including heat and massage, helps reduce muscle cramps and relieve tension headaches caused by the rigidity of neck muscles. The person is aided by psychological support while learning to cope with the disability. Additionally, a new method of "deep brain stimulation" with electrodes implanted into the thalamus is showing promise. The person may turn on or off the "pulse generator," a small pacemaker-like-device implanted under the collarbone, by passing a magnet over it.

The cause of Parkinson's disease in unknown, but a hereditary factor may be involved.

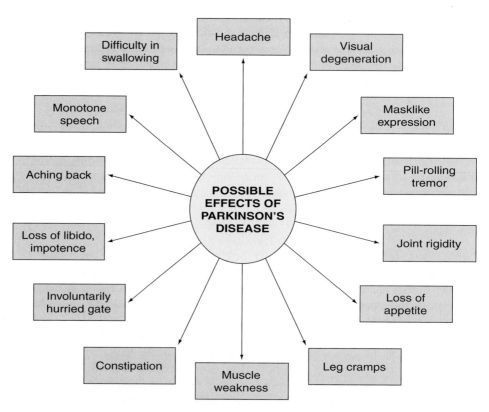

Figure 16–9
Summary of Parkinson's disease effects.

Huntington's Disease (Huntington's Chorea) Huntington's disease is an inherited disease, but symptoms may not appear until middle age. If either parent has the disease, all their children will have a 50% chance of inheriting it. (See Chapter 5 for the manner of transmission). **Huntington's chorea** is a progressive degenerative disease of the brain that results in the loss of muscle control. The word *chorea* means ceaseless, rapid, jerky movements, which are involuntary—an appropriate description of Huntington's symptoms. Some abnormality of the neurotransmitters causes bizarre transmission of nerve impulses.

The disease affects both the mind and body. Personality changes include carelessness, poor judgment, and impaired memory, ultimately deteriorating to total mental incompetence, **dementia.** The physical disabilities include speech loss and a difficulty in swallowing coupled with involuntary jerking, twisting, and muscle spasms. There is no cure for Huntington's chorea. In families afflicted with this disease, the risk for the offspring being affected should be clearly understood. Genetic engineering has now identified the dominant gene on chromosome 4 that is responsible for Huntington's chorea. Families with a history of this disease may choose to be tested for its presence.

Huntington's chorea
(hŭnt′-ĭng-tŭnz kō-rē′-ǎ)

dementia
(dē-měn′-shē-ǎ)

➤ ALZHEIMER'S DISEASE

The underlying cause of Alzheimer's disease is genetically based. The two prominent genes being surveyed are the apo E-3 and apo E-4. Their names indicate the respective proteins each is responsible for: apolipoprotein E-3 and apolipoprotein E-4. Apo E-4 protein binds to beta amyloid deposited in neuritic plaque as noted in Alzheimer victims. Problems arise depending on the number of genes for the apolipoproteins or their absence. More recent research indicates that it is more imperative to have the presence of the apo E-3 gene relative to the absence of apo E-4. Confirmation of Alzheimer's disease is subject only to autopsy.

The resultant impact leading to this devastating disease is the characteristic brain lesion called neuritic plaque, composed of a fibrous protein known as beta amyloid. These plaque formations surround nerve cell bodies that have acquired dense bundles of neurofibrillary tangles within them. This combination results in a reduction or loss of the chemical signal acetylcholine and the dysfunction of synaptic junctions necessary to carry out the message designated by the nerve(s).

Disease by the Numbers   x + ÷

Currently, about 4 million Americans have the age-related condition known as Alzheimer's disease. Individuals with one afflicted parent are three times as likely to develop Alzheimer's disease compared with individuals in families without a history of the disease. By the middle of this century, 14 million Americans will have this disease unless preventative measures are found.

Of people 75 to 84 years of age, 19% have Alzheimer's disease and beyond age 85 the percentage jumps to 30% to more than 40%. With 70% of Alzheimer victims living at home, the annual care cost is about 80 billion dollars. Correspondingly, the number four cause of death for adult Americans is Alzheimer's disease.

Some symptoms of Alzheimer's disease may start as early as the 40s or 50s. Manifestations of this primarily elderly condition are forgetfulness, confusion, emotional outbursts, and personality changes. These characteristics are startling discoveries for the victims and their families.

➤ CONVULSION

A convulsion is a sudden, intense series of involuntary contractions and relaxations by muscles. Numerous factors, often involving a chemical imbalance within the body, can cause convulsions. The accumulation of waste products in the blood resulting from uremia, toxemia of pregnancy, drug poisoning, and withdrawal from alcohol are all capable of causing convulsions.

Various irritations to the nerve cells can lead to convulsions. Infectious diseases of the brain such as meningitis and encephalitis are frequently accompanied by convulsions. These erratic contractions may also occur in infants and young children with high fevers.

The basis of convulsions is that abnormal electrical discharges spread over the brain. The hyperexcitation of nerves abnormally stimulate muscles to contract. Prevention of injury to the person during a convulsion is the primary concern.

Epilepsy

Epilepsy is a group of uncontrolled cerebral discharges that recurs at random intervals. The seizures associated with **epilepsy** are a form of convulsion. Brain impulses are temporarily disturbed, with resultant involuntary convulsive movements. Epilepsy can be acquired as a result of injury to the brain, including birth trauma, a penetrating wound, or depressed skull fracture. A tumor can irritate the brain, causing abnormal electrical discharges to be released. Alcoholism can also lead to the development of epilepsy. Most cases of epilepsy are idiopathic, but a predisposition to epilepsy may be inherited.

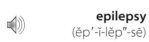
epilepsy
(ĕp′-ĭ-lĕp″-sē)

Epilepsy may manifest itself mildly, particularly in children. Loss of consciousness may last only a few seconds, during which time the child appears absent-minded. Some muscular twitching may be noticed around the eyes and mouth, and the child's head may sway rhythmically. The child does not fall to the floor. This form of epilepsy is known as **petit mal** and usually disappears by the late teens or early 20s.

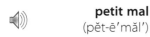
petit mal
(pĕt-ē′mǎl′)

Major seizures of epilepsy involve a loss of consciousness during which the person falls to the floor. Generalized convulsions are mild to severe, with violent shaking and thrashing movements. Hypersalivation causes a foaming at the mouth. The individual loses control of urine and sometimes feces. These features are characteristic of grand mal epilepsy.

aura
(aw′-rǎ)

Individuals sometimes have a warning of an approaching seizure that gives them time to lie down or reach for support. This warning, known as an **aura,** may come as a ringing sound in the ears, a tingling sensation in the fingers, spots before the eyes, or various odors. The signs described are characteristic of grand mal epilepsy. After a seizure, the person is groggy and unaware of what happened. Seizures last for varying lengths of time and appear with varying frequencies.

Epileptic seizures may take different forms. The classification system adopted by the World Health Organization is called the International Classification of Epileptic Seizures. It classifies seizures into four categories.

1. Partial seizures begin locally and may or may not involve a larger area of brain tissue.
2. Generalized seizures are bilaterally symmetrical and without local onset.

3. Unilateral seizures generally involve only one side of the brain.

4. Unclassified epileptic seizures.

Diagnosis of epilepsy can be made on the results of an **electroencephalogram (EEG),** a recording of brain waves. X-ray films are also used to identify any brain lesions. Family histories of epilepsy are very important in diagnosing the condition. The diagnosis of epilepsy and the seizure type has become more accurate with new techniques for imaging the brain. Computerized tomography (CT) using x-rays and magnetic resonance imaging (MRI) using magnetic fields visualize brain anatomy.

Medication is very effective in controlling epilepsy, particularly the anticonvulsant drugs, such as Dilantin. Alcohol must be avoided with these types of medication. Molecular neurobiology research is providing new information on how nerve cells control electrical activity, thus making development of more effective antiepileptic drugs possible. It is now known which drugs are best for treating the various kinds of seizures. Assistance or treatment during a seizure is directed toward preventing self injury to the individual. Finally, epilepsy does not appear to interfere with mental prowess or creative talents for those afflicted.

electroencephalogram
(ē-lĕk″-trō-ĕn-sĕf′-ă-lō-grăm)

➤ DEVELOPMENTAL ERRORS

Fetal development is so complex that the relatively small number of abnormalities is miraculous. Some developmental errors are minor and cause no problem, but some systemic errors can cause severe problems.

Spina Bifida

Spina bifida is a condition in which one or more vertebrae fail to fuse, leaving an opening in the vertebral canal. The word *bifid* means a cleft or split into two parts, which is the condition of the vertebra in spina bifida. The consequences of spina bifida depend on the extent of the opening and the involvement of the spinal cord.

One form of spina bifida, spina bifida occulta (hidden), may not be apparent at birth. Other malformations, such as hydrocephalus, cleft palate, cleft lip, club foot, and **strabismus** (crossed eyes) that tend to accompany this developmental error may point to this disorder. The spinal cord is affected, and muscular abnormalities appearing later— such as incorrect posture, inability to walk, or lack of bladder and bowel control—may signal spina bifida occulta. A slight dimpling of the skin and tuft of hair over the vertebral defect indicates the site of the lesion. Most lesions are located in the lower part of the vertebral column. The opening can be seen on x-ray films.

One form of spina bifida noticeable at birth is a **meningocele.** In this condition, meninges protrude through the opening in the vertebra as a sac filled with cerebrospinal fluid. The spinal cord is not involved in this defect.

Meningomyelocele is a serious anomaly in which the nerve elements protrude into the sac and are trapped, thus preventing proper placement and development. The child with this defect may be mentally retarded, fail to develop, lack sensation, or be paralyzed. The consequences of the defect depend on the part of the spinal cord affected. Surgical correction of various forms of spina bifida have been very effective. Some procedures are intrauterine, to repair the defect of the fetus, and these new operations look promising.

The most severe form of spina bifida is **myelocele,** in which the neural tube itself fails to close and the nerve tissue is totally disorganized. This condition is usually fatal. The various forms of spina bifida are shown in Figure 16–10.

spina bifida
(spī′-nă bĭf′-ĭ-dă)

strabismus
(stră-bĭz′-mŭs)

meningocele
(mĕn-ĭn′-gō-sēl)

meningomyelocele
(mĕn-ĭn″-gō-mī-ĕl′-ō-sēl)

myelocele
(mī′-ĕ-lō-sēl)

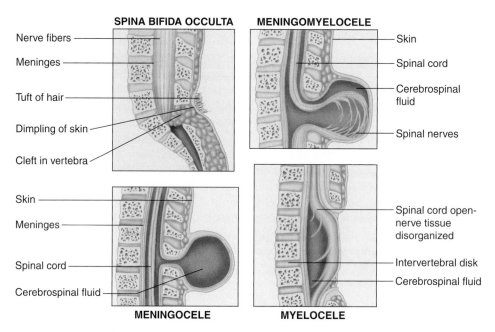

Figure 16–10
Forms of spina bifida.

PREVENTION *PLUS!*

Spina bifida and associated congenital malformations may be prevented by a dietary supplement of folic acid (folate) at a dose of 0.4 mg or 400 μg per day. In addition, the insistence of no smoking or consumption of alcohol by the pregnant woman will assure the best chances of normal spinal cord and cranial development.

Hydrocephalus

The name **hydrocephalus** means water or fluid on the brain or head. The formation, circulation, and absorption of cerebrospinal fluid is described previously in this chapter. In hydrocephalus this fluid accumulates abnormally, causing the ventricles to enlarge and push the brain against the skull.

An obstruction in the normal flow of cerebrospinal fluid is the usual cause of hydrocephalus. A congenital defect like stenosis of an opening from the ventricles or an acquired lesion can block the cerebrospinal fluid flow. Meningitis, a tumor, or birth trauma may result in acquired hydrocephalus. The error may also be a failure to absorb the fluid into the circulatory system.

There are two types of hydrocephalus, called *communicating* and *noncommunicating*. In the communicating type, the increased cerebrospinal fluid enters the subarachnoid space. In the noncommunicating hydrocephalus, the increased pressure of the cerebrospinal fluid is confined within the ventricles and is not evident in a lumbar puncture.

The head of a child born with hydrocephalus may appear normal at birth, but it will enlarge rapidly in the early months of life as the fluid accumulates. The brain is compressed, the cranial bones are thin, and the sutures of the skull separate under the pressure. The appearance of a hydrocephalic infant is typical; the forehead is prominent and

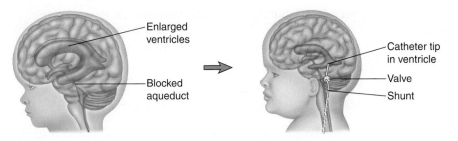

Figure 16–11
Hydrocephalus.

the eyes bulge, giving a frightened expression. The scalp is stretched and the veins of the head are prominent. The weight of the excessive fluid in the head makes it impossible for the baby to lift its head. The infant fails to grow normally and is mentally retarded.

There have been cases of self-arrested hydrocephalus in which expansion of the head stops. A balance is reached between production and absorption of the fluid. The cranial sutures fill in and the skull bones thicken. The extent of brain damage before the arrest determines the degree of retardation.

Success in relieving the excessive cerebrospinal fluid has been achieved by placing a shunt between the blocked cranial ventricle and the veins (Figure 16–11), to the heart, or peritoneal cavity. This connection allows the fluid to enter the general circulation.

➤ BRAIN INJURY

The impact of damage to the brain depends on the location and extent of the injury. Manifestations of brain damage include mental retardation and muscular disorders, such as the lack of coordination and partial paralysis.

Cerebral Palsy

Cerebral palsy is a motor function disease of the brain manifested by motor impairment and perhaps varying degrees of mental retardation that become apparent before age 3. The brain damage may be due to injury at or near the time of birth, a maternal infection such as rubella (German measles), or infection of the brain even after birth. Lack of oxygen or incompatible blood cause brain injury. An Rh⁻ mother may produce antibodies against the blood of an Rh⁺ fetus. The result is excessive destruction of fetal blood cells that causes hyperbilirubinemia, which is toxic to the brain. Often cerebral palsy is idiopathic.

There are three forms of cerebral palsy: spastic, athetoid, and atactic. The largest number of cerebral palsy victims have the spastic type of condition; muscles are tense, and reflexes are exaggerated. In the athetoid form, there are constant, purposeless movements that are uncontrollable. A continuous tremor or shaking of the hands and feet is present. Cerebral palsy sufferers with the atactic form have poor balance and are prone to fall. Poor muscular coordination and a staggering gait is characteristic of this disease.

Depending on the area of the brain affected, there may be seizures along with visual or auditory impairment. If the muscles controlling the tongue are affected, speech defects result. Intelligence may be normal, but often there is mental retardation. Treatment depends on the nature of the brain injury. Muscle relaxants can relieve spasms; anti-convulsant drugs reduce seizures; casts or braces may aid walking; and traction or surgery is helpful in some cases. Muscle training is the most important therapy, and the earlier it is started, the more effective it is.

➤ CEREBROVASCULAR ACCIDENT (STROKE) (CVA)

stroke
(strōk)

Vascular disturbances are the most frequent causes of brain lesions. The term **stroke** is used broadly to include cerebral hemorrhages and blood-clot formation within cerebral blood vessels. Nerves damaged by the lack of blood flow or hemorrhage do not regenerate and are replaced by scar tissue and would be considered a secondary neurologic incident/condition.

Cerebral Hemorrhage

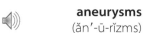

aneurysms
(ăn'-ū-rĭzms)

The main cause of cerebral hemorrhage is hypertension. Prolonged hypertension tends to result from atherosclerosis, which leads to arteriosclerosis, explained in Chapter 9. The combination of high blood pressure and hard, brittle blood vessels is a predisposing condition for cerebral hemorrhage. **Aneurysms,** weakened areas in vascular walls, are also susceptible to rupture (Figure 16–12). Subsequent hemorrhage into the brain tissue damages the neurons, causing a sudden loss of consciousness. Death can follow, or, if the bleeding stops, varying degrees of brain damage can result. Another potential site for aneurysms is in the inferior descending aorta. When detected, surgical repairs of aortic aneurysms may save lives.

Thrombosis and Embolism

Blood clots that block the cerebral arteries cause infarction of brain tissue. Thromboses develop on walls of atherosclerotic vessels, particularly in the carotid arteries. The clots take time to form, and some warning may precede the occlusion of the vessel. The person may experience blindness in one eye, difficulty in speaking, or a generalized state of confusion. When the cerebral blood vessel is completely blocked, the individual may lose consciousness.

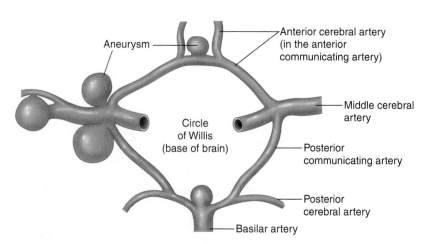

Figure 16–12
Aneurysms.

Because an embolism is a traveling clot, it may suddenly occlude a blood vessel. The embolism is most frequently a clot from the heart, aorta, or carotid artery, but it can travel from another part of the body. Consciousness is generally lost suddenly.

Tissue plasminogen activator (TPA), called a "clot buster," may be used to dissolve clots and restore blood flow. However, if TPA is given in hemorrhagic cases of cerebrovascular accidents, intracranial bleeding may continue and the individual could die. Crucial decisions must be made in acute cases and because most cerebrovascular accidents are of the ischemic form, TPA is a ready agent for the physician.

The site and extent of the brain damage, regardless of its cause, determines the outcome for the patient. Consciousness is usually regained, but immediately after the stroke, speech is often impaired. Loss of speech (**aphasia**) requires therapy, but the ability to speak is often restored.

aphasia
(ă-fā′-zĭ-ă)

Damage to the motor nerves at the point passing down the spinal cord causes weakness (paresis) or paralysis on the side of the body opposite the brain lesion due to the crossover of nerve fibers in the brain stem. Paralysis on one side of the body is referred to as **hemiplegia.**

hemiplegia
(hĕm″-ĭ-plē′-jĭ-ă)

Various procedures make it possible to determine the site of blockage in a cerebral blood vessel. Angiography, a process in which radiopaque material is injected into cerebral arteries, allows x-rays to locate the lesion.

A blockage in a carotid artery can be treated surgically. **Endarterectomy,** the more common procedure, removes the thickened area of the inner vascular lining. Carotid bypass surgery removes the blocked vascular segment, and a graft is inserted to allow blood flow to the brain.

endarterectomy
(ĕnd″-ăr-tĕr-ĕk′-tō-mē)

Transient Ischemic Attack (TIA)

Transient ischemic attacks are caused by brief but critical periods of reduced blood flow in a cerebral artery. The reduced flow may be due to an atherosclerotic narrowing of the blood vessel or to small emboli that temporarily lodge in the vessel. The attacks may last for a minute or two or up to several hours, with the average attack lasting 15 minutes. Manifestation is often abrupt and can include visual disturbances, transient hemiparesis (muscular weakness on one side), or sensory loss on one side. Lips and tongue may become numb, causing slurred speech. TIAs often precede a complete stroke and often serve as warning of a cerebral vascular disturbance. Further diagnostic testing such as a cerebral angiogram or CT scan may be indicated.

➤ TRAUMATIC DISORDERS

Physical injury to the head can damage the brain by causing a cerebral hemorrhage, that results in increased pressure from edema, or by creating a route for bacterial invasion.

Concussion of the Brain

A **concussion** is a transient disorder of the nervous system resulting from a violent blow on the head, or a fall. The person typically loses consciousness and cannot remember the events of the accident. Although the brain may not actually be damaged, the whole body is affected; the pulse rate is weak, and when consciousness is regained the person may experience nausea and dizziness. A severe headache may follow, and the person should be watched closely as a coma may ensue.

concussion
(kŏn-kush′-ŭn)

A person suffering from a concussion should be kept quiet, and drugs that stimulate or depress the nervous system, such as painkillers, are contraindicated. The condition will usually correct itself with rest.

Contusion

contusion
(kŏn-too′-zhŭn)

In a **contusion** there is an injury, a bruise, to brain tissue without a breaking of the skin at the site of the trauma. The brain injury may be on the side of the impact or on the opposite side, where the brain is forced against the skull. Blood from broken blood vessels accumulates in the brain, causing swelling and pain. The blood clots and necrotic tissue form and block the flow of cerebrospinal fluid, causing a form of hydrocephalus.

Skull Fractures

The most serious complication of a skull fracture is damage to the brain. A fracture at the base of the skull is likely to affect vital centers in the brain stem. The pressure that increases due to accumulation of cerebrospinal fluid must be reduced by medications. Another danger of skull fractures is that bacteria may be able to access the brain.

Hemorrhages

Hemorrhages can occur in the meninges, causing blood to accumulate between the brain and the skull. A severe injury to the temple can cause an artery just inside the skull to rupture. The blood then flows between the dura mater and the skull: This is called an **extradural** or **epidural** hemorrhage (Figure 16–13). The increased pressure of the blood causes the patient to lose consciousness. Surgery is required immediately to tie off the bleeding vessel and remove the blood. No blood is found in a lumbar puncture because the blood accumulation is outside the dura mater.

extradural
(ĕks-tră-dū′-răl)

epidural
(ĕp″-ĭ-dū′-răl)

subdural
(sŭb-dū′-răl)

A hemorrhage under the dura mater, a **subdural** hemorrhage (Figure 16–14), is from the large venous sinuses of the brain rather than an artery. This may occur from a severe blow to the front or back of the head. The blood clots, and cerebrospinal fluid accumulates into a cystlike formation. Intracranial pressure increases, but the cerebral symptoms may not develop for a time. Subdural hemorrhages are sometimes chronic in alcoholics and abused children.

subarachnoid
(sŭb″-ă-răk′-noyd)

The surface membrane of the brain may be torn by a skull fracture, causing a **subarachnoid** hemorrhage. Blood flows into the subarachnoid space where cerebrospinal fluid circulates. Blood is found in the cerebrospinal fluid with a lumbar puncture. Rupture of an aneurysm can also cause a subarachnoid hemorrhage.

➤ BRAIN TUMORS

Tumors of the brain may be malignant or benign. Because benign tumors may grow and compress vital nerve centers, they are considered serious disorders. Benign tumors are usually encapsulated and they can be completely removed surgically. Malignant tumors have extensive roots and are extremely difficult or impossible to remove in their entirety. Most malignant tumors of the brain are metastatic from other organs. Primary malignant tumors of the brain are called **gliomas,** tumors of the glial cells that support nerve tissue rather than of the neurons themselves. Figure 16–15 shows a glioma in the corpus callosum of the brain.

gliomas
(glī-ō′-măs)

Brain tumors manifest themselves in different ways depending on the site and growth rate of the tumor. **Astrocytomas** are basically benign, slow-growing tumors. **Glioblastomas** are highly malignant, rapid-growing tumors. Brain function is affected by the increased intracranial pressure. Blood supply to an area of the brain may be reduced by an infiltrating tumor or by edema causing the tissue to become necrotic.

astrocytoma
(ăs″-trō-sī-tō′-mă)

glioblastomas
(glī″-ō blăs-tō′-măs)

Symptoms of brain tumors may include a severe headache because of the increased pressure of the tumor. Personality changes, loss of memory, or development of poor judgment may signal a brain tumor. Visual disturbances, double vision, or partial blindness

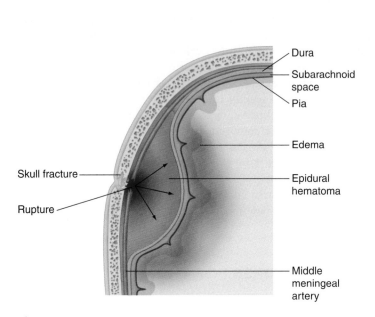

Dura
Subarachnoid space
Pia
Edema
Skull fracture
Epidural hematoma
Rupture
Middle meningeal artery

Figure 16–13
Extradural hematoma.

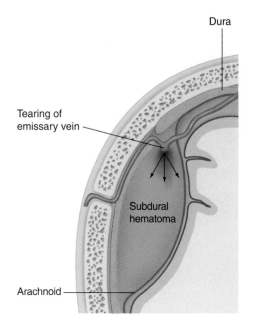

Dura
Tearing of emissary vein
Subdural hematoma
Arachnoid

Figure 16–14
Subdural hematoma.

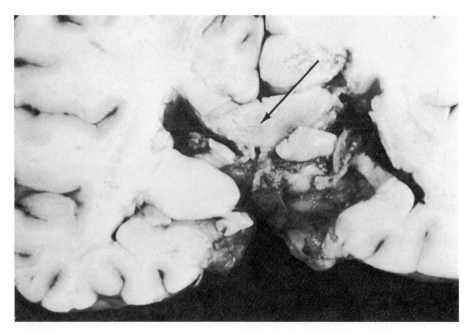

Figure 16–15
A glioma in the corpus callosum of the brain (arrow) (*courtesy of Dr. David R. Duffell*).

often occur, and the ability to speak may be impaired. The person may be unsteady while standing and develop seizures. A drowsy condition can progress to a coma.

Individual cranial nerves may be affected by degeneration or unknown causes and thus involved with various ailments. The fifth (V) cranial nerve, or trigeminal nerve, may become inflamed causing severe intermittent pain on one side of the face. This condition is known as trigeminal neuralgia or *tic douloureux* (Figure 16–16). This recurring pain may or may not respond readily to drugs. Bell's palsy involves the inflammation of the seventh (VII) cranial nerve, or facial nerve. This nerve may also be traumatized, compressed, or invaded by pathogens. Because the seventh cranial nerve innervates facial muscles and salivary glands, the attacks cause sagging of the facial muscles, and the person may drool and have slurred speech (Figure 16–17). In these cases, massage or heat treatment may help. Time seems to work best; and this may take weeks. Although the exact cause for these ailments may not be apparent, prior conditions like viral infections are suspect. Therefore, relief of symptoms may not always be quick or simple.

➤ DIAGNOSTIC PROCEDURES FOR THE NERVOUS SYSTEM

cerebrospinal
(sĕr″-ĕ-brō-spī′-năl)

Neurologic laboratory tests include **cerebrospinal** fluid (CSF) examination obtained by a lumbar spinal tap as previously described. Angiography allows visualization of the cerebral circulation through the injection of radiopaque material. Computed tomographic (CT) scans are particularly valuable for diagnosing pathologic conditions such as tumors, hemorrhages, hematomas, and hydrocephalus. Electromyelography (EMG) is a ra-

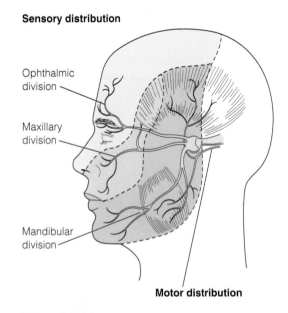

Sensory distribution

Ophthalmic division

Maxillary division

Mandibular division

Motor distribution

Figure 16–16
Sensory and motor distribution of the trigeminal nerve. There are three sensory divisions: ophthalmic, maxillary, and mandibular.

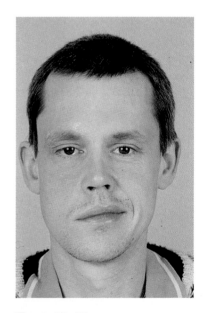

Figure 16–17
This man with Bell's palsy shows typical drooping of the one side of the face.

diographic process by which the spinal cord and spinal subarachnoid space are viewed and photographed after injection of contrast medium into the lumbar subarachnoid space. Myelography is used to identify spinal lesions caused by trauma or disease, such as amyotrophic lateral sclerosis (ALS). Electroencephalography (EEG) records the electrical activity of the brain (brain waves). It is used to diagnose lesions or tumors, **seizures,** and impaired consciousness. Magnetic resonance imaging (MRI) uses magnetic fields in conjunction with a computer to view and record tissue characteristics at different planes. MRI is excellent for visualizing brain soft tissue, spinal cord, white matter diseases, tumors, and hemorrhages.

seizures
(sē′-zhŭrs)

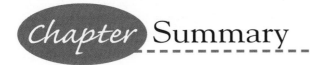 Summary

The nervous system enables the human body to respond to changes in the external and internal environment. This system is affected by diseases in numerous ways. Microorganisms that enter the nervous system by various routes cause infectious diseases, such as meningitis, encephalitis, polio, tetanus, rabies, Reye's syndrome, and shingles.

A degeneration of nerves and brain tissue results in multiple sclerosis, amyotrophic lateral sclerosis, Parkinson's disease, and Huntington's chorea. A manifestation of these progressively degenerative diseases is abnormal functioning of the muscles.

Convulsions often result from some chemical imbalance that causes irritation to nerve cells. The seizures of epilepsy are a form of convulsions resulting from abnormal electrical discharges in the brain.

Hydrocephalus and the various forms of spina bifida are caused by developmental errors, obstruction to the flow of cerebrospinal fluid, and failure of the vertebral column to close. Damage to the brain during fetal life or at birth can result in cerebral palsy, which is manifested by various forms of muscular abnormalities. Cerebrovascular accidents, cerebral hemorrhages, and blood clots damage brain tissue. The results of the damage depend on the site and extent of the brain lesion.

A severe head injury that causes hemorrhaging within the brain or in the meninges has serious effects on the nerve tissue and may even be fatal. Tumors of the brain, both malignant and benign, strangle nerve fibers and obstruct blood flow. No other tissue of the body depends on a continuous supply of oxygenated blood as does the brain.

Diseases at a Glance: Nervous System

Categories	* Disease	Signs and Symptoms
Malignancies	* Glioma, * Glioblastoma	Severe headache, personality changes, loss of memory, visual disturbances, impaired speech, unsteady movement, seizures, coma
Infections	* Meningitis	High fever, chills, severe headache, stiff neck, nausea, vomiting, rash, delirium, convulsions, coma
	* Encephalitis	Mild to severe, headache, fever, cerebral dysfunction, disordered thought, seizures, persistent drowsiness, delirium, coma
	* Poliomyelitis	Stiff neck, fever, headache, sore throat, GI disturbances, paralysis may develop
	* Tetanus	Rigidity of muscles, painful spasms and convulsions, stiff neck, difficulty swallowing, jaws clenched
	* Rabies	Fever, pain, mental derangement, rage, convulsions, paralysis, profuse sticky saliva, throat muscle spasm produces hydrophobia
	* Shingles	Painful rash of small water blisters with red rim, lesions follow a sensory nerve, confined to one side of body, severe itching, scarring
	* Reye's Syndrome	Persistent vomiting, rash, lethargy about 1 week after a viral infection, may progress to coma; link with use of aspirin
	* Abscess	Fever, headache
Degenerative	* Multiple sclerosis (MS)	Muscle impairment, double vision, nystagmus, loss of balance, poor coordination, tingling and numbing sensation, shaking tremor, muscular weakness, emotional changes, remission and exacerbation
	* Amyotrophic lateral sclerosis (ALS) Lou Gehrig's disease	Disturbed motility, fasciculations, atrophy of muscles in hands, forearms, legs, impaired speech and swallowing, death from pulmonary failure in 3 to 4 years
	* Parkinson's disease (PD)	Bradykinesia, tremor, rigidity; pill-rolling tremors, nodding of head, frequent falling, slow and difficult muscle movement, stooped posture, forward-leaning, short shuffling gait

Affected Organ/Body Region	Diagnostic Procedures	Treatment
Brain	CT scan, MRI	Surgery, chemotherapy, radiation
Meninges	Lumbar puncture (spinal tap)	Antibiotics, if bacterial infection
Brain and meninges	Lumbar puncture (spinal tap)	Control fever, fluid and electrolyte balance, monitoring respiratory and kidney function
Spinal cord and brain	Physical exam	Supportive; preventive vaccination
Toxin affects motor nerves	Physical exam, patient history	Antitoxin, supportive preventive vaccination
Central nervous system	Physical exam, history of animal bite	Vaccination before disease develops; fatal once CNS involved
Sensory nerve	Physical exam	Alleviation of symptoms and pain relief, steroids
Brain and liver	Patient history, liver enlargement, hypoglycemia, ammonia in blood	Supportive, close monitoring necessary
Brain	Lumbar puncture (spinal tap)	Surgical draining of abscess, antibiotics
Central nervous system	Physical exam, patient history, MRI	None effective; physical therapy and muscle relaxants, steroids, counseling
Motor neurons	Electromyelography (EMG)	Supportive
Basal ganglia	Patient history and physical exam	Prescribed exercise, physical therapy, L-dopa

Nervous System (continued)

Categories	* Disease ❑ Condition ● Congenital ❖ Injury	Signs and Symptoms
	* Huntington's disease (Huntington's chorea)	Involuntary, rapid, jerky movements, speech loss, difficulty swallowing, personality changes, carelessness, poor judgment, impaired memory, mental incompetence
Other abnormal structure/function	❑ Convulsion	Involuntary contractions, or series of contractions; a seizure is a sign of illness, not a disease
	* Epilepsy	Petit mal—brief loss of consciousness, "absence seizure"
		Grand mal—often preceded by aura (various sensations), total loss of consciousness, generalized convulsions, hypersalivation, incontinence may occur
	● Spina bifida	Opening in vertebral canal Spina bifida occulta is hidden Meningocele—meninges protrude Meningomyelocele—nerve elements protrude Myelocele—nerve tissue disorganized
	● Hydrocephalus	Enlarged head develops
Brain Damage	* Cerebral palsy	Seizures, visual or auditory impairment, speech defects, 3 types: Spastic—muscles tense, reflexes exaggerated Athetoid—Uncontrollable, persistent movements, tremor Atactic—Poor balance, poor muscular coordination, staggering gait
	* Transient ischemic attacks (TIA), "mini strokes"	Visual disturbances, transient muscle weakness on one side, sensory loss on one side, slurred speech; attacks last minutes to hours, average 15 minutes
	* Cerebrovascular accident (CVA), stroke, brain attack	Severe, sudden headache, muscular weakness or paralysis, disturbance of speech, loss of consciousness
	❖ Concussion	Transient loss of consciousness due to trauma, nausea, dizziness, headache
	❖ Contusion	Trauma resulting in immediate loss of consciousness, lasting 5 minutes or less, loss of reflexes, briefly stops breathing, slow return to full consciousness

Affected Organ/Body Region	Diagnostic Procedures	Treatment
Brain	Patient history (inherited disease) & physical exam	No cure; genetic counseling for family
Voluntary muscles	Observation of seizure	Removal of cause once detected
Brain, voluntary muscles	Electroencephalogram (EEG), x-ray, family history, CT scan, MRI	Anticonvulsive drugs
Vertebral canal, spinal cord	Physical exam, CT scan, MRI, EEG	Surgical, physical therapy
Meninges, CSF	Physical exam, CT scan, MRI, spinal tap	Implanting shunt to drain CSF
Brain	Physical exam	Muscle relaxants, anticonvulsive drugs, casts, braces, traction, surgery, physical therapy
Brain	Cerebral angiogram, CT scan	Depends on cause, surgical treatment of blocked vessels
Brain	Angiography, CT scan, MRI	Clot-dissolving drugs, surgery; endarterectomy
Brain	Patient history, physical exam	Observation, avoid drugs
Brain	Patient history, physical exam, x-ray, CT scan, MRI	Surgery to relieve pressure, remove blood, monitoring

Nervous System (continued)

Category	* Disease ❖ Injury	Signs and Symptoms
	❖ Skull fracture	Blow to head, broken bone
	❖ Hemorrhages	Severe headache, loss of consciousness Epidural (extradural) hemotoma—arterial bleeding outside of dura mater Subdural hemorrhage—venous bleeding under dura mater Subarachnoid hemorrhage—into subarachnoid space

Affected Organ/Body Region	Diagnostic Procedures	Treatment
Skull, sometimes brain	Patient history, physical exam, x-ray, CT scan, MRI	Surgery, control of intracranial pressure, monitoring
Arteries, venous sinuses in meninges	Patient history, physical exam, x-ray, CT scan, MRI	Surgery, control of intracranial pressure, monitoring

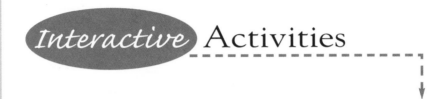

Interactive Activities

CASE FOR CRITICAL THINKING

A 65-year-old woman named Alice visited her physician because her family was concerned about her. A family member told the physician that Alice had become confused, forgot where she put things, and even put things in the wrong place. Last week she put the iron in the freezer. The family member reported that memory loss is getting more severe.

1. What might a possible diagnosis be for Alice's condition?
2. What measures are available for preventing these kinds of conditions?

MULTIMEDIA EXTENSION ACTIVITIES

www.prenhall.com/mulvihill
Use the above address to access the free, interactive companion Website created for this textbook. Included in the features of this site are chapter specific activities, internet links, and an audio-glossary.

Audio Glossary
Use the CD-ROM disk enclosed with your textbook to hear the pronunciation of the key terms in this chapter.

Diseases at a Glance: Nervous System

Use the chart on page(s) 362–367 to answer the following questions.

1. List 5 types of diseases or conditions that affect the nervous system.

2. What are the major signs and symptoms of the diseases or conditions you named?

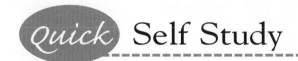 Self Study

MULTIPLE CHOICE

1. Rabies is primarily a disease of warm-blooded animals such as dogs, cats, raccoons, skunks, wolves, foxes, and bats; but it can be transmitted to humans through bites or scratches from _____.
   a. rabid animal
   b. an elderly cat
   c. a cancerous animal
   d. a tuberculin-tested animal

2. Epilepsy can be acquired as a result of _____.
   a. a birth trauma
   b. injury to the brain
   c. a penetrating wound
   d. a, b, or c

3. Infectious neural diseases have numerous causes, such as _____.
   a. an infection elsewhere in the body
   b. a contaminated puncture wound
   c. a dog or insect bite
   d. a, b, or c

4. An acute inflammation of the first two meninges of the brain and spinal cord, the pia mater and the arachnoid, is known as _____.
   a. thrombophlebitis
   b. meningitis
   c. prostatitis
   d. encephalitis

TRUE OR FALSE

_____ 1. Rabies is a viral infection.

_____ 2. The Sabin vaccine works in the digestive tract.

_____ 3. Oxygen under high pressure would be effective in treating rabies.

_____ 4. Blood is not normally found in cerebrospinal fluid.

_____ 5. Dopamine deficiency causes epilepsy.

_____ 6. Transient ischemic attacks are characterized by loss of consciousness.

FILL-INS

1. _____, commonly called "lockjaw," is an infection of nerve tissue caused by the tetanus bacillus that lives in the intestines of animals and human beings.

2. Amyotrophic lateral sclerosis is diagnosed by _____.

3. _____ is a major disorder of the central nervous system; it is a chronic, progressive disease of unknown origin.

4. _____, also known as shaking palsy, is a disease of brain degeneration that appears gradually and progresses slowly.

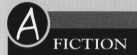 FICTION

Benign tumors tend to grow and crowd out precious cranial space and, thus, apply pressure or restrict blood flow to particular brain regions. If these benign growths are inoperable or uncontrolled, they will kill the victim.

Malignant brain tumors may be lethal, but they may also be surgically removed or reduced with beams of high-powered mediation. All brain tumors require attention and may be lethal. If they tend to grow slowly, are encapsulated, and /or are surgically removable, then skill and technology may restore a healthy state for those affected.

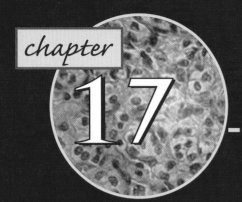

Diseases of the Bones, Joints, and Muscles

All bodily movements are the result of muscular contractions. These movements range from the wink of an eye to the acrobatic performance of a gymnast. All facial expressions—happiness, sorrow, anger, or surprise—are the result of muscle action.

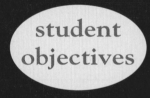

student objectives

After studying this chapter, students should be able to

➤ Define osteomyelitis and list causes

➤ Define infectious arthritis and list examples

➤ Know causes and differences between rickets and osteomalacia

➤ Compare osteoporosis to Paget's disease

➤ Define osteoarthritis and describe its impact on health

➤ Relate rheumatoid arthritis to its pathogenesis and treatment versus osteoarthritis

➤ Discuss causes, symptoms, and treatment for gout

➤ Describe muscular dystrophy, in particular Duchenne's form, as to its causes and manifestations

➤ Describe myasthenia gravis and its treatment

➤ List potential causes and treatments for bone cancer

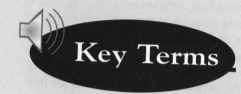

Key Terms

Ankylosis

Arthritis

Autoimmune

Bursae

Bursitis

Creatine phosphate

Dystrophin

Dystrophy

Electromyography

Gout

Intervertebral disk

Ligaments

Medullary cavity

Myasthenia gravis

Osteitis fibrosa cystica

Osteoarthritis

Osteogenic sarcoma

Osteoma

Osteomalacia

Osteomyelitis

Osteopenia

Osteoporosis

Periosteum

Reduction

Rhabdomyosarcoma

Rickets

Sprains

Spurs

Strains

Synovial

Tendons

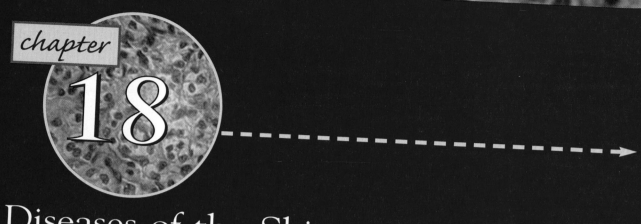

18

Diseases of the Skin

Skin comes in a variety of colors—white, yellow, red, brown and black—but it always performs the same functions.

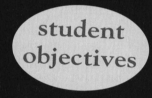

student objectives

After studying this chapter, students should be able to

➤ Describe the structure and function of the skin

➤ Provide a description of the following lesions: bullae, pustules, macule, papule, and vesicles

➤ Describe causes, symptoms and lesions associated with impetigo, erysipelas, cellulitis, folliculitis, furuncle, carbuncle, and abscess

➤ Describe the characteristics of benign neoplasms: verruca, moles

➤ Describe the attributes of the various types of ringworm infections and *Candida* infections

➤ Distinguish among parasitic infestations

➤ Describe the response of the skin to allergens

➤ Compare and contrast the immune response that results in urticaria, eczema, and poison ivy

➤ Depict the various skin lesions commonly associated with drug eruptions

➤ Compare and contrast the nature of basal cell carcinoma, squamous cell carcinoma, and malignant melanoma

➤ Identify the causes of acne vulgaris

➤ Describe the abnormalities that result from seborrheic dermatitis, acne vulgaris, and acne rosacea

➤ Describe the lesions associated with psoriasis

➤ Describe the methods used to diagnose skin conditions

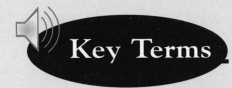

Key Terms

Acne	Pallor
Albinism	Papular
Dermatitis	Pediculosis
Dermatophyte	Plantar warts
Eczema	Pruritis
Erysipelas	Psoriasis
Erythema	Pustules
Erythematous	Ringworm
Furuncles	Scabies
Genital warts	Sebaceous
Herpes simplex	Seborrheic dermatitis
Hypersensitivity	Sebum
Impetigo	Squamous
Keratin	Urticaria
Keratinocytes	Verruca vulgaris
Macular	Vesicles
Melanin	Vitiligo
Melanocytes	Wheals
Nevus	

➤ CHAPTER OUTLINE

- Functions of the Skin
- Structure of the Skin
- Classification of Skin Diseases
- Infectious Skin Diseases
  Bacterial Skin Infections
  Viral Skin Infections
  Parasitic Infections
  Fungal Skin Infections
  Ringworm
  Candidiasis
  Parasitic Infestations
- Hypersensitivity or Immune Diseases of the Skin
  Insect Bites
  Urticaria (Hives)
  Eczema
  Poison Ivy
  Drug Eruptions
- Benign Tumors
  Nevus (Mole)
- Skin Cancer
  Basal Cell Carcinoma
  Squamous Cell Carcinoma
  Kaposi's Sarcoma
  Malignant Melanoma
- Sebaceous Gland Disorders
  Acne (Vulgaris)
  Seborrheic Dermatitis
  Sebaceous Cysts
  Acne Rosacea
- Metabolic Skin Disorder
  Psoriasis
- Pigment Disorders
  Albinism
  Vitiligo
- Diagnostic Tests for Skin Diseases
- Chapter Summary
- Diseases at a Glance
- Interactive Activities
- Quick Self Study

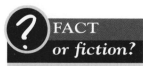

pallor
(păl′-ŏr)

➤ FUNCTIONS OF THE SKIN

The skin or the integument is a vital organ and a protective wrap. As an organ, the skin regulates body temperature, senses pain, keeps substances and microorganisms from entering the body, and provides a shield from the harmful effects of the sun.

The skin indicates malfunction within the body through color changes. Cyanosis, a blue coloration of the skin in the extremities signals a lack of oxygen—a cardiovascular or pulmonary problem. Jaundice indicates liver disease, bile obstruction, or hemolysis of red blood cells, in which case an accumulation of the bilirubin in the blood produces the yellowish coloration. An abnormal redness accompanies polycythemia (Chapter 7), carbon monoxide poisoning, and fever. **Pallor,** or whitening of the skin, may indicate anemia.

Skin color, texture, and folds identify people as individuals. Anything that goes wrong with the skin function or appearance can have important consequences for physical and mental health.

on the Practical Side

Corns and Calluses a Value?
Corns and calluses are layers of firm thick tissue that protect skin exposed to friction. They may become enlarged or painful but can usually be treated with over-the-counter products.

keratin
(kĕr′-ă-tĭn)

keratinocytes
(kĕ-răt′-ĭ-nō-sīts)

➤ STRUCTURE OF THE SKIN

Each layer of the skin performs specific tasks. The outermost layer of the skin is the epidermis, consisting of stratified or layered squamous epithelium. The top portion of the epidermis, the stratum corneum contains keratin. **Keratin** is a tough, fibrous protein produced by cells called **keratinocytes** and protects the skin from harmful substances. At the bot-

on the Practical Side

Evaluation of Burn Depth
Burns are classified on the depth of skin involved. First degree burns affect the epidermis and are caused by sunburn or low-intensity flash. Recovery is complete within a week, and peeling of the dead epidermis occurs.

Second-degree burns are caused by scalds or flash flame and affect the dermis or true skin. The epidermis is blistered, red, and broken, and the area is very painful. Recovery requires 2 to 3 weeks and some scarring and depigmentation usually occurs. If infection develops, a major problem with burns, it may convert to a third-degree burn.

Third-degree burns result from fire and prolonged exposure to hot liquids. Subcutaneous tissue is affected and the burn appears pale or charred. Broken skin exposes underlying fat issue. The patient shows symptoms of shock. Healing requires time and grafting is necessary. Scarring and loss of contour results.

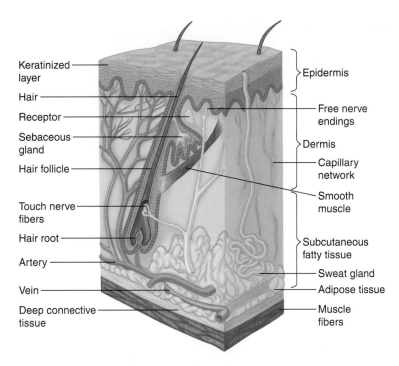

Keratinized layer
Hair
Receptor
Sebaceous gland
Hair follicle
Touch nerve fibers
Hair root
Artery
Vein
Deep connective tissue

Epidermis
Free nerve endings
Dermis
Capillary network
Smooth muscle
Subcutaneous fatty tissue
Sweat gland
Adipose tissue
Muscle fibers

Figure 18–1
Structure of the skin.

tom of the epidermis are the **melanocytes,** or the cells that produce **melanin.** Melanin is the dark pigment of the skin that protects the body from the harmful rays of the sun.

The dermis, or "true skin" lies below the epidermis. The dermis is composed of connective tissue that supports blood and lymph vessels, elastic fibers, nerves, hair follicles, sweat glands, and **sebaceous** or oil glands.

The subcutaneous tissue lies under the dermis and connects the skin to underlying structures. Adipose tissue or fat cells are in the subcutaneous tissue and help insulate the body from heat and cold. Figure 18–1 shows the structure of the skin.

➤ CLASSIFICATION OF SKIN DISEASES

Skin diseases are identified and classified according to characteristic lesions. Revealing characteristics of skin lesions include the size, shape, color, and location as well as the presence or absence of other signs and symptoms. **Pruritis** (itching), edema (swelling), **erythema** (redness), and inflammation usually accompany lesions and are helpful in making a diagnosis.

Lesions may be small, blisterlike eruptions, called **vesicles,** or larger fluid-containing lesions, called bullae. Lesions containing pus are referred to as **pustules,** and nodules and tumors are lesions that are hard to the touch. Lesions that are flat are called **macular,** whereas those that are raised are termed **papular.** An area of skin reddened by congested blood vessels resulting from injury or inflammation is said to be **erythematous.** Pruritus, or itching, accompanies many skin diseases, especially those caused by allergies or parasitic infestation. Figure 18–2 shows various skin lesions.

melanocytes
(měl′-ăn-ō-sīts)

melanin
(měl′-ă-nĭn)

sebaceous
(sē-bā′-shŭs)

pruritis
(proo-rī′-tŭs)

erythema
(ěr″-ĭ-thē′-mă)

vesicles
(věs′-ĭ-kls)

pustules
(pŭs′-tūls)

macular
(măk′-ū-lăr)

papular
(păp′-ū-lěr)

erythematous
(ěr″-ĭ-thěm′-ă-tŭs)

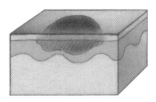

A macule is a discolored spot on the skin; freckle

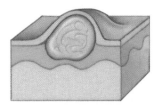

A pustule is a small, elevated, circumscribed lesion of the skin that is filled with pus; varicella (chickenpox)

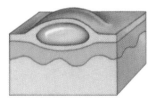

A wheal is a localized, evanescent elevation of the skin that is often accompanied by itching; urticaria

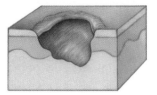

An erosion or ulcer is an eating or gnawing away of tissue; decubitus ulcer

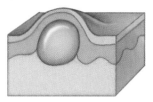

A papule is a solid, circumscribed, elevated area on the skin; pimple

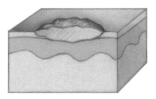

A crust is a dry, serous or seropurulent, brown, yellow, red, or green exudation that is seen in secondary lesions; eczema

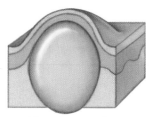

A nodule is a larger papule; acne vulgaris

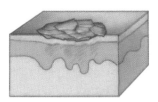

A scale is a thin, dry flake of cornified epithelial cells; psoriasis

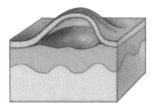

A vesicle is a small fluid filled sac; blister. A bulla is a large vesicle.

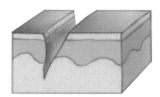

A fissure is a crack-like sore or slit that extends through the epidermis into the dermis; athlete's foot

Figure 18–2

Skin signs are objective evidence of an illness or disorder. They can be seen, measured, or felt.

➤ INFECTIOUS SKIN DISEASES

Bacteria, viruses, fungi, and parasites may cause infections of the skin. Normal microbes that reside on the skin cause the most common skin infections. Infections from less common microbes may develop in high-risk individuals (immunocompromised or diabetic people), and those who reside in nursing homes and hospitals. Most skin infections are not serious unless systemic involvement occurs.

Bacterial Skin Infections

Impetigo Impetigo is an acute, contagious skin infection common in children. It is caused by streptococcal and staphylococcal organisms carried in the nose that are passed to the skin. The face and hands are most frequently affected. Erythema, a reddened area, develops and oozing vesicles and pustules form. These rupture, and a yellow crust covers the lesion. Fever and enlarged lymph nodes may accompany the infection. The lesions should be washed with soap and water, kept dry, and exposed to the air. Antibiotic ointment may be used, and oral antibiotics are sometimes prescribed to treat the infection systemically.

impetigo
(ĭm″-pĕ-tī′-gō)

Erysipelas Erysipelas is an inflammatory skin infection caused by streptococcus bacteria. Most commonly, the infections appear on the face, arm, or leg. Sometimes the infection begins where skin is broken. A shiny, swollen, and red rash may develop initially and is often accompanied with small blisters. The erythematous rash is hot to touch and tender. Fever and chills develop when the infection is severe. Mild erysipelas is self-limiting; however, when the infection is severe, treatment with antibiotics is required.

erysipelas
(ĕr″-ĭ-sip′-ĕ-lăs)

Cellulitis Cellulitis is a spreading infection of the skin that is most often caused by streptococcus bacteria. The infection is most common on the legs and begins with skin damage. The involved area is generally swollen, red, and tender. Symptoms of the infection may include fever and chills. Prompt treatment prevents the spread of the infection to the blood and vital organs (Figure 18–3).

Folliculitis, Furuncles, and Carbuncles Folliculitis is an inflammation of hair follicles caused by infection with staphylococci. A small number of pustules develop in the hair follicle. This condition commonly occurs in young men and affects the thighs, buttocks, beard, and scalp (Figure 18–4).

Boils or **furuncles** are large, tender, swollen raised lesions caused by staphylococci. The infection appears in hair follicles located on the face, neck, breasts, or buttocks. The core of the furuncle becomes necrotic and liquefies forming pus (Figure 18–5).

furuncles
(fū′-rŭng-k′ls)

Carbuncles are clusters of boils. These lesions arise in a cluster of hair follicles. Carbuncles develop and heal more slowly than boils. They appear mostly in men and are commonly located on the back of the neck.

Boils and furuncles are effectively treated with application of moist heat, antiseptic skin cleansing, oral antibiotic administration, and incision and drainage. Folliculitis is effectively treated with daily cleansing with an antiseptic soap. Severe cases of folliculitis require treatment with oral antibiotics.

Viral Skin Infections

Many types of viruses invade the skin. The most common viruses cause cold sores or fever blisters and warts. Cold sores or fever blisters are caused by the virus **herpes simplex.**

herpes simplex
(hĕr′-pēz
sim′-plĕks)

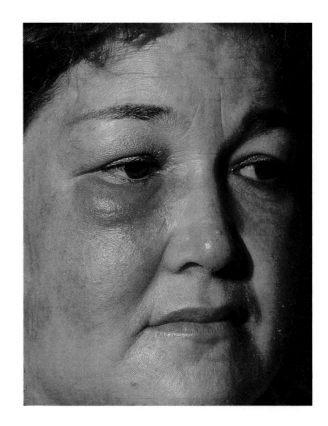

Figure 18–3
Cellulitis is a bacterial infection localized in the dermis and
subcutaneous tissue. The involved area is red, swollen, and painful.

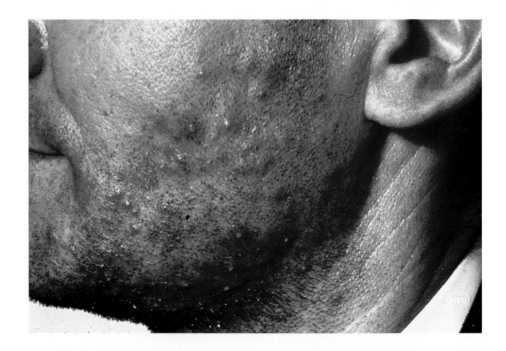

Figure 18–4
The lesions of folliculitis
are pustules surrounded by
areas of erythema.

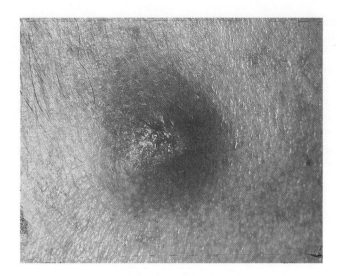

Figure 18–5
A furuncle (or boil) is a
deep, firm, red, painful
nodule.

The lesions generally form near the mouth or lips, as in Figure 18–6. The virus may be
harbored in the body for a long time with no ill effect, but suddenly it becomes active
and the infection develops. Cold sores frequently form when a person's resistance to infection is low or at a time of emotional stress. They often accompany a respiratory infection such as the common cold, or they develop during menstruation. A bad sunburn
sometimes triggers the formation of cold sores. Antiviral drugs are effective for certain
viral infections such as cold sores, and antibiotics are sometimes applied topically to
treat secondary bacterial invasion.

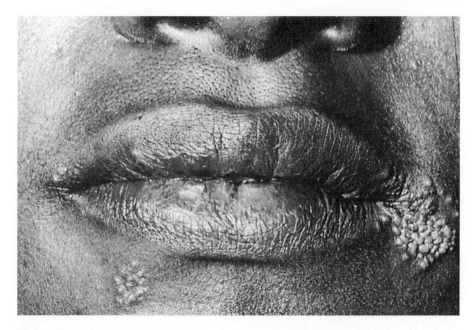

Figure 18–6
Typical cold sores or fever blisters caused by the virus herpes simplex. (*From Feinstein,*
Dermatology. *Courtesy of Robert J. Brady Co.*)

verruca vulgaris
(vĕr-roo'-kă
vŭl-gā'-rĭs)

Warts, called **verucca vulgaris,** are caused by viruses affecting the keratinocytes of the skin, causing them to proliferate. A benign neoplasm develops with a rough keratinized surface. Warts are most common in children and young adults, developing particularly on the hands. They are often multiple and are contagious, being spread by scratching. Warts sometimes disappear spontaneously, but they should be removed only by a physician. If the virus remains in the body, the warts tend to recur (Figure 18–7).

plantar warts
(plăn'-tăr worts)

Warts are not serious or painful except when they form on the soles of the feet. These warts are called **plantar warts,** and, in contrast to warts elsewhere on the body, which appear as an elevation from the skin, plantar warts grow inward. Pressure on the soles of the feet make them very painful, and they are often difficult to remove permanently. Venereal or **genital warts** (Chapter 15) are very serious and difficult to remove.

genital warts
(jĕn'-ĭ-tăl worts)

Fungal Skin infections

dermatophytes
(dĕr″-mă-tō-fī-ts)

Fungi or **dermatophytes** that infect the skin tend to live on the dead, top layer of the skin. Fungal infections may or may not cause symptoms. Serious infections generally cause itching, swelling, blisters, and severe scales. Minor infections cause mild irritation and swelling.

Fungi usually reside on moist areas of the body where skin surfaces touch. The skin folds of the breast, groin, and toes are the most common areas affected. Obese people, with excessive skin folds, are more susceptible to fungal infections.

Ringworm

ringworm
(rĭng'-wŭrm)

Ringworm or tinea is caused by many different fungi and is classified by its location on the body (Table 18–1). The fungi particularly reside in warm moist areas of the body, but may also occur with hairy skin on the head, groin, arms, and legs. The fungi can produce symptoms ranging from mild scales, cracking skin, to painful raw rashes. Treatment includes keeping the affected area clean and dry, and application of topical antifungal creams, powders, and solutions.

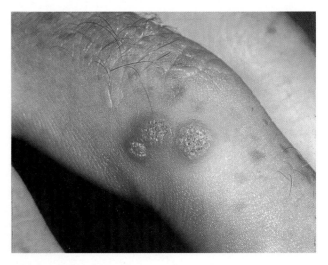

Figure 18–7
The common wart is a lesion of the skin caused by a virus. It commonly appears as a raised, dome-shaped lesion.

TABLE 18–1. RINGWORM CLASSIFICATION AND SYMPTOMS	
Tinea corporis	Body ringworm; affects smooth areas of skin on the arms, legs and body; produces a pink to reddish rash that sometimes forms round patches with clear areas in the center
Tinea pedis	Most commonly known as "athlete's foot"; scales and fissures occur on the soles of the feet, between the toes, or toenail; a foul odor and pruritis usually accompany lesions
Tinea cruris	Most commonly known as "jock itch"; because it occurs on the skin around the groin and over the upper, inner thighs; is more common in men than women and develops more frequently in warm weather; the fungi produce red, ringlike areas with blisters, (Figure 18–8)
Tinea capitis	"Scalp ringworm"; is highly contagious and most commonly occurs in children; may produce a mild scaly rash or a patch of hair loss without a rash

Candidiasis

Candidiasis is a fungal infection that is caused by the fungus *Candida*. This infection appears on the skin, mucous membranes, or fingernail. Candidiasis on the skin may produce patches of itchy red blisters and pustules. Candida growing on the nail bed produces redness and swelling. The nail may turn white or yellow in color and separate from the finger or toe.

Vaginal Candida infections are common in pregnant women, diabetics, or those who are immunocompromised. Vaginal candidiasis is commonly known as a "yeast infection" and frequently occurs after antibiotic therapy. Oral antibiotics suppress resident

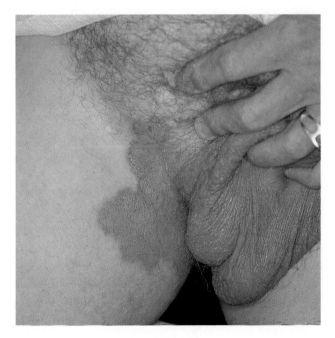

Figure 18–8
Tinea cruris (jock itch) is a fungal infection of the groin and inner thighs.

vaginal bacterial flora that normally inhibits overgrowth of Candida. Symptoms include a white "cottage cheese"-like discharge from the vagina accompanied by burning, itching, and redness. Vaginal candidiasis is effectively treated with vaginal antifungal creams, or oral antifungal agents (Figure 18–9).

Creamy white patches on the tongue or side of the mouth often characterize a Candida infection of the mouth or thrush. The patches are often painful and can easily be scraped off. Thrush is common in young healthy children, immunosuppressed adults, and diabetics. Long-term treatment of oral thrush with topical liquids or oral antifungals is generally required.

Parasitic Infestations

pediculosis
(pě-dǐk″-ū-lō′-sǐs)

Pediculosis or louse infestations are classified into three categories: head lice, pubic lice, and body lice.

Head lice are common among school children, and although annoying, these parasites are not dangerous and do not carry epidemic disease. Lice are spread from head to head directly or indirectly by shared combs, scarves, hats, and bed linen. Itching, the first symptom, results from the saliva of lice as they penetrate the scalp and engorge on human blood. The scratching that follows can open the skin to other invading organisms. Adult head lice are difficult to see, but their white eggs, called nits, can be located on the hair shaft. Treatment includes use of medicated shampoos followed by use of a fine-toothed comb. Over-the-counter medications are also available.

Pubic lice infest pubic hair of both men and women and are generally spread by sexual contact. The lice do not spread other sexually transmitted diseases. Treatment includes use of a prescription cream.

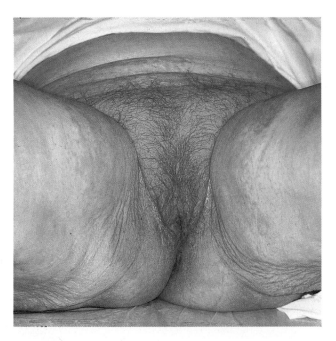

Figure 18–9
Candida albicans, a fungus, causes a skin infection characterized by erythema, pustules, and a typical white substance covering the area.

Body lice are most common among underprivileged, transient people. This type of infestation can be prevented with good grooming and hygiene. Body lice can spread serious disease, and they have been responsible for typhus epidemics among soldiers during wartime.

Scabies, commonly called "the itch," is a contagious skin disease usually associated with poor living conditions. It is caused by a parasite called a mite. The female mite burrows into skin folds in the groin, under the breasts, and between fingers and toes. As she burrows, she lays eggs in the tunnels, the eggs hatch, and the cycle starts again. The intense itching is caused by hypersensitivity to the mite. Blisters and pustules develop, and the tunnels in the skin appear as grayish lines. Scratching opens the lesions to secondary bacterial infection. Scabies is transmitted by close personal contact and can be linked to a venereal disease. Epidemics of scabies are common in camps and barracks.

To recover from scabies, the mites and eggs must be totally destroyed by hot baths, scrubbing, and medications to eliminate them. Underwear and bedding that harbor the eggs must be changed frequently. The itch may persist while treatment is being administered.

scabies
(skā′-bēz)

➤ HYPERSENSITIVITY OR IMMUNE DISEASES OF THE SKIN

Allergic or **hypersensitivity** reactions are frequently manifested by the skin. This fact serves as the basis for the patch tests given to determine specific allergies. Some diseases of the skin develop in atopic people, persons with a genetic predisposition to allergies. Others occur in anyone who has been sensitized to an allergen such as poison ivy. Emotional stress frequently triggers or exacerbates an allergy-caused skin disease.

hypersensitivity
(hī″-pĕr-sĕn″-sĭ-tĭv′-ĭ-tē)

Insect Bites
Insect bites and stings can produce local inflammatory reactions that may vary in appearance. Acute reactions may appear as hives whereas more chronic reactions may appear as papules (solid elevation of the skin) or bullous (blisters).

Urticaria (Hives)
Urticaria, or hives, results from a vascular reaction of the skin to an allergen. The word *urticaria* is derived from a Latin word that means "plants covered with stinging nettles." The lesions are **wheals,** rounded elevations with red edges and pale centers. Wheals develop most often at pressure points like those under tight clothing, but they may appear anywhere on the skin or mucous membranes. The lesions are extremely pruritic, or itchy.

urticaria
(ŭr-tĭ-kā′-rē-ă)
wheals
(hwēlz)

The allergic response causes damage to mast cells, which then release histamine. Histamine causes blood vessels to dilate and become more permeable. Blood proteins and fluid ooze out of the capillaries into the tissues and result in edema. This irritation to the tissues causes intense itching.

Urticaria is generally treated with steroids, antihistamines, and calamine lotion applied topically to reduce the itching. If the cause of the allergic reaction can be determined, that allergen should be avoided. Foods that are a common cause of hives include certain berries, chocolate, nuts, and seafood. Other allergens discussed in Chapter 2 frequently cause hives in the hypersensitive person. An attack of hives can also be brought on by emotional stress.

Eczema

eczema
(ĕk′-zĕ-mă)

dermatitis
(dĕr″-mă-tī′-tĭs)

Eczema, also called contact **dermatitis,** is a noncontagious inflammatory skin disorder. Eczema results from sensitization that develops from skin contact with various agents, plants, chemicals, and metals. Poison ivy (to be described) and poison oak, dyes used for hair or clothing, and metals, particularly nickel, used in costume jewelry are examples of allergens that can cause eczema.

Eczema is a delayed type of allergic response in which lymphocytes are sensitized by an antigen, such as poison ivy, and react with it on subsequent exposure. The typical inflammatory reaction occurs: dilated blood vessels, reddened skin, and edema. Vesicles and bullae develop from the excess tissue fluid, and the lesions are very itchy. Scratching causes the vesicles to burst and ooze, and the eczema is thus spread. Scaly crusts form on the ruptured lesions. A patient with contact dermatitis is shown in Figure 18–10.

Contact dermatitis can affect anyone and is not limited to the genetically allergic person. Skin that has been damaged is more easily sensitized by contact with allergens than healthy skin. Emotional stress can also be a factor in sensitization. Corticosteroids are sometimes used to reduce the inflammatory reaction.

Poison Ivy

Contact with poison ivy can cause an extremely itchy rash with blisters and hive-like swelling; the response is a typical example of allergic contact dermatitis. Severity of the condition depends on the amount of plant resin on the skin and the individual's sensitivity to it. Some people are apparently immune to the resin. An initial exposure to the poison ivy plant produces no visible effect but sensitizes the person to subsequent exposure. The rash usually develops a few hours or a few days after contact. Treatment to lessen the inflammation is use of a topical cortisone-type cream, gel, or spray.

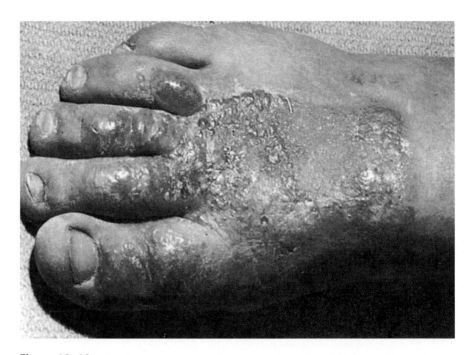

Figure 18–10
A patient with contact dermatitis from leather shoes. (*From Feinstein,* Dermatology. *Courtesy of Robert J. Brady Co.*)

Drug Eruptions

Adverse drug reactions manifest more often on the skin than any other organ system. Topical drug reactions vary in severity from mild pimples over a small area to peeling of the entire skin. Skin reactions may be serious enough to cause anaphylaxis, shock, or death. The most common offending drugs are penicillin, sulfa, anticonvulsants, tetracycline, morphine, codeine, and anti-inflammatory medications. Table 18–2 summarizes the most common rashes caused by drugs.

TABLE 18–2. COMMON RASHES CAUSED BY DRUGS		
SKIN ERUPTION	**DESCRIPTION OF LESION**	**MEDICATION COMMONLY ASSOCIATED WITH ERUPTION**
Acneiform	• Appear like acne on any part of the body • Unlike common acne, these lesions appear suddenly	Prednisone, Oral contraceptives, anticonvulsant medications, lithium
Exfoliative dermatitis	• Large areas of skin become erythematous and scaly and slough off (Figure 18–11) • May follow other drug eruptions • Associated with systemic infections and reactions	Sulfa drugs, penicillin, gold compounds, vitamin A
Epidermal necrolysis	• Painful red area that may develop blisters (Figure 18–12) • Top layer of skin peels in sheet • Skin appears scalded • Is the most serious skin eruption, 30% of cases result in death from fluid loss or secondary infection	Ibuprofen, penicillin, sulfa drugs
Fixed drug eruption	• Caused exclusively by drugs • Red lesions with sharp borders that appear darker in color than the surrounding unaffected skin • Have a propensity to reappear at the same site each time the causative drug is reintroduced	Aspirin, acetaminophen, penicillin, tetracycline, sulfa, codeine, morphine
Urticaria	• Hives with intense itching • Sudden onset, resolves within 24 hours after the offending drug has been stopped • Edematous, flat lesions	Aspirin, penicillin, sulfa, codeine, morphine, ibuprofen
Maculopapular	• Flat, red lesions involve extensive areas and appear within a week after the causative drug has been started • Pruritus may or may not be present • Resolve 7 to 14 days after the offending drug has been stopped	Ampicilin, amoxicillin, allopurinol, sulfa
Photosensitive	• Require the presence of light and the offending drug to occur • Manifest as fluid-filled lesions and sunburn (Figure 18–13)	Sulfa, tetracycline, anticonvulsant medications, antipsychotic medications, ibuprofen, naproxen
Purpura	• Characterized by small hemorrhages under the skin • Lesions are purplish in color (Figure 18–14)	Diuretics, penicillin, sulfa, coumadin
Stevens–Johnson	• Small hivelike blisters that most commonly occur on mucous membranes • May be accompanied by fever, fatigue • Most common type of severe drug eruption • Mortality is estimated in the range of 5% to 18%	Sulfa, barbiturates, penicillin, lithium

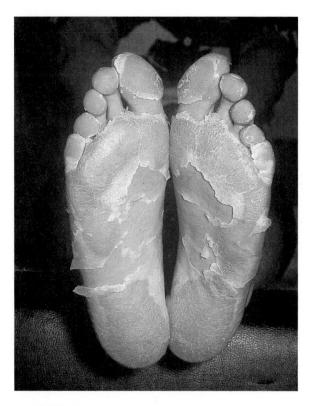

Figure 18–11
Exfoliative dermatitis is an inflammatory skin disorder causing excessive skin peeling.

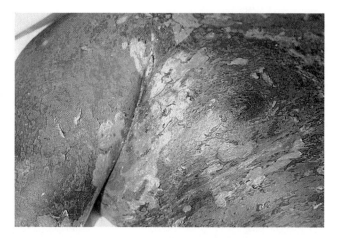

Figure 18–12
Toxic epidermal necrolysis (TEN) is a life-threatening skin disease characterized by the sloughing of large skin surfaces.

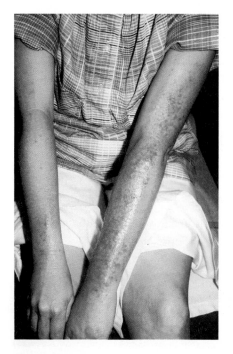

Figure 18–13
Photodermatitis (*Courtesy of Jason L. Smith, MD*).

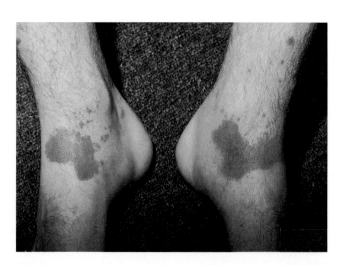

Figure 18–14
Purpura (*Courtesy of Jason L. Smith, MD*).

➤ BENIGN TUMORS

Nevus (Mole)

A **nevus** is a small, dark skin growth that develops from pigment-producing cells or melanocytes. Moles may be flat or raised and vary in size. Most people have about 10 moles. The moles themselves are usually harmless, but they can become malignant. Sudden changes in moles such as enlargement with an irregular border, darkening, inflammation, and bleeding are warning signs of malignant melanoma (Figures 18–15 and 18–16).

nevus
(nē'-vŭs)

PREVENTION *PLUS!*

Basal and squamous cell skin cancers are increasing in incidence at a rate of 2% to 3% annually. Sun exposure is the main risk factor. Overexposure to ultraviolet B rays is the primary carcinogen. Fair-skinned people are the most vulnerablie; however, with enough exposure, anyone's skin will change.

Basal Cell Carcinoma

The most common skin cancer is basal cell carcinoma—a slow-growing, generally non-metastasizing tumor. It generally develops on the face of people with light skin who do not tan in the sun but have been exposed to the sun. Figures 18–17, 18–18, and 18–19 show patients with basal cell carcinoma. The lesion begins as a pearly nodule with rolled edges that may bleed and form a crust. Ulceration occurs and size increases if it is neglected. This tumor is treated by surgical removal, cauterization, or radiation therapy.

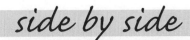

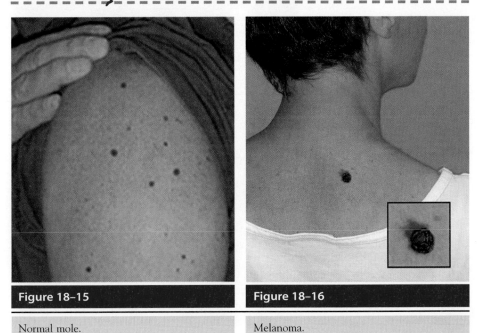

Figure 18–15

Normal mole.

Figure 18–16

Melanoma.

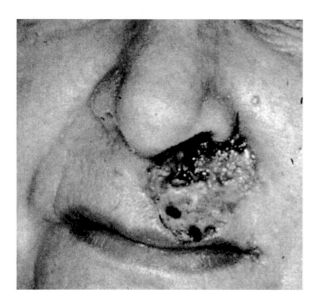

Figure 18–17
Basal cell carcinoma. *(Courtesy of Dr. Barry A. Goldsmith.)*

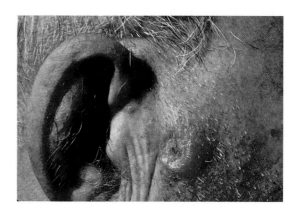

Figure 18–18
As a squamous cell cancer grows, it tends to invade surrounding tissue. It also ulcerates, may bleed, and is painful.

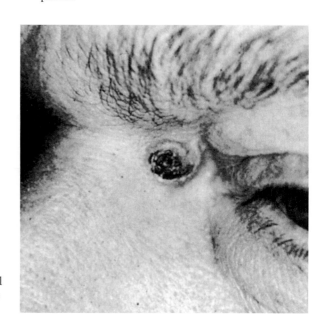

Figure 18–19
A 62-year-old man with basal cell carcinoma. *(Courtesy of Dr. Barry A. Goldsmith.)*

Squamous Cell Carcinoma

squamous
(skwā'-mŭs)

Squamous cell carcinoma is more serious than basal cell carcinoma because it grows more rapidly, infiltrates underlying tissues, and metastasizes through lymph channels. Squamous cell carcinoma is a malignancy of the keratinocytes in the epidermis of people who have been excessively exposed to the sun. The lesion is a crusted nodule that ulcerates and bleeds. This cancer develops in any squamous epithelium of the body, including the skin or mucous membranes lining a natural body opening. It should be completely excised surgically or treated with radiation.

Disease by the Numbers x + ÷

SKIN CANCER

Skin cancer is the most common type of cancer. More than 500,000 new cases of skin cancer are diagnosed each year. The development of skin cancer is frequently linked to excessive sun exposure in the fair-skinned person. The most common skin cancer is the basal cell carcinoma, and the most deadly is malignant melanoma. Malignant melanoma accounts for 74% of all skin cancer deaths.

Kaposi's Sarcoma

Classic Kaposi's sarcoma is a purplish neoplasm of the lower extremities. The lesions are classically described as red-to-purple lesions varying from macules to nodules. This cutaneous cancer has been epidemic in persons with AIDS. Kaposi's sarcoma is quoted as a cause of AIDS-related death in 11% of cases.

Malignant Melanoma

The most serious skin cancer is malignant melanoma, which arises from the melanocytes of the epidermis. It is highly malignant and metastasizes early. A malignant melanoma of the skin is seen in Figure 18–20. Melanoma sometimes develops from a mole that changes its size and color and becomes itchy and sore. It is usually excised with the surrounding lymph nodes to reduce metastasis. Prognosis depends on the depth of infiltration, previous spread, and how completely the tumor is excised. Figure 18–21 shows a malignant melanoma that metastasized to the brain.

➤ SEBACEOUS GLAND DISORDERS

Hyperactivity of the sebaceous glands causes acne and chronic dandruff. Raised, horny lesions result from an excessive production of keratinocytes.

Acne (Vulgaris)

Many adolescents suffer at some time or another from **acne:** blackheads, pimples, and pustules. About 80% or the population between the ages 12 and 25 develop some form of acne. Most teens get the mild form, called noninflammatory acne, and just get a few whiteheads and blackheads. Some suffer from inflammatory acne and have a constant

acne
(ăk′-nē)

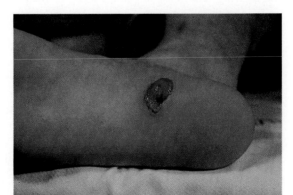

Figure 18–20
Malignant melanoma is a serious skin cancer that arises from melanocytes.

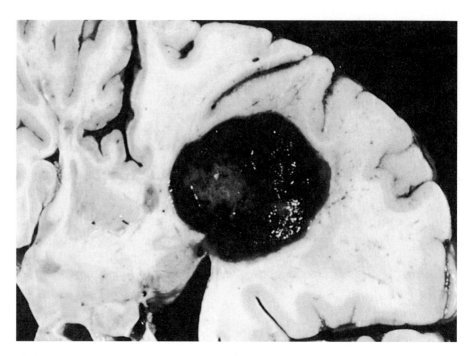

Figure: 18–21
Malignant melanoma that metastasized to the brain. (*Courtesy of Dr. David R. Duffell.*)

breakout of pus-filled pimples and cysts that cause deep pitting and scarring. Acne is the result of hormonal changes that occur at puberty. The increased level of estrogen and testosterone stimulates not only growth at this time but also glandular activity. The **sebaceous** glands increase their secretions of **sebum,** the oily fluid that is released through the hair follicles. If the duct becomes clogged by dirt or make-up, the sebaceous secretion accumulates, causing a little bump or whitehead. Sebaceous accumulation at the surface becomes oxidized and turns black, causing the familiar blackhead. Blackheads should not be squeezed or picked because the broken skin offers an entry to bacteria that are always present on the skin surface. Once pyogenic bacteria enter the skin, pus forms and a pimple or pustule results. Squeezing the pimple spreads the infection.

There is no cure for acne, but various treatments can control the lesions. Acne generally corrects itself with maturity, but it may persist as a chronic condition that is aggravated by stress. Severe chronic acne as seen in Figure 18–22, can lead to disfiguring and scarring. The most important measure for controlling acne is frequent, thorough washing of the skin to remove excess oil and bacteria. Creams and heavy make-up that clog the pores should be avoided. Severe cases of acne are best treated by a dermatologist, who may prescribe topical or oral antibiotics, and comedolytic agents.

Seborrheic Dermatitis (Chronic Dandruff)

The cause of dandruff is similar to that of acne: the excessive secretion of sebum from the sebaceous glands. The person with **seborrheic dermatitis** has an oily scalp, and the excessive secretion of sebum forms the familiar scales of dandruff. This condition can spread to the face and ears, and the eyebrows are often affected. Frequent shampooing, particularly with medicated shampoo, is the most effective treatment. Thorough brushing of the hair loosens the dandruff scales, and they will wash out easily.

sebaceous
(sē'-bā'-shŭs)

sebum
(sē'-bŭm)

**seborrheic
dermatitis**
(sĕb"-ō-rē'-ik
dĕr"-mă-tī'-tĭs)

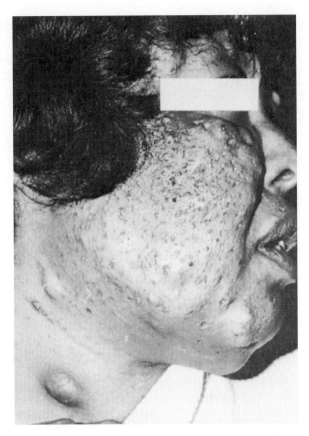

Figure 18–22
A patient with severe chronic acne. Note deep scarring and
prominent cysts. *(From Feinstein,* Dermatology. *Courtesy of
Robert J. Brady Co.)*

Sebaceous Cysts

Sebaceous cysts form when a sebaceous gland duct becomes blocked, and the sebum
accumulates under the surface of the skin, forming a lump. Sebaceous cysts are not considered serious, but they can rupture, allowing bacteria to enter the body. These cysts
can be incised and drained, although they tend to recur, or they can be removed surgically.

Acne Rosacea

Acne rosacea is a condition that appears during or after middle age in persons with fair skin.
Usually the cheeks, chin, and nose develop tiny pimples and broken blood vessels that eventually thicken and gives the nose a bulbous appearance. The cause of rosacea is not known,
although this condition responds well to topical antibiotic treatment (Figure 18–23).

➤ METABOLIC SKIN DISORDER

Psoriasis

Psoriasis is a superficial recurring idiopathic skin disorder characterized by an abnormal rate of epidermal cell production and turnover. Rapid replacement of epidermal cells
results in formation of red, round, raised lesions with silvery scales. The lesions typically occur on the elbows, knees, and scalp. Psoriasis on the scalp may be mistaken as

psoriasis
(sō-rī′-ă-sĭs)

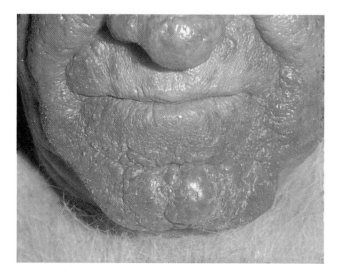

Figure 18–23
Acne rosacea is more common in the middle-aged to older adult. It causes changes in skin color, enlarged pores, and in some cases, thickening of the soft tissues of the nose.

severe dandruff. The cause of psoriasis is not known although there tends to be a familial basis. Psoriasis may flair up for no apparent reason and follow with periods of remission and exacerbation. Typical lesions in psoriasis are seen in Figure 18–24.

There is no cure for psoriasis. The formation of lesions can be controlled by application of emollient cream, topical and oral steroids, coal tar cream, and ultraviolet light. Severe psoriasis can be treated with anticancer medication. Psoriasis can be aggravated by injury to the skin, stress, drugs, and lack of sunlight.

➤ PIGMENT DISORDERS

The main skin pigment, melanin, is interspersed among other cells in the epidermis. Skin color varies from light to dark depending on the number of melanocytes present. Melanin production normally increases with exposure to sunlight causing tanning.

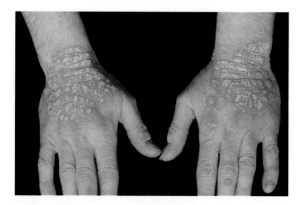

Figure 18–24
The characteristic lesions of psoriasis are raised, red, round plaques covered with thick, silvery scales.

Hypopigmentation is an abnormally low amount or absence of melanin. The skin may be pale white to various shades of pink caused by the blood flowing through it.

Albinism

Albinism is a rare inherited disorder in which no melanin is formed. The person has white hair, pale skin, and pink eyes. Because melanin protects the skin from the sun, albinos are prone to sunburn and skin cancer.

albinism
(ăl'-bĭn-ĭsm)

Vitiligo

Vitiligo is a loss of melanin resulting in white patches of skin. The white patches are usually well demarcated and may cover large parts of the body. Hypopigmentation is most striking in dark-skinned persons. As in albinism, the unpigmented skin is prone to sunburn. There is no cure for vitiligo. Small areas of skin may be covered with tinted make-up, and sunscreen should always be applied to the skin to prevent sunburn.

vitiligo
(vĭt-ĭl-ī'-gō)

➤ DIAGNOSTIC TESTS FOR SKIN DISEASES

Skin conditions are usually identified by looking at them. Revealing characteristics include size, shape, color, and location as well as the presence or absence of systemic signs and symptoms.

Culturing the purulent lesion usually identifies bacterial, fungal, and viral infections. The culture is allowed to grow, and the specimen is identified under a microscope.

Biopsies are the usual tests for neoplastic lesions, chronic eruptions, and nodular lesions. The removed piece of skin is about 1/8 inch in diameter and is examined under a microscope.

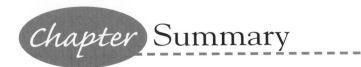

Chapter Summary

The skin sometimes reveals a medical condition of the entire body. To rule out systemic conditions, blood tests and other laboratory tests may be performed.
The skin, which protects the body from various elements in the environment, can become diseased in numerous ways. Streptococci and staphylococci cause such bacterial infections as impetigo, erysipelas, cellulitis and folliculitis. Cold sores and warts result from viral infections. Tinea and candidiasis are caused by fungus. Parasites such as the louse and mite can infest the skin.

Skin diseases frequently manifest allergies. Hives and eczema are examples of skin eruptions caused by hypersensitivy to various antigens, insect bites or drugs. Abnormal growth or neoplasia of the skin cells causes malignant and benign tumors, ranging from the common mole to malignant melanoma. Hyperactivity of the sebaceous glands results in acne, sebaceous cysts and seborrheic dermatitis. A patchy loss or complete absence of melanin is evidence of pigment disorders. Hyperactivity in epidermal cell production results in characteristic silvery lesions of psoriasis.

Skin lesions take many forms, each of which is significant in diagnosing the disease. The lesions may be reddened areas indicating inflammation, or fluid filled indicating edema. Pus-filled lesions result from pyogenic bacterial infections. The location of the lesion, whether it tends to recur, and whether it itches, are also factors in the diagnosis.

Diseases at a Glance: Skin

Categories	* Diseases	Signs and Symptoms
Infections ■ Bacterial ◆ Viral	■ Impetigo	Erythema, oozing vesicles, pustules that crust, fever, swollen lymph nodes
	■ Erysipelas	Shiny, swollen red rash, tender, hot to touch, adults
	■ Cellulitis	Red, swollen, tender, spreading lesions follow skin damage
	■ Folliculitis	Inflammation of hair follicle, pustules appear
	■ Furuncles	"Boil," large, tender, swollen, pus-filled lesion
	■ Carbuncles	A cluster of boils (furuncles)
	◆ Herpes simplex	"Cold sore," "fever blister," small blisters
	◆ Verucca vulgaris	Wart, raised lesion of dead keratinocytes
	◆ Plantar wart	Wart on sole of foot, grows inward, pressure, pain
✓ Fungal	✓ Ringworm (Tinea)	T. corporis, "body ringworm," pink-red, rash with round patches that are clear in center
		T. pedis, "athlete's foot," scales and fissures
		T. cruris, "jock itch," itchy, red ringlike patches with blisters in groin
		T. capitis, "head ringworm," mild scaly rash, patchy hair loss
	✓ Candidiasis	Body: itchy red blister, pustules Vaginal: white creamy "cottage cheese" discharge, intense itching Mouth: "thrush," creamy white painful patches
❖ Parasitic infestations	❖ Lice	Affected areas itchy, nits visible on hair shafts
	❖ Scabies	Mites burrow into skin folds; intense itching with blisters and pustules

Mostly Commonly Affected Region	Diagnostic Procedures	Treatment
Face and hands	Exam, culture	Antibiotics
Face, arm, leg	Exam, culture	Antibiotics
Legs	Exam, culture	Antibiotics
Thighs, buttocks, beard, scalp	Exam, culture	Cleansing, antibiotics
Face, neck, breasts, buttocks	Exam, culture	Moist heat, cleansing, antibiotics, surgical
Back of neck	Exam, culture	Moist heat, cleansing, antibiotics, surgical
Lips, mouth	Exam, culture	Self-limiting, antiviral medication
Hands	Exam, culture	Removal (cryosurgery, laser, surgery)
Sole of foot	Exam, culture	Removal (cryosurgery, laser, surgery)
Arms, legs, body, smooth areas of skin	Exam, culture	Antifungals
Soles of feet, between toes, toenails	Exam, culture	Antifungals
Groin, upper inner thighs	Exam, culture	Antifungals
Scalp	Exam, culture	Antifungals
Skin, mucous membranes, fingernails	Exam, culture	Antifungals
Body, head, pubic area	Physical exam	Medicated shampoo, nit removal
Anywhere on skin	Physical exam	Hot bath, scrubbing, medication

Skin (continued)

Categories	* Diseases	Signs and Symptoms
Malignancies	* Basal cell carcinoma	Slow-growing pearly nodule, rolled edges, lesion bleeds, forms crust
	* Squamous cell carcinoma	Crusted nodule, ulcerates and bleeds, infiltrates underlying tissue
	* Malignant melanoma	Mole undergoes color change, size change, irregular border, bleeds, itches
	* Kaposi's sarcoma	Red or purple lesions, varying from macules to nodules, itchy, painful
Inflammations	Urticaria	Hives, itchy wheals, rounded elevations, red, pale center
	Eczema	Contact dermatitis, red itchy lesions, swelling, blisters
	Drug allergy reactions	Acneiform, exfoliative dermatitis, epidermal necrolysis, fixed eruptions, urticaria, maculopapular, photosensitive, purpura, Stevens-Johnson lesions see Table 18-2
Other abnormal structure/ function	Acne vulgaris	Whiteheads, blackheads, cysts with increased sebum
	Seborrheic dermatitis	"Dandruff," oily scales
	Sebaceous cyst	Lump under skin surface from blocked oil gland
	Acne rosacea	Reddened skin, broken blood vessels, nose and chin develop bulbous appearance
	Nevus	Mole, "beauty mark," flat or raised, dark-colored mass of melanocytes
	Psoriasis	Round, red raised lesions with slivery scales
	Albinism	Lack of melanin, skin white, eyes pink, light sensitivity
	Vitiligo	White, well-demarcated areas of skin with lost pigment

Mostly Commonly Affected Region	Diagnostic Procedures	Treatment
Sun or UV-exposed skin	Biopsy	Surgical
Sun or UV-exposed skin	Biopsy	Surgical
Sun or UV-exposed skin	Biopsy	Surgical
Lower extremities; persons with AIDS	Patient history, biopsy	Surgery, radiation, chemotherapy
Skin, mucous membranes	Physical exam	Antihistamine, calamine lotion, steroids
Area contacting irritant	Physical exam	Steroids
Anywhere on skin	Patient history, physical exam	Change medication
Face, neck, back	Physical exam	Antibiotics, comedolytic agents
Scalp, ears, eyebrows, face	Physical exam	Medicated shampoo
Oil glands	Physical exam	Surgical
Cheeks, chin, nose	Physical exam	Antibiotic
Anywhere	Exam, biopsy	Cryosurgery, excision
Elbows, knees, scalp	Exam, biopsy	Medicated creams, steroids, UV
Entire skin surface	Physical exam	Sunscreen
Patchy	Physical exam	Sunscreen, make-up

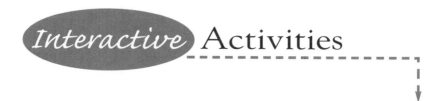

CASES FOR CRITICAL THINKING

1. A 17-year-old young man presents to an outpatient clinic with complaints of an itchy rash. The rash is mostly on his elbows and behind his knees. The patient mentioned that he had this type of rash before, and the doctor had treated him with pills and topical creams. The patient is allergic to penicillin, sulfa, and was recently on a camping trip. What types of skin diseases should we consider in this patient?

2. A 52-year-old man recently returned from a business trip with an acute flare-up of itchy, erythematous plaques. The plaques are covered with silvery white scales and are located on his scalp. He has used an antidandruff shampoo with poor results. He also states that he has lost much hair in the areas of the lesions. Describe the possible causes and treatment of this condition.

3. A 4-year-old girl presents to the pediatrician's office with "scabs under her nose." According to mom, the scabs appeared shortly after she developed a cold. The child has red lesions with crust under her nose and on her cheek. On examination, the doctor notes that her "glands are still swollen." Should the doctor culture these lesions? Why or why not? What skin diseases should we consider in this child?

4. A 25-year-old man complains of intense "jock itch." On examination, the doctor observes raised lesions on his penis and red circular patches on his groin. He lives in a transient hotel, and his hygiene is poor. What are the possible causes for this rash? What diagnostic tests should the doctor order?

5. A 39-year-old woman notices a mole on the tip of her ear that has recently started to bleed. She has a fair complexion and suntan lines on her shoulders. What condition should be considered? What type of diagnostic test should be ordered? Should systemic involvement be considered? Why or why not?

MULTIMEDIA EXTENSION ACTIVITIES

www.prenhall.com/mulvihill
Use the above address to access the free, interactive companion Website created for this textbook. Included in the features of this site are chapter specific activities, internet links, and an audio-glossary.

Audio Glossary
Use the CD-ROM disk enclosed with your textbook to hear the pronunciation of the key terms in this chapter.

Diseases at a Glance: Skin

Use the chart on page(s) 416–419 to answer the following questions.

1. List 5 types of diseases or conditions that affect the skin.

2. What are the major signs and symptoms of the diseases or conditions you named?

Quick Self Study

MULTIPLE CHOICE

1. Bacterial infections on the skin are caused by _____.
   a. tinea   b. herpes simplex
   c. staphylcocci

2. Round elevations of the skin with red borders and pale centers are lesions called

   _____.
   a. acne   b. macules
   c. wheals

3. Sulfa, tetracycline, and antipsychotic medications can cause a _____
   reaction on the skin upon exposure to sunlight.
   a. photosensitive   b. exfoliative
   c. urticarial

4. A _____ carcinoma grows rapidly and metastasizes through
   lymph channels.
   a. basal cell   b. squamous cell
   c. melanocyte

TRUE OR FALSE

_____ 1. Impetigo can involve a systemic infection.

_____ 2. Basal cell carcinoma metastasizes rapidly.

_____ 3. Fever blisters are examples of a bacterial infection.

_____ 4. Seborrheic dermatitis is a malignant skin tumor.

_____ 5. Warts are benign neoplasms.

_____ 6. A mole is a nevus.

_____ 7. Ringworms are viral infections.

FILL-INS

1. Urticaria, also known as _____, results from a vascular reaction of the skin to an allergen.

2. Scabies, also known as _____ _____,
   is a contagious skin disease usually associated with poor living conditions.

3. A person with seborrheic dermatitis has an oily scalp, and the excessive secretion of
   sebum forms scales of _____.

4. The dark-colored pigment of the skin that protects the body from the harmful rays
   of the sun is called _____.

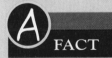

FACT

Most teens get the mild form, called noninflammatory acne, and just get a few whiteheads and blackheads. Some suffer from inflammatory acne and have a constant breakout of pimr' and cysts.

Stress, Aging, and Wellness

Stress, aging, and wellness are all connected because each plays a part of the other. Many diseases have been described throughout this book. Many of the diseases have been described as stress related. It is known that chronic stress can ruin our health and stress influences the manner in which aging occurs. Wellness is the condition of good physical health and mental health. In the following chapters, you will learn more about the interdependent relationship of stress, aging, and wellness.

Part

III

chapters

Microscopic Image of a Kidney Carcinoma

chapter

19

Stress and Aging

Under "stress," and "stressed out" are common terms in today's
fast-paced society, but few people realize the toll that stress takes on
the human body.

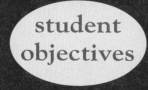

student
objectives

After studying this chapter, students should be able to
➤ Discuss the stress hormones and their effects on the body
➤ Describe the function of the autonomic nervous system in response to stress
➤ Describe the effect of stress on the cardiovascular, respiratory, integumentary,
  digestive, nervous, and immune systems
➤ Discuss stress and sexuality
➤ Describe supportive therapies for stress
➤ List and describe common diseases of the elderly
➤ Discuss care of the elderly

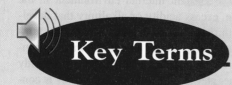

Key Terms

Alzheimer's disease

Analgesics

Anti-inflammatory
hormone

Aura

Beta-amyloid

Cataracts

Geriatrics

Gerontology

Homeostasis

Photophobia

Plaque

Senility

Serotonin

to the point of opacity. The patient experiences blurred and dimmed vision and may see double. These symptoms do not necessarily signal a cataract, but the eyes should be examined. Removal of cataracts has become a simple procedure, one that can often be performed on an outpatient basis. Intraocular lens implants have been very successful, eliminating the need for thick glasses.

senility
(sě-nǐl′-ǐ-tē)

In addition to the physical diseases that are common to the elderly, **senility** often causes a loss of memory, disorientation, and personality changes. Senility is defined as the loss of mental, physical, or emotional control and is manifested by delusions of persecution, apathy, slovenliness, and at times, sudden emotional outbursts. The patient's recent memory may be poor but long-standing memories are very vivid. The past is confused with the present, and the patient may fail to recognize loved ones.

on the Practical Side

Cataracts

Some degree of cataract formation affects about 50% of adults over 65. Several conservative procedures often eliminate the need for surgical removal. New prescription lenses, better lighting, and in some cases, eyedrops may be adequate treatment.

If surgery is chosen, the procedure is fast, simple, and requires only local anesthesia. A small incision allows the removal of the clouded lens.

The cause of senility may be physical, such as brain damage resulting from inadequate blood flow through hardened cerebral arteries. Psychological factors may also foster senility. A feeling of worthlessness, loss of interests, and the stress of worrying about health and future security may be underlying causes of senility. Lack of interest and attention can account for the failure to recall recent events.

Many of the problems of aging can be prevented through preparation for retirement time. Maintaining an interest in life by engaging in hobbies, community service activities, and part-time employment are effective in preventing withdrawal from society and in fulfilling the need to be useful.

Disease by the Numbers x + ÷

EPIDEMIOLOGY

Alzheimer's disease is the most common form of senility, affecting about 4 million Americans. Alzheimer's disease strikes 10% of people over 65 and 50% of people over 85. The cost of caring for Alzheimer's patients in the United States is $80–$100 billion a year.

Alzheimer's disease
(ahlts′-hǐ-merz dǐ-zēz′)

Alzheimer's disease is the most common form of senility and is unique to humans. It is named for Dr. Alzheimer who first described it in 1907. The disease usually is diagnosed in persons over age 65, but it can occur in the late 40s or 50s. Women are slightly more susceptible than men. Nearly 100% of Down's syndrome patients develop Alzheimer's by age 40. Alzheimer's disease manifests itself in the early stages by forgetfulness, failing attention, and declining mathematical ability, such as the inability to balance a checkbook. Later, the person exhibits personality changes, speech difficulties, and general confusion. There is a tendency toward depression, irritability, and severe anxiety. Symptoms may be more noticeable to the casual observer than to family members. When the disease becomes severe, the person experiences hallucinations at night, and the resulting sleeplessness causes the person to wander aimlessly. Early-onset Alzheimer's has a shorter duration and is more severe. Risk factors include age and genetics.

Extensive research on the changes that take place in the nerve cells of these patients' brains has been done on autopsy findings. Abnormalities include loss of neurons in regions essential for memory and understanding as well as accumulations of twisted filaments and nerve tangles in the cortex. Aggregates of protein interfere with cerebral circulation, and degenerating nerve endings, referred to as **plaque,** disrupt transmission of nerve impulses. The plaque is created by a protein fragment called **beta-amyloid,** a byproduct of cell formation. Beta-amyloid is constantly being produced and cleared from the brain, but in Alzheimer's victims, disposal is inhibited. Scientists believe the problem could lie with two enzymes involved in the production of the protein. Recently, scientists have identified an enzyme that sparks the formation of the plaque deposits.

How is Alzheimer's disease diagnosed? A laboratory diagnosis cannot be made, the brain would have to be dissected for that. Family histories and interviews with family members are used. Tests are used to determine the patient's orientation and mood, recent and long-term memory, and the ability to solve problems and make judgments. The diagnosis remains a question until autopsy.

There is no known prevention, treatment, or cure for Alzheimer's disease. Symptoms may be reduced through physical activity to reduce the patient's restlessness. Counseling and support for family members is extremely important in dealing with this irreversible and progressive disease that leads to complete mental and physical disability of loved ones. The identification of the new enzyme may offer hope for new treatments for Alzheimer's victims. Other treatment ideas on the horizon include immune system mobilizers, vaccines, and anti-inflammatory drugs.

plaque
(plăk)

beta-amyloid
(bā'-tă ăm'-ĭ-loyd)

Care of the Elderly

Advances in medical science enabling people to live longer than in the past, and a decrease in the birth rate, have raised the median age in western society. A higher percentage of people are in an older age bracket and require proper attention and health care. **Geriatrics** is the branch of medicine that deals with the problems of aging and the diseases of the elderly.

Research in **gerontology,** the study of aging problems, has revealed the need for psychological support and counseling as well as physical care of the elderly. The aging patient must experience a sense of dignity, worth, and acceptance, whether the person is living with relatives or friends, at home, or in a healthcare facility. The elderly should be supervised carefully to prevent accidents and should be kept alert and aware of their surroundings.

An important physical need of the elderly is proper nutrition: a diet that includes an adequate supply of protein, vitamins and minerals, fruits, vegetables, and milk. If a digestive problem exists, small and more frequent meals may be desirable. Food may have to be chopped or strained because of the inability to chew.

Another need of the aged is a rest and exercise program that helps maintain circulation. The elderly person should be encouraged to engage in a walking program that takes into account the person's strength limitations and does not cause exhaustion. Rest should include short naps or sitting in a chair with the feet elevated. Staying in bed for long periods is harmful, and anemia can develop in the absence of exercise because the mechanism for red blood cell production is not stimulated (Chapter 7).

geriatrics
(jār-ē-ăt'-rĭks)

gerontology
(jār-ŏn-tŏl-ō-jē)

A good understanding of the changes that occur in the aging process makes one better able to give proper healthcare to the elderly patient. The slowed rate of metabolism, with its decreased production of energy, makes the aged very sensitive to temperature changes. The elderly may require warmer clothing or extra blankets.

Resistance to infection is reduced in the elderly as the activity of lymphoid tissue decreases. Bronchopneumonia caused by staphylococci and pneumococci commonly develops in the aged after the flu. A vaccine against bacterial pneumonia has been developed that confers temporary inumunity. Early signs of infection should be noted and the proper medication should be prescribed. The chance of death naturally increases with age, and although many of the diseases that have been mentioned in this chapter do not cause death themselves, they can, in combination with stress, bring about premature death.

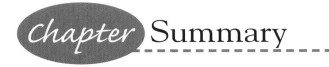

Chapter Summary

The body responds to stress in a variety of ways in the attempt to maintain homeostasis or adapt to the stress. The autonomic nervous system is extensively stimulated, and its response provides the body with additional energy to meet the emergency. Blood pressure is elevated, heart activity is increased, and blood rich in oxygen is provided to active muscles. The liver releases stored glucose needed by the actively metabolizing cells. Adrenalin is secreted by the adrenal medulla, enhancing the effect of the sympathetic nervous system.

The hypothalamus responds to stress by stimulating hormonal activity of the pituitary gland, which in turn, stimulates the thyroid gland and the adrenal cortex. The rate of cellular metabolism and that of concurrent energy production is greatly increased by the elevated thyroxine level.

The glucocorticoids, such as cortisol, increase the level of circulating glucose and prevent an unnecessary inflammatory and immune response. Cortisol also suppresses the immune system. Excessive cortisol can cause the spread of infection by reducing the protective barrier around an infectious agent and preventing the symptoms that signal an infection.

Many diseases are aggravated by stress, particularly those of the cardiovascular system, the skin, the respiratory, and digestive systems. Psychological and emotional factors, as well as physical factors, can trigger the alarm reaction, and the response to it exacerbates the disease. The treatment of these diseases includes identification of the source of stress and removing it where possible, which can enable the patient to adapt to the stress. Medication is prescribed as warranted.

Physiologic changes that are part of the aging process begin early in life. Heredity and environment significantly affect the rate at which these changes occur. A person's ability to withstand stress or adapt to it influences the manner in which aging occurs.

Elderly persons often suffer from cardiovascular problems: heart conditions, hypertension, and arteriosclerosis, which are interrelated. Wear and tear on the body causes degenerative diseases such as osteoarthritis, the pain and stiffness of which decrease mobility and predispose to circulatory problems, muscle atrophy, and anemia. The incidence of cancer is high among the elderly, although many malignancies are detected only at autopsy.

Mental changes also occur with aging. Memory may fail in the elderly patient, and the person then becomes disoriented. Personality changes, inappropriate behavior, and the inability to recognize loved ones indicate the altered mental state of senility. Senility can have a physical basis of brain damage owing to the lack of blood flow through cerebral arteries or Alzheimer's disease, or it can stem from psychological factors such as depression, worry, or a sense of uselessness.

Interactive Activities

CASE FOR CRITICAL THINKING

A patient comes to the clinic complaining of severe diarrhea with blood and mucus. As the patient's history is taken, one notices that the diarrheal episodes are aggravated by stress. What is the diagnosis? What treatment options are available? Are there risks associated with any of the treatment options? What possible side effects are associated with the treatment options? Please explain them to the patient.

MULTIMEDIA EXTENSION ACTIVITIES

www.prenhall.com/mulvihill
Use the above address to access the free, interactive companion Website created for this textbook. Included in the features of this site are chapter specific activities, internet links, and an audio-glossary.

Audio Glossary
Use the CD-ROM disk enclosed with your textbook to hear the pronunciation of the key terms in this chapter.

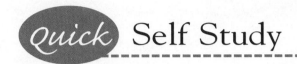

Self Study

MULTIPLE CHOICE

1. The portion of the peripheral nervous system that regulates involuntary motor activity is the _____.
   a. central nervous system
   b. somatic nervous system
   c. autonomic nervous system
   d. parasympathetic nervous system

2. The portion of the autonomic nervous system that triggers the alarm reaction is the

   _____.
   a. sympathetic nervous system
   b. parasympathetic nervous system
   c. central nervous system
   d. peripheral nervous system

3. The alarm reaction causes an increase in _____.
   a. heart rate
   b. respiration rate
   c. blood pressure
   d. all of the above

4. Returning the body to homeostasis after the alarm response is the function of the

   _____.
   a. sympathetic nervous system
   b. parasympathetic nervous system
   c. central nervous system
   d. peripheral nervous system

TRUE/FALSE

_____ 1. Blood sugar level rises when the body is subjected to stress.

_____ 2. Stress triggers increased glucocorticoid production.

_____ 3. Cortisol stimulates the immune system.

_____ 4. Gonadotropin production may decrease during stress.

FILL-INS

1. The _____ gland is regulated by the hypothalamus.

2. Clouding of the eye lens is called _____.

3. The body's ability to maintain internal constancy is called

   _____.

4. The most common form of senility is _____.

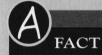

FACT

Vitamin C may be the most essential anti-stress nutrient. Studies on rats show large doses of vitamin C reduce the levels of stress hormones in the blood. These stress hormones weaken the immune system, leaving the body vulnerable to disease and infection.

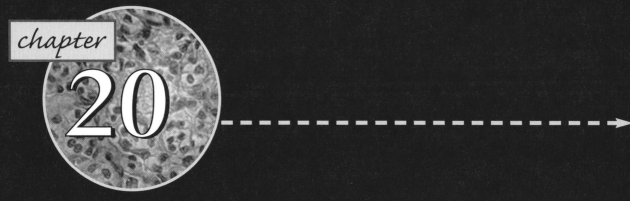

chapter

20

Wellness

We hear much today about health and wellness. What do these terms really mean?

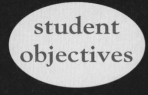

student objectives

After studying this chapter, students should be able to
➤ Define health and wellness
➤ Describe a healthful, well-balanced meal
➤ List important vitamins and their functions
➤ Compare and contrast good and bad cholesterol
➤ Compare the benefits of aerobic and anaerobic exercise

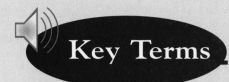

Key Terms

Aerobic exercise

Anaerobic exercise

Antioxidants

Beta carotene

Cholesterol

Cruciferous

Free radicals

Health

High-density
lipoproteins (HDL)

Lipoproteins

Low-density
lipoproteins (LDL)

Phytochemicals

Polyunsaturated

Saturated

Triglycerides

Unsaturated

Very-low-density
lipoproteins (VLDL)

Wellness

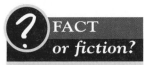

FACT
or fiction?

Human beings need only one tablespoon of vegetable oil per day.

Read this chapter to find the answer.

health
(hĕlth)

wellness
(wĕl'-nĭs)

➤ HEALTH AND WELLNESS

When someone says "at least I have my **health,**" what is meant by the term health? Health is a state of relative equilibrium in which the body's many organ systems function adequately. It is freedom from disease. An individual's health is greatly influenced by genetic make-up, family environment, and psychological characteristics. If this is health, what is **wellness?** Wellness is the condition of good physical and mental health, especially when maintained by proper diet, exercise, and habits. The term wellness describes a state that includes not just physical health but fitness and emotional well-being.

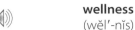

on the Practical Side

Corporations and communities are getting on the wellness bandwagon. A wellness program called Body Smart was started in 1998 in Fresno, California. The program included a media partnership. A local news program featured weekly segments and promotional spots. To encourage people to learn their health status, the program provided free quarterly blood pressure, cholesterol, and body fat screenings. Local grocery stores participated by giving away healthful recipe cards. More than 4,000 people enrolled in Body Smart, double the projected enrollment. Participants exercised more, lost weight, controlled blood pressure, controlled blood sugar levels, and lowered cholesterol. Because Body Smart was so successful, six local employers have incorporated Body Smart into their health and wellness initiatives. Corporations have realized that wellness programs are a great investment. Healthier employees require less medical care, so health care costs are kept down.

on the Practical Side

Skin Patch or Medication to Stop Smoking

The stick-on nicotine patch is helping many smokers quit the habit. The patch is available over the counter. It reduces the craving for cigarettes and reduces withdrawal symptoms by delivering nicotine through the skin in decreasing doses over time. A prescription drug is also available that does not contain nicotine but reduces the withdrawal symptoms.

➤ NUTRITION

Nutrition is a vitally important component of wellness. Diet affects energy levels, well-being, and overall health. Diet can also be closely linked with certain diseases and health problems. Of particular concern is the connection between lifetime nutritional habits and the risk of the major chronic diseases, including heart disease, cancer, and diabetes. Scientists estimate that 30% to 40% of all cancers in men and up to 60% of all cancers in women are linked to the foods we eat. On the more positive side, good nutrition in conjunction with exercise can help prevent such conditions or even reverse some of them.

The Food Pyramid

The best way to eat for good health is to follow the daily food guide pyramid (Figure 20–1). Eat more foods at the bottom of the pyramid and fewer at the top. The key is to get a balance of nutrients by choosing from a wide variety of foods and eating moderate portions.

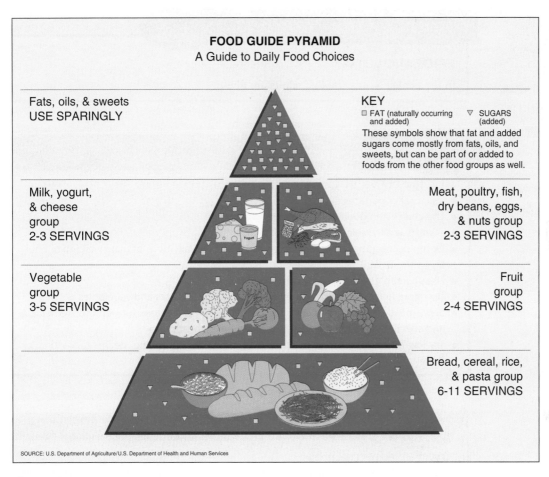

FOOD GUIDE PYRAMID
A Guide to Daily Food Choices

Fats, oils, & sweets
USE SPARINGLY

KEY
□ FAT (naturally occurring   ▽ SUGARS
  and added)   (added)
These symbols show that fat and added
sugars come mostly from fats, oils, and
sweets, but can be part of or added to
foods from the other food groups as well.

Milk, yogurt,
& cheese
group
2-3 SERVINGS

Meat, poultry, fish,
dry beans, eggs,
& nuts group
2-3 SERVINGS

Vegetable
group
3-5 SERVINGS

Fruit
group
2-4 SERVINGS

Bread, cereal, rice,
& pasta group
6-11 SERVINGS

SOURCE: U.S. Department of Agriculture/U.S. Department of Health and Human Services

Figure 20–1
The Food Guide Pyramid is a guide for selecting a wide variety of foods daily.

High-Fiber/Low-Fat Diet

The most healthful diets are high in fiber and low in fat. Fats, also known as lipids, are stored in the body to insulate and cushion organs and to provide energy. Triglyceride is the chemical name for fat. Body fat, for instance, is a triglyceride deposit. Animal fats such as lard and butter as well as fat in meat, poultry, and fish are triglycerides. Triglycerides are compounds formed by joining fatty acids to glycerol. If three fatty acids are joined, the compound is a triglyercide; if only one fatty acid is attached, it is a monoglyceride; if two, a diglyceride. These terms appear on common food labels. The terms **saturated, unsaturated,** and **polyunsaturated** refer to the component fatty acids in a triglyceride. Fatty acids are long chains of carbon atoms connected together, and when the carbon atoms hold all the hydrogen atoms they can, they are saturated and tend to be solid fats. When hydrogen atoms are missing they are called unsaturated fatty acids; polyunsaturated means that several hydrogen atoms are missing, and these tend to be more liquid. Eating too much saturated fat raises blood cholesterol levels in many people, increasing their risk for heart disease. Fat should be limited to 30% of a person's total calorie intake.

saturated
(săt′-ū-rā″-tĕd)

unsaturated
(ŭn-săt′-ū-rāt″-ĕd)

polyunsaturated
(pŏl″-ē-ŭn-săch′-ĕ-rā-tĕd)

Disease by the Numbers x + ÷

EPIDEMIOLOGY

In the United States, 18% of adults are obese.

on the Practical Side

Tips for Low-Fat Cooking

- Use smaller portions of meat
- Use choice and good grades of meat
- Trim away all visible fats on cuts of meat
- Decrease consumption of red meat—red meats contain more fat than most fish or poultry (without skin)
- Use vegetable cooking sprays instead of frying in fat
- Use more herbs and spices, rather than fats to flavor meats and vegetables
- Serve meatless dishes regularly, such as dried beans and peas or tofu with cooked grains and starched like brown rice, bulgur, and whole wheat pasta
- Try low-fat cooking methods like baking, simmering, poaching, steaming, roasting, or broiling

PREVENTION *PLUS!*

Low-Fat Alternatives

The average American eats the fat equivalent of a stick of butter every day, but needs only a single tablespoon of vegetable oil per day. Try switching to some low-fat alternatives to cut down on fat consumption.

- Use skim milk instead of whole, and save 8 grams of fat
- Choose two slices of cheese pizza instead of pepperoni, and save 7 grams of fat
- Eat a regular hamburger instead of a cheeseburger, and save 15 grams of fat
- Eat broiled chicken with the skin removed instead of fried chicken breast, and save 22 grams of fat
- Eat a fudge bar instead of an ice cream bar, and save 12 grams of fat

Commonly known as "bulk" or "roughage," dietary fiber consists of carbohydrate plant substances that are difficult or impossible for humans to digest. Instead, fiber passes through the intestinal tract and provides bulk for feces in the large intestine, which in turn, facilitates elimination. In the large intestine, some types of fiber are broken down by bacteria into acids and gases, which explains why consuming too much fiber can lead to intestinal gas. A diet high in fiber can help manage diabetes, high blood pressure, diarrhea, constipation, hemorrhoids, diverticulitis, and colon and rectal cancer. The average American would benefit from an increase in daily fiber intake. Currently, most Americans consume about 16 grams of fiber a day, whereas the recommended daily amount is 20–35 grams per day. Dietary fiber is found in fruits, vegetables, beans, and whole grains.

Functions of Vitamins

In addition to providing fiber, fruits and vegetables provide a variety of vitamins, minerals, and other chemicals that may be related to cancer protection. One such example is **beta carotene,** which the body uses to make vitamin A. It is contained in deep yellow and dark green vegetables. Good sources are carrots, spinach, sweet potatoes, winter squash, and tomatoes.

Vitamins C and E are **antioxidants** that fight **free radicals,** molecules that may cause disease by injuring cells. Vitamin C is present in oranges and grapefruit, strawberries, baked potatoes, and broccoli. Vegetable oils, leafy greens, and whole grains contain vitamin E.

Vitamin D is necessary for proper absorption of calcium and phosphorus from the gastrointestinal tract. These are the minerals that give hardness to bone. Calcium may be adequate in the diet, but in the absence of vitamin D, it cannot be utilized. Vitamin D-fortified milk is a good source of this vitamin. Exposure to sunlight also provides a source of vitamin D because ultraviolet light converts a substance in the skin (a sterol) to vitamin D.

The B vitamins are water-soluble and many play an essential part in the body's enzyme system. The B vitamins include thiamine, riboflavin, pyridoxine, niacin, pantothenic acid, cobalamin (vitamin B_{12}), and folic acid.

Vitamin B_{12} and folic acid are essential in the formation of red blood cells. Vitamin B_{12} is obtained only from animal products or from supplements derived from microbes. Lack of this vitamin over a number of years leads to severe anemia and neurologic damage. By including lean meat, eggs, or dairy products in the diet, the deficiency can usually be prevented. Folic acid is important in preventing certain birth defects; bread and cereal are enriched with folic acid.

The B vitamins are widely distributed in nature and, therefore, eating a balanced diet, as mentioned, prevents any deficiency. Many breakfast cereals are fortified to provide the recommended daily allowance (RDA), and fruits and vegetables are rich sources of vitamins.

Occasionally, severe vitamin deficiencies occur in the elderly who live alone and stop eating, and in drug addicts and chronic alcoholics in the absence of adequate nutrition. Vitamin B deficiencies most seriously affect the nervous system causing "pins and needles" sensations, mental confusion, and an unsteady walk. Signs of the deficiency can be reversed with an improved diet and appropriate doses of vitamin supplements, but acute brain damage is irreversible.

Most nutritionists recommend using a multivitamin. It should be noted that vitamins are not regulated by the Food and Drug Administration.

Hypervitaminosis

Severe liver damage, even cirrhosis, can result from extremely high consumption of the fat-soluble vitamins, A and D. The current RDA for vitamin A is 5000 IU (international units) for adult men or pregnant women, 4000 for other women, and 2500 for young children. It is almost impossible for adults to achieve toxic levels of vitamin A from food, but supplements, which come in a wide range of dosages, some far exceeding the RDA, should never be used for extended periods of time without medical supervision. A nutritious diet coupled with normal intestinal function never needs a vitamin A or beta carotene supplement. Common side effects of taking too much vitamin A include itching, hair loss, dry skin and mouth, nausea, fatigue, and headaches.

Phytochemicals

Phytochemicals are substances contained naturally in fruits, vegetables, and grains that may be related to cancer protection. **Cruciferous** vegetables (those with cabbage-like

beta carotene
(bā'-tă kăr'-ō-tēn)

antioxidants
(ăn"-tē-ōk'-sĭ-dănts)

free radicals
(frē răd'-ĭ-kăls)

phytochemicals
(fī"-tō-kĕm'-ĭ-kăls)

cruciferous
(kroo-sĭ'-fĕr-ŭs)

odors)—brussels sprouts, cauliflower, broccoli, cabbage, kale, turnips, and rutabaga—are good sources of these chemicals.

Preliminary studies have shown that people who have survived a heart attack may minimize chances of a second heart attack with a diet high in fruits, vegetables, grains, and fish. These foods provide large amounts of soluble fiber, antioxidant vitamins, and beta carotene. Essential minerals such as magnesium and potassium are also contained in these foods.

Cholesterol: Good and Bad

cholesterol
(kō-lĕs′-tĕr-ŏl)

Cholesterol is not a fat, chemically, but rather an alcohol. The large size of the cholesterol molecule gives it the solid, waxy characteristic. The name means "bile solid," and it is this that makes up most of the fatty cholesterol deposits (plaque) that block arteries. Cholesterol is an animal product found in meats and dairy products.

Total cholesterol values refer to the amount of cholesterol found in blood serum or plasma. Laboratory methods differ in accuracy, and an individual's cholesterol level may be affected by various factors. Recommended values have differed, however, it is generally agreed that a reduction in the total cholesterol level significantly reduces the risk of heart attacks and strokes.

triglycerides
(trī-glĭs′-ĕr-īds)

lipoproteins
(lĭp-ō-prō′-tēns)

A person's total cholesterol value is not sufficient to evaluate cardiovascular risk. A breakdown into "good" and "bad" cholesterol levels is essential. To appreciate the difference one has to understand how cholesterol is transported through the blood. Lipids, fats (including **triglycerides**), and fatty-like substances (cholesterol) are not water-soluble and, therefore, cannot mix with blood plasma. To be water-soluble, they are packaged into particles that contain blood proteins, which do mix with water. These particles, called **lipoproteins,** are classified according to their size—small, large, and very large. The size varies according to the amount of triglycerides they contain. The smallest lipoprotein particles containing the smallest amount of triglycerides are dense and therefore, are called **high-density lipoproteins (HDL).** These particles do not contribute to the fatty cholesterol deposits in the arteries. They help carry cholesterol and fat to the liver for reprocessing and, thus, reduce the amount of circulating fat. This HDL component is called "good" cholesterol.

**high-density
lipoproteins (HDL)**
(hī-dĕn′-sĭ-tē
lĭp″-ō-prō′-tē-ĭns)

The larger lipoprotein particles containing more triglycerides are less dense and are called **low-density lipoproteins (LDL).** These molecules tend to lodge in arterial walls forming the plaque that leads to heart attacks, strokes, and other problems, Hence, LDL cholesterol is called "bad" cholesterol. Lipoproteins that contain the most triglycerides are the largest and least dense and are known as **very-low-density lipoproteins (VLDL).**

**low-density
lipoproteins (LDL)**
(lō-dĕn′-sĭ-tē
lĭp″-ō-prō′-tē-ĭns)

**very-low-density
lipoproteins (VLDL)**
(vĕr′-ī-lō-dĕn′-sĭ-tē
lĭp″-ō-prō′-tēins)

An individual's HDL cholesterol measurement indicates the number of smaller fatty-cholesterol particles present in a serum sample, and the LDL measurement indicates the number of larger fatty particles. The higher the LDL cholesterol, the greater the risk of coronary artery disease. The higher the HDL cholesterol, the lower the risk.

There are three risk groups associated with cholesterol levels

Desirable risk: Total Cholesterol <200
                 LDL Cholesterol <130

Borderline risk: Total Cholesterol 200–239
                  LDL Cholesterol 130–159

High risk: Total Cholesterol >240
            LDL Cholesterol >160

Dietary cholesterol in the small intestine is absorbed into the bloodstream, but not all cholesterol in the body comes from food. The major source is the liver that manufactures it. The chief way the body rids itself of cholesterol is through the bowel with the elimination of feces.

The best way to reduce the "bad" cholesterol (LDL) level is by diet and exercise. Dietary fat enhances the absorption of cholesterol and stimulates the liver to form more of it; therefore, fat intake should be restricted. Regular endurance-type exercise, walking, running, swimming, and so forth, tends to reduce LDL and increase HDL cholesterol. This is the greatest protection against fatty deposits in the arteries. Medications are prescribed to reduce the cholesterol level for some individuals with various risk factors.

➤ VALUE OF EXERCISE

Regular aerobic exercise improves the body's ability to use oxygen, which is necessary to burn calories for the production of energy. The efficiency of the heart and lungs is improved; the resting heart rate is lowered, and blood pressure is reduced.

Oxygen, unlike food, cannot be stored, but it is readily available for ordinary action. The secret is to distribute it throughout the entire body, often to meet increased demands for it. During exercise the lungs are working hard to take in more oxygen, the heart is pumping strongly to circulate the blood, and the blood vessels are carrying the blood to active muscles for the energy production that is needed. How well these systems function determines endurance fitness.

When the body is not used, it deteriorates. Symptoms of inadequate exercise include fatigue, falling asleep after a heavy meal, and experiencing shortness of breath with minimal activity. Like nutrition, think of exercise in pyramid form and one can add more activity into the daily routine. Find enjoyable activities; set realistic goals. Be consistent and change the routine if boredom develops (Figure 20–2).

There are two basic types of exercise: aerobic and anerobic.

Aerobic Exercise

Aerobic exercise forces the body to take in and distribute oxygen. It includes running, walking, swimming, and cycling. Exercise of this type enables the lungs to process more air with less effort. The heart becomes stronger, pumping out more blood with each stroke and, therefore, reducing the number of strokes per minute. The conditioned athlete has a very low resting heart rate because of the heart's efficiency. The number and size of blood vessels is increased to better distribute blood. As calories are being burned for energy, weight loss follows with the development of a leaner body.

Walking for fitness is the fastest growing participant sport in the country. Brisk walking on a regular schedule offers cardiovascular benefits, promotes weight loss, improves muscle tone, and prevents age-related illnesses. The walking must be brisk, last for at least 20 to 30 minutes without interruption, and be done at least three days a week to attain the aerobic benefits. The walk must be brisk enough to elevate the heart and respiratory rate sufficiently. Kenneth H. Cooper, M.D., the father of aerobics, provides tables in his book, *Aerobics,* which give the amount of exercise optimum for one's age, sex, and conditioning. Before beginning an exercise program, a person should check with his or her medical doctor to assure that it is appropriate. This applies even to children who may have a condition that would preclude the exercise.

aerobic exercise
(ĕr-ō'-bĭk ĕk'-sĕr-sīz)

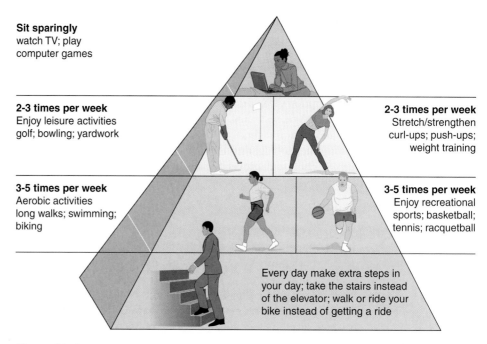

Sit sparingly
watch TV; play
computer games

2-3 times per week
Enjoy leisure activities
golf; bowling; yardwork

2-3 times per week
Stretch/strengthen
curl-ups; push-ups;
weight training

3-5 times per week
Aerobic activities
long walks; swimming;
biking

3-5 times per week
Enjoy recreational
sports; basketball;
tennis; racquetball

Every day make extra steps in
your day; take the stairs instead
of the elevator; walk or ride your
bike instead of getting a ride

Figure 20–2
The Activity Pyramid may be used as a guide for adding more activity into one's daily life.

Anaerobic Exercise

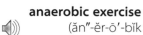

anaerobic exercise
(ăn″-ĕr-ō′-bĭk
ĕk′-sĕr-sĭz)

Anaerobic exercise focuses on specific muscles and their size, endurance, and strength. Weight-lifting is an example of anaerobic exercise. This form of exercise will not provide as many benefits as aerobic exercise, but it is a good supplement to an aerobic workout and may also increase bone density.

Remember, there are many benefits to exercise. It can help one sleep better, be more alert, handle stress better, prevent osteoporosis and even look and feel better. An exercise program should fit the individual's particular needs; however, a complete program should include some form of both aerobic and anaerobic exercise. Talk to a doctor before starting an exercise program.

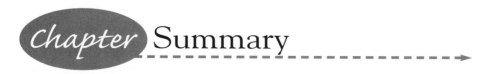

Chapter Summary

The meaning of the terms health and wellness were discussed. The importance of nutrition was reviewed and suggestions for a healthful diet were given. The major vitamins and their functions were discussed. The danger of excessive fat intake was described, and "good" and "bad" cholesterol were distinguished. The value of regular aerobic exercise to increase the efficiency of the heart and lungs was explained.

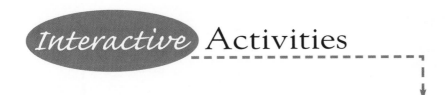

CASE FOR CRITICAL THINKING

A patient comes into the clinic for a check-up. She has lost 25 pounds in two months. You ask her how she lost the weight. She says she is eating a no-carbohydrate, high protein and fat diet, with no exercise routine. Using your knowledge from the chapter, what possible risks in terms of overall health, nutrition, and wellness would you discuss with her? What type of diet and exercise routine might you suggest for her?

MULTIMEDIA EXTENSION ACTIVITIES

www.prenhall.com/mulvihill
Use the above address to access the free, interactive companion Website created for this textbook. Included in the features of this site are chapter specific activities, internet links, and an audio-glossary.

Audio Glossary
Use the CD-ROM disk enclosed with your textbook to hear the pronunciation of the key terms in this chapter.

Quick Self Study

MULTIPLE CHOICE

1. _____ is essential in the formation of red blood cells.
   a. Thiamine   b. Riboflavin
   c. Vitamin B_{12} d. Vitamin D

2. Vitamin B deficiency most seriously affects the _____ system.
   a. Digestive   b. Nervous
   c. Urinary   d. Reproductive

3. Severe liver damage can result from excessive consumption of _____ vitamins.
   a. Fat-soluble   b. Water-soluble

4. _____ fats tend to be solid.
   a. Saturated   b. Unsaturated

TRUE/FALSE

_____ 1. Folic acid can prevent certain birth defects.

_____ 2. Vitamin A is necessary for proper absorption of calcium and phosphorus from the digestive tract.

_____ 3. High-density lipoproteins (HDL) contribute to plaque deposits within arterial walls.

_____ 4. Exercise can reduce blood pressure levels.

FILL-INS

1. _____ exercise increases the size, strength, and endurance of muscles.

2. Vitamins _____ are antioxidants.

3. _____ are substances found in fruits, vegetables, and grains that may be related to cancer prevention.

4. _____ is a state of relative equilibrium in which the body's many organ systems function adequately.

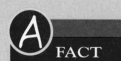

FACT

The average American eats the fat equivalent of a stick of butter every day but needs only one tablespoon of vegetable oil per day.

Glossary

Abdominal. Special muscles of expiration, utilized with difficult breathing.

Achlorhydria. A condition in which hydrochloric acid is absent in the stomach.

Achondroplasia. A disorder resulting from one defective dominant allele. Cartilage formation in the fetus is defective.

Achondroplastic dwarfism. A condition caused by defective cartilage formation that results in improper bone development.

Acidosis. The condition in which the production of acids lowers the body's pH.

Acne. Blackheads, pimples, and pustules, that result from hormonal changes that occur at puberty.

Acquired immunodeficiency syndrome (AIDS). The deadly disease caused by HIV that destroys an individual's immune system, making them remarkably susceptible to infection.

Acromegaly. The condition that results if an excessive production of growth hormone occurs after puberty. The word *megaly* means enlargement.

Activated lymphocytes. White blood cells that have been stimulated by antigens which include B and T cells.

Active immunity. A type of artificial immunity; the person is given a vaccine or toxoid as the antigen, and he or she forms antibodies to counteract it.

Acute. A disease is one that has a sudden onset and is short term.

Adenocarcinomais. Cancer of the pancreas.

Adenocarcinomas. Cancerous glandular tumors.

Adenohypophysis. The anterior and larger portion of the hypophysis, it is truly glandular and is in direct communication with the hypothalamus of the brain.

Adenoma. A benign tumor of glandular tissue which often develops in the breast, thyroid gland, or in mucous glands of the intestinal tract.

Adenoma. A tumor.

Adhesions. Connective tissue fibers that anchor adjacent structures together; a kinking of the intestines.

Adrenalin. The most vital therapy in treatment of allergy and can be self injected in an emergency.

Adrenocorticotropic hormone. The tropic that affects the adrenal cortex.

Androgenital syndrome. A form of hyperadrenalism caused when the male hormone is secreted in excess.

Aerobic exercise. Exercise that forces the body to take in and distribute oxygen such as running, walking, swimming, and cycling.

Agglutinate. Term meaning "to clump together."

Albinism. A rare inherited disorder in which no melanin is formed causing a person to have white hair, pale skin, and pink eyes.

Albuminuria. The presence of the plasma protein albumin in urine.

Aldosterone. The principle hormone in the group of steroid hormones that cause sodium retention and potassium secretion by the kidneys.

Alkalosis. The condition in which the blood is too alkaline; the pH is higher than 7.45.

Alleles. Alternative forms of a gene.

Allergy. Abnormal immunologic response to allergens such as pollens, dust, dog hair, and certain foods.

Allogenic. The transplant of tissue or organs from one human to another.

Alveoli. Small air sacs.

Alzheimer's disease. A common form of senility unique to humans usually over age 65.

Amenorrhea. The absence of menstruation, always accompanies anorexia nervosa.

Amoeboids. A form of protozoa, a single-celled eukaryotic microorganism.

Amphetamines. Appetite depressants which may be prescribed at the beginning of a diet regimen.

Amylase. A digestive enzyme which breaks down carbohydrates.

Amyotrophic (ALS). Also known as Lou Gehrig's disease, a chronic terminal neurologic disease.

Anaerobic exercise. Exercise that focuses on specific muscles and their size, endurance and strength. Weightlifting is an example of this type of exercise.

Anaerobic. Thrives in the absence of oxygen.

Analgesics. Medications that reduce pain.

Anaphylactic shock. Accompanies a severe inflammation that accompanies a severe antigen-antibody reaction, such as occurs in an incompatible blood transfusion.

Anaphylaxis. The condition of anaphylactic shock which is a life-threatening state in which blood pressure drops and airways become constricted.

Anaplasia. Term used to describe lack of form in rapidly growing tumors.

Androgenital syndrome. A form of hyperadrenalism, often called *adrenal virilism.*

Androgens. The sex hormone in males.

Anemia. A condition caused by a reduction of oxygen-carrying hemoglobin.

Aneurysm. A localized dilation caused by a weakening in the wall of a blood vessel.

Angina pectoris. The temporary chest pain or sensation of chest pressure that is caused by transient oxygen insufficiency.

Angiocardiography. An x-ray of the heart and great vessels in which a contrast indicator (dye) is injected into the cardiovascular system.

Angioma. A type of benign tumor, composed of blood vessels such as red birthmark or "port-wine" stain.

Angioplasty. A procedure by which a balloon-tip catheter is inserted into the coronary arteries and expanded to break and crush the plaques.

Ankylosis. Scar tissue that can turn to bone develops between the bone ends, causing the ends to fuse.

Anorexia. A loss of appetite.

Anorexia nervosa. A disease of psychoneurotic origin in which the aversion to food leads to emaciation and malnutrition found to be most common in teenage girls.

Antibiotic resistance. Resistance arising when bacteria adapt to antibiotics and the adaptation becomes common in the bacterial population, soon rendering the antibiotics ineffective.

Antibiotics. Drugs that are used to treat bacterial infections.

Antibodies. Proteins secreted by plasma cells that aid in defense against infectious agents.

Anticoagulant. Medication used to prevent intravascular clotting.

Antidiuretic hormone. One of two hormones secreted by the posterior pituitary.

Antigen. The foreign element that triggers the immune response.

Antihistamine. A drug to counteract the unpleasant effects caused by the release of histamines in the body due to allergies. It has a drying effect on the mucous membranes of the mouth and throat.

Anti-inflammatory hormone. Hormones having an inhibitory effect on the inflammatory response. Certain drugs are described as anti-inflammatories.

Antioxidants. The substances like vitamins C and E that fight free radicals.

Antitoxin. A type of immunization.

Anuria. The total stoppage of urine production.

Aorta. The largest artery that carries blood away from the heart to the arteries.

Aortic stenosis. The narrowing of the valve leading into the aorta.

Aphasia. Loss of speech.

Aplasia. Developmental failure leading to the absence of a structure or tissue.

Aplastic anemia. A type of anemia in which the bone marrow fails to function.

Arrhythmia. A deviation from the normal rhythm of the heart beat.

Arthritis. The inflammation of a joint.

Ascites. Fluid that develops as a result of liver failure and accumulates in the peritoneal cavity.

Aseptic. The absence of infection or contamination.

Aspermia. Caused when there is no formation or emission of sperm caused by the absence of the gonadotropic hormones in a male before puberty.

Astrocytoma. Basically benign, slow-growing tumors of the brain.

Atherosclerosis. The accumulation of fatty material under the inner lining of the arterial wall.

Atresia. The absence or closure of a normal body opening or tubular structure.

Atrophic. A degenerating, wasting condition.

Atrophy. The decrease in size or function of an organ.

Aura. A warning signal such as the symptoms that precede an epileptic seizure.

Auscultation. Listening through a stethoscope for abnormal sounds.

Autoimmune. Antibodies are produced against the body's own tissue.

Autoimmune diseases. These occur when immune tolerances fail and activated T cells and antibodies attack the body's own tissue.

Autologous. A type of transplant in which the patient donates to themselves his/her own tissue.

Autosomes. Name for 44 of the 46 chromosomes.

Azotemia. An increase in the blood urea nitrogen (BUN) caused when the kidneys are unable to excrete urea normally and it accumulates in the blood causing toxicity.

B lymphocytes. One of two types of lymphocytes that provide immunity.

Bacilli. Rod-shaped bacterial cells.

Bacteria. A single-celled organism with simple structure and lacking a nucleus.

Barium. A substance used to provide contrast when producing an x-ray of hollow internal organs such as the stomach or intestine.

Basal ganglia. Nerve cell bodies deep within the white matter of the brain, which help control position and automatic movements.

Basophils. A type of white blood cell that promotes inflammation and participates in allergic responses.

Benign. The term used to describe a noncancerous neoplasm or tumor.

Beta carotene. Substance that body uses to make vitamin A, found in deep yellow and dark green vegetables.

Beta-amyloid. A protein fragment that creates plaque.

Bile. Substance secreted by the liver and necessary for fat digestion. It consists of water, bile salts, cholesterol, and bilirubin.

Biliary calculi. Also called gallstones and form when bile substances that are normally soluble precipitate out of solution. They consist mainly of cholesterol, bilirubin, and calcium.

Biliary cirrhosis. Another form of cirrhosis when bile accumulates in the bile ducts of the liver as a result of cholecystitis causing necrosis and fibrosis of the liver cells lining the ducts.

Bilirubin. A colored pigment that is produced when hemoglobin breaks down.

Binary fission. Process in which bacteria grow rapidly reproduce by splitting in half.

Biopsy. Procedure in which a small sample of a tissue is surgically removed and examined microscopically for abnormalities.

Bowman's capsule. A sac containing the glomerular capillaries.

Bradycardia. When the heart rate is abnormally slow.

Bradykinesia. Slowness of movement.

Bradykinin. The substance released by damaged tissue that promotes inflammation.

Bronchi. The passageway that leads from the trachea to the lung.

Bronchioles. Small tubules located in the lung cavity.

Bronchitis. Inflammation of the bronchi, may be acute or chronic.

Bronchogenic carcinoma. The most common type of lung cancer that arises from the bronchial tree, posing the danger of airway obstruction.

Bronchopneumonia. A type of pneumonia that may develop as a result of small bronchi becoming obstructed because of infection or aspirated gastric contents.

Bulbourethral glands. A pair of glands that secrete into the urethra as it enters the penis.

Bulimia. A gorge-purge syndrome, is the opposite of, yet similar to, anorexia nervosa.

Bundle of His. The specialized tissue in heart muscle capable of sending the impulse for contraction to the ventricles.

Bursae. Sacs of fluid situated near the joint to reduce friction on movement.

Bursitis. Inflammation of the bursae, small, fluid-filled sacs located near the joints that reduce friction on movement.

Cachexia. Condition caused when a patient becomes weak and emaciated in appearance due to the rapid growth of a malignant tumor. The condition of weakness and emaciation that accompanies many chronic diseases like cancer, HIV/AIDS, and tuberculosis.

Capsid. A protein coat of viruses.

Carcinogenesis. The development of cancer.

Carcinogens. Various chemicals that promote cancer development.

Carcinoma. A type of cancer affecting epithelial tissues, skin, and mucous membranes lining body cavities. Also the malignancy of glandular tissue such as the breast, liver, and pancreas.

Carcinoma in situ. A premalignant lesion, the earliest stage of cancer in which the underlying tissue has not yet been invaded.

Cardiac catheterization. Procedure in which a catheter is passed into the heart through appropriate blood vessels to sample the blood in each chamber for oxygen content and pressure.

Cardiac cycle. The alternate contraction and relaxation of atria and ventricles.

Cardiac sphincter. Muscular gateway between the esophagus and stomach.

Cardiogenic shock. The result of extensive myocardial infarction, it is often fatal, but drugs to combat it are sometimes effective.

Carotene. A plant pigment from which vitamin A is derived.

Carotid audiofrequency analysis. An extension of auscultation in which special microphones are placed over areas of abnormal sounds that are heard with a stethoscope.

Caseous. The term used to describe soft and cheese-like tissue in the lungs.

Casts. Molds of kidney tubules consisting of coagulated protein and blood.

Cataracts. Clouding of the eye lens to the point of opacity.

Cell walls. A rigid layer of organic material surrounding delicate cell membranes of bacteria.

Cell-mediated immunity. Protection from infection provided by T cells.

Cerebral vascular accident (CVA). A stroke.

Cerebrospinal. A term pertaining to the brain and spinal cord, cerebrospinal fluid bathes these organs.

Cervix. A part of the female reproductive system, the lowest part of the uterus.

Chancre. An ulceration on the genitals, in the primary stage of infection.

Chemotaxis. The attraction of white blood cells to the site of inflammation.

Cholecystectomy. The surgical removal of the gallbladder.

Cholecystitis. Inflammation of the gallbladder usually caused by an obstruction, a gallstone or tumor.

Cholelithiasis. The formation or presence of gallstones.

Cholesterol. An animal product found in meats and dairy products.

Chorionic gonadotropin. The hormone that indicates a positive pregnancy test.

Chromosome. A molecule of DNA found in the human cell. Each human cell contains 46 chromosomes divided into 23 pairs.

Chronic. A disease that may begin insidiously and be long-lived.

Chronic fatigue syndrome. A disease that produces flulike symptoms including severe and persistent fatigue, muscle and joint pain, and fever.

Chronic obstructive pulmonary disease (COPD). The term used to describe a number of conditions including chronic bronchitis and emphysema in which the exchange of respiratory gases in ineffective.

Chronic ulcerative colitis. A serious inflammation of the colon, the origin of which is unknown.

Chymotrypsin. A digestive enzyme which digests protein.

Cilia. The hairlike projections found in the mucous membrane that lines the respiratory tract.

Ciliates. A form of protozoa, a single-celled eukaryotic microorganism.

Cirrhosis. A chronic destruction of liver cells and tissues with a nodular, bumpy regeneration.

Clitoris. A tuft of erectile tissue, similar to that of the penis located at the anterior junction of the labia minora.

Coarctation. A narrowing, or stricture of the aorta that provides blood to the entire body.

Cobalamin. A component of vitamin B_{12}.

Cocci. Spherical, round bacterial cells.

Collagen. A fibrous protein found in connective tissues, causing wounds to heal poorly.

Colostomy. An artificial opening in the abdominal wall with a segment of the large intestine attached.

Communicable. An infectious disease transmitted from human to human.

Complications. When another disease develops in a patient already suffering from a disease.

Compression sclerotherapy. A treatment for spider veins in which a strong saline solution is injected into specific sites of the varicose veins.

Computerized tomography (CT Scan). A diagnostic-imaging technique used to make a diagnosis and to determine the shape and size of an aneurysm.

Concussion. A transient disorder of the nervous system resulting from a violent blow on the head, or a fall.

Congenital. Abnormalities occurring at or shortly after birth.

Congenital birth defects. Defects, mental or physical, due to developmental error resulting from a maternal infection such as rubella or German measles during pregnancy, the use of certain drugs, or the mother's excessive consumption of alcohol.

Congenital diseases. Diseases that appear at birth or shortly after, but are not caused by genetic or chromosomal abnormalities.

Conjunctiva. The membrane that lines the eyelids and covers the eyeball.

Contagious. An infectious disease transmitted from human to human.

Contusion. An injury, bruise, to brain tissue without a breaking of the skin at the site of the trauma.

Cor pulmonale. A serious heart condition in which the right side of the heart fails as a result of long-standing chronic lung disease.

Coronary arteriography. The selective injection of contrast material into coronary arteries for a film recording of blood vessel action.

Coronary thrombosis. A blood clot on the inner wall of the coronary artery.

Corpus luteum. The structure that develops from the ovarian follicle after ovulation.

Cortisol. The principle hormone in the group of steroid hormones, also known as hydrocortisone.

Cortisone. A hormone of the adrenal gland that has anti-inflammatory properties.

Creatinine. Nitrogen-containing waste products of protein metabolism.

Creatine phosphate. Assists in providing the necessary energy for muscle contraction.

Cretinism. A congenital thyroid deficiency in which thyroxine is not synthesized.

Crohn's disease. An inflammatory disease of the intestine in which the intestinal walls become thick and rigid. A cause of vitamin B_{12} deficiency.

Cruciferous. Refers to a type of vegetable (with cabbage-like odors—brussels sprouts, cauliflower, and broccoli) that are a good source of phytochemicals.

Cryptorchidism. The failure of the testes to descend from the abdominal cavity, where they develop during fetal life, to the scrotum.

Curettage. Part of the procedure known as dilatation and curretage (D&C), the removal of tissue from the uterus.

Cushing's syndrome. A condition resulting from excessive levels of glucocorticoids hormones.

Cyanosis. Blue color in the body tissues.

Cyst. A sac or capsule containing fluid and is usually harmless.

Cystic fibrosis. A disease that affects all the exocrine glands of the body, the glands of external secretion usually affecting children.

Cystitis. An inflammation of the urinary bladder, commonly called a "bladder infection."

Cystoscope. An endoscope through which tumors of the bladder can be seen.

Cytotoxic T cells. One of several types of T cells, often called *killer cells* because of their capability to kill invading organisms.

Defibrillator. A machine that delivers electrical shocks used to re-establish normal heart rhythm.

Delirium tremens. A medical emergency caused by heavy drinking over a long period of time and may occur after withdrawal from heavy alcohol intake.

Dementia. Organic loss of intellectual functions.

Deoxyribonucleic acid (DNA). The blueprint for protein synthesis within the cell.

Dermatitis. A noncontagious skin disorder.

Dermatophytes. Fungi that infect the skin and tend to live on the dead, top layer.

Dermoid cyst. A peculiar benign tumor of the ovary, it may contain many kinds of tissues.

Desensitize. A procedure for causing tolerance to allergens so that they do not trigger allergic reactions.

Diabetes insipidus. A disease that results from a deficiency of ADH.

Diabetes mellitus. An endocrine disease in which the beta cells fail to secrete insulin or target cells fail to respond to insulin.

Diabetic nephropathy. A kidney disease resulting from diabetes mellitus.

Diagnosis. The determination of the nature of a disease based on many factors, including signs, symptoms, and, often, laboratory results.

Dialysis. The artificial cleansing of blood.

Diaphragm. The main muscle of inspiration.

Diastole. The period of the heartbeat when the heart relaxes and fills with blood.

Diethylstilbestrol (DES). A synthetic hormone which was used to prevent spontaneous abortion.

Dilation. Scraping of the uterus.

Discoid. The mild form of lupus erythematosus in which red, raised, itchy lesions develop.

Disease. A state of functional disequilibrium that may be resolved by recovery or death.

Disinfection. Reducing the risk of infection or contamination.

Diuretic. A substance that causes the kidneys to excrete water. Diuretics can lower blood pressure.

Diverticula. Little pouches or sacs formed when the mucosal lining pushes through the underlying muscle layer.

Diverticulitis. Inflammation of the diverticula, usually occurring in the colon or small intestines.

Dominant. A gene that is expressed when inherited.

Dopamine. A neuronal transmitter substance.

Doppler imaging. Instrument that uses echoes of moving blood columns to produce images of the vessel wall outline; the velocity of the blood is measured and the degree of carotid thenosis is determined.

Down's syndrome. A disorder caused by the presence of an extra autosomal chromosome.

Duodenal ulcers. Ulcers of the small intestine caused by an excessive secretion of hydrochloric acid.

Dysentery. An acute inflammation of the colon, a colitis.

Dysmenorrhea. Painful menstruation.

Dyspareunia. Painful sexual intercourse.

Dysphagia. The term for difficult or painful swallowing.

Dysplasia. An abnormal development, such as a congenital heart defect.

Dyspnea. Shortness of breath.

Dystrophin. A skeletal protein that is missing in Duchene's muscular dystrophy.

Dystrophy. Muscle degeneration that disables an individual.

Dysuria. Painful urination.

Ecchymoses. A large hemorrhagic area.

Ecchymosis. Hemorrhagic spots that develop on the skin and in mucous membranes, causing discoloration.

Echocardiography. A noninvasive procedure (ultrasound cardiography) that utilizes high-frequency sound waves to examine the size, shape, and motion of heart structures.

Eclampsia. Convulsions and coma that follow untreated pregnancy-induced hypertension.

Ectopic pregnancy. A pregnancy in which the fertilized ovum implants in a tissue other than the uterus, most commonly in the fallopian tubes.

Eczema. A noncontagious inflammatory skin disorder known as "contact dermatitise."

Edema. Swelling caused by leakage of plasma into tissues.

Ejaculatory duct. An accessory gland near the base of the urinary bladder where the vas deferens joins a duct of the seminal vesicle.

Electrocardiogram (ECG). An electrical recording of the heart action that aids in the diagnosis of coronary artery disease, myocardial infarction, valvular heart disease, and some congenital heart diseases.

Electroencephalogram. A recording of brain waves.

Electrolyte balance. The proper balance of salts, like potassium, and calcium.

Electromyogram (EMG). The method used to diagnose muscle disorders.

Electromyography. An electrodiagnostic test used to confirm the presence of carpal tunnel syndrome.

Encephalitis. The inflammation of the brain and meninges, caused by a viral infection.

Embolism. A circulating blood clot.

Emphysema. A crippling disease which is not contagious but one of chronic lung obstruction and destruction.

Encephalopathy. Chronic, destructive, or degenerative condition of the brain.

Endarterectomy. A common surgical procedure used to treat a blockage in a carotid artery by removing the thickened area of the inner vascular lining.

Endemic. Describes a disease which always occurs at low levels in a population.

Endocarditis. Inflammation within the heart.

Endocardium. A smooth delicate membrane that lines chambers of the heart.

Endometriosis. A disease condition in which endometrial tissue from the uterus becomes embedded elsewhere.

Endoscope. An instrument consisting of a hollow tube with a lens and light system used to view the inner surface of the digestive tract.

Endoscopic sclerotherapy. A procedure in which a retractable needle is guided into the esophagus by means of a fiberoptic endoscope.

Endospores. Structures produced by bacteria and formed to cope with harsh environmental conditions.

Endotoxin. A potent toxin from certain bacteria that causes life-threatening shock.

Eosinophils. A type of white blood cell that kill parasites and are involved in allergic responses.

Epidemic. Describes a disease that occurs in unusually large numbers over a specific area.

Epidermoid carcinomas. Tumors of the skin.

Epididymis. A coiled tube that lies along the outer wall of the testis and leads into the vas deferens.

Epidural. A hemorrhage between the dura mater and the skull.

Epilepsy. A group of uncontrolled cerebral discharges that recurs at random intervals.

Epinephrine. The hormone secreted by the adrenal medulla when additional energy and strength are needed; a drug used to treat an allergy attack.

Epistaxis. Bleeding from the nose.

Erysipelas. An inflammatory skin infection caused by streptococcus bacteria. Most commonly, the infections appear on the face, arm, or leg.

Erythema. A reddened area of skin.

Erythematous. An area of skin reddened by congested blood vessels resulting from injury or inflammation.

Erythrocytes. A cellular component of red blood cells.

Erythropoiesis. The process of red cell formation that takes place in the red marrow of flat bones such as the sternum, hip bones, ribs, and skull bones.

Erythropoietin. A hormone synthesized principally by the kidney that stimulates red blood cell development.

Esophageal varices. Varicose veins of the esophagus.

Esophagitis. Inflammation of the esophagus caused by acid reflux.

Estrogen. The sex hormone in females.

Etiology. The cause of a disease.

Exacerbation. The period of a chronic disease when signs and symptoms recur in all their severity.

Exfoliative cytology. A means of obtaining cells for microscopic examination through scrapings, washings, and secretions from suspected areas.

Exocrine glands. The glands of external secretion. They secrete mucus, perspiration, and digestive enzymes.

Exophthalmos. The condition in which the eyeballs protrude outward, characteristic of a person with Graves' disease.

External intercostals. The muscles found between the ribs, the main muscles of inspiration.

Extradural. A hemorrhage between the dura mater and the skull.

Fallopian tubes. A part of the female reproductive system, they extend laterally from each side of the uterus.

Familial polyposis. A hereditary disease in which numerous polyps develop in the intestinal tract.

Fibrin. A plasma protein essential for blood-clotting.

Fibroblasts. Connective tissue cells that produce fibers to aid in healing damaged tissue.

Fibrocystic disease. The formation of numerous lumps in the breast that are fluid-filled.

Fimbriae. Fingerlike projections at the outer ends of the fallopian tubes, they propel ova into the tube.

Flagellates. A form of protozoa; a single-celled eukaryotic microorganism.

Flatus. Gas.

Flatworm. A worm-like animal that has a flattened body.

Fluoroscopy. A diagnostic procedure that permits visualization of the lungs and diaphragm during respiration.

Foramen ovale. A small opening that allows blood from the right side of the heart to enter the left directly, bypassing the nonfunctional fetal lungs.

Fragile X syndrome. A genetic condition associated with mental retardation. It is identified by a break, or weakness, on the long arm of the X chromosome.

Free radicals. The molecules that may cause disease by injuring cells.

Friable. Easily broken modules or vegetations.

Fulminating. Having a rapid or severe onset.

Functional. Condition is one in which there is no organic change.

Furuncles. Large, tender, swollen raised lesions, boils, caused by staphylococci.

Galactosemia. The disease in which the enzyme necessary to convert galactose, a sugar derived from lactose in milk to glucose is lacking.

Gangrene. Condition in which bacteria infects and destroys dead tissue.

Gastric ulcers. Ulcers of the stomach.

Gastritis. Inflammation of the stomach caused by irritants such as aspirin, excessive coffee, tobacco, alcohol or an infection.

Gastroscopy. A procedure in which a camera is attached to a gastroscope, and the entire inner stomach is photographed.

Genes. Found in chromosomes, each is responsible for the synthesis of one protein.

Genital warts. Venereal warts that are very serious and difficult to remove.

Geriatrics. The branch of medicine that deals with the problems of aging and the diseases of the elderly.

Gerontology. The study of aging problems.

Gigantism. Usually the result of a tumor of the anterior pituitary.

Glioblastomas. Highly malignant, rapid-growing tumors of the brain.

Gliomas. Primary malignant tumors of the brain.

Glomerulonephritis. A common disease primarily affecting children and young adults. It usually results from a previous streptococcal infection.

Glomerulus. A tuft of capillaries situated inside Bowman's capsule.

Glucagon. A hormone that works antagonistically to insulin and is released when the blood sugar level falls below normal.

Glucocorticoids. The group of steroid hormones that helps regulate carbohydrate, lipid, and protein metabolism.

Glycogen. A form of glucose that is stored in the liver.

Glycosuria. The condition in which excess glucose is excreted in the urine. It is a major sign of diabetes mellitus.

Goiter. An enlargement of the thyroid gland that may be caused by hypoactivity or hyperactivity of the thyroid or a deficiency in iodine.

Gonadotropins. Hormones of the anterior pituitary that regulate sexual development and function.

Gout. Often called "gouty arthritis," it affects the joints of the feet, particularly those of the big toe and is very painful.

Graafian follicles. Ovarian follicles stimulated at the beginning of each monthly cycle so that they begin to grow and develop by a pituitary gonadotropic hormone.

Gram stain. The staining technique that permits the identification of bacteria.

Gynecomastia. A condition in which the breasts become enlarged.

Health. A state of relative equilibrium in which the body's many organ systems function adequately and are free from disease.

Heart block. When the impulse for contraction within the heart fails to spread from the atria to the ventricles, and pulse is drastically reduced.

Heart murmurs. Characteristic sounds of the heart that indicate the presence of valve defects.

Helicobacter pylori. A bacterium associated with ulcers.

Helper T cells. One of several types of T cells, they help the immune system by increasing the activity of killer cells and stimulating the suppressor T cells.

Hematemesis. Vomiting of blood.

Hematocrit. The ratio of red blood cell-volume to whole blood.

Hematoma. A bruise caused by an injection.

Hematuria. Blood in the urine.

Hemiplegia. Paralysis on one side of the body.

Hemoglobin. A protein containing iron and serves as the oxygen-carrier protein that enables red blood cells to carry oxygen from the lungs to all body tissues.

Hemolysis. The rupture of red blood cells.

Hemolytic streptococci. A type of bacteria that cause a variety of infectious diseases, including infections of throat, skin, ear, and heart valves.

Hemolyze. Term meaning "to rupture."

Hemorrhage. A large loss of blood in a short period of time, either internally or externally.

Hemorrhoids. Varicose veins of the rectum or anus.

Hemostasis. Lack of blood flow.

Heparin. An anticoagulant.

Hepatic coma. Develops in the final stages of advanced liver disease: it is caused by an accumulation of ammonia in the blood, which has a toxic effect on the brain and may be a cause of death.

Hepatocarcinoma. Cancer of the liver.

Hermaphrodites. Individuals who have both testes and ovaries.

Herpes simplex. The virus that causes cold sores or fever blisters.

Heterozygous. A person having 2 different alleles of a certain gene.

Hiatal hernia. The protrusion of part of the stomach through the diaphragm at the point where the esophagus joins the stomach.

High-density lipoproteins (HDL). The smallest lipoprotein particles containing the smallest amount of triglycerides. This HDL component is called "good" cholesterol.

Hirsutism. Term to describe the condition in which hair develops on the face of a woman.

Histamine. A substance that causes the capillary walls to become more permeable.

Hodgkin's disease. A type of lymphoma, it is distinguished by the presence of characteristic *Reed-Sternberg* cells in affected lymph nodes.

Homeostasis. The maintenance of a steady state within the body.

Homozygous. A person having the same two alleles of a particular gene.

Horizontal transmission. The route by which an infectious disease is transmitted directly from an infected human to a susceptible human.

Human immunodeficiency virus (HIV). The causative agent of AIDS; a retrovirus, i.e., it carries its genetic information as RNA rather than DNA.

Human papillomavirus (HPV). The type of virus responsible for genital warts that seems to be the causative agent in uterine cervical carcinoma.

Humoral immunity. Protection from infection provided by antibodies.

Huntington's chorea. A progressive degenerative disease of the brain that results in the loss of muscle control.

Hydatidiform mole. A benign tumor of the placenta, consisting of multiple cysts and resembling a bunch of grapes.

Hydrocephalus. The accumulation of cerebrospinal fluid in the brain.

Hydrolithotripsy. A procedure using sonic vibrations to crush kidney stones while the patient is immersed in a tank of water.

Hydronephrosis. A condition when the kidney is extremely dilated with urine.

Hydrosalpinx. Inflammation that subsides after an infection when treated with antibiotics, and the fallopian tube is filled with a watery fluid.

Hydroureters. The condition caused when the ureters above a kidney obstruction dilate.

Hymen. A membranous fold that partly or completely closes the vaginal opening.

Hyperactive. The term used to describe when a gland produces an excessive amount of its secretion.

Hypercalcemia. A condition in which too much calcium occurs in the blood.

Hyperemia. Increased blood flow to an injured area causing heat and redness associated with inflammation.

Hyperglycemia. A condition resulting from deposits of calcium in organs such as kidneys, heart, lungs and the walls of the stomach.

Hyperkalemia. An excess of potassium which causes muscle weakness and can slow the heart to the point of cardiac arrest.

Hypernephroma. Carcinoma of the kidney, causes enlargement of kidney and destroys the organ.

Hyperparathyroidism. The condition in which an overactive parathyroid gland hypersecretes too much parathormone, which raises the level of circulating calcium above normal.

Hyperpituitarism. Conditions associated with hypersecretion of the pituitary, usually manifested as the effects of excessive growth hormone, which retards the normal closure of bones at puberty.

Hyperplasia. Also known as fibrocystic disease, the formation of numerous lumps in the breast that are fluid-filled cysts.

Hypersensitivity. An abnormal immune response and sensitivity to allergens such as pollens, dust, dog hair, and certain foods.

Hypertrophy. Abnormal enlargement of an organ.

Hyperthyroidism. A condition of excessive amount of thyroxine.

Hypervitaminosis. A toxic condition caused by an excess of vitamins.

Hypoactive. The term used to describe when a gland fails to secrete its hormone or secretes an inadequate amount.

Hypoalbuminemia. An albumin deficiency.

Hypochromic. Red blood cells appear lighter than normal, caused by an iron deficiency.

Hypophysis. Another name for the pituitary gland. It has two parts, each of which acts as a separate gland.

Hypoplasia. Incomplete or underdevelopment of an organ or tissue.

Hypothalamus. An extremely important coordinating center for the brain that directs which hormones the anterior pituitary gland should secrete at a particular time.

Hypothyroidism. A condition in which there is an inadequate level of thyroxine.

Hypovolemic shock. Results from fluid volume loss after severe hemorrhage or loss of plasma in burn patients.

Hypoxia. An insufficient oxygenation of the tissues in the lungs as a result of swelling and increased mucous.

Idiopathic thrombocytopenia purpura. Bleeding caused by low platelet levels. The cause is unknown.

Idiopathic. Term used to describe a disease for which the cause is not known.

Immunoglobulin. Antibodies; Bind to foreign antigens and provide protection from infection.

Impetigo. An acute, contagious skin infection common in children most frequently affecting face and hands.

Incidence. The number of new cases of a disease in a population.

Infarct. Dead tissue that occurs when an area of the myocardium is suddenly deprived of blood.

Infectious diseases. Diseases caused by pathogenic microorganisms.

Infestations. Infections involving wormlike animals called helminths.

Inflammatory exudate. Fluid composed of plasma and white cells that escape from capillaries.

Influenza. A viral infection of the upper respiratory system.

Initiation. The first stage of cancer in which there is a genetic change in a cell, an altering of the DNA by some agent, chemical, radiation, or an oncogenic virus.

Insulin. A hormone that is secreted when the blood sugar level rises.

Internal intercostal muscles. Special muscles of the rib cage that assist difficult breathing.

Intima. The inner lining of the arterial wall.

Intravenous pyelogram. Allows the visualization of the urinary system by means of contrast dyes injected into the veins followed by an x-ray examination.

Intrinsic factor. Produced in the stomach, it carries vitamin B_{12} to the small intestine where it is absorbed in to the bloodstream.

Intussusception. A type of organic obstruction in which a segment of intestine telescopes into the part forward of it.

Irritable bowel. A functional condition of the colon with diarrhea, constipation, abdominal pain and gas.

Irritable colon. A functional disorder of the colon that results in diarrhea and cramping.

Ischemia. A deficiency of blood supply to any organ.

Isolation. Keeping an infected person in the hospital or staying at home in bed when suffering from a disease as a way of controlling the transmission of infectious diseases.

Jaundice. A yellow-orange discoloration of the skin, tissues, and the whites of the eyes caused when bilirubin (an orange pigment) accumulates in the plasma.

Juxtaglomerular apparatus. Specialized cells within the arterioles leading to the functional kidney area.

Karyotype. The chromosomal composition of the nucleus of the cell.

Keloid. The healing that occurs after surgery or a severe burn consisting of a scar that is hard and raised.

Keratin. Contained in the epidermis; a tough, fibrous protein produced by cells called keratinocytes and protects the skin from harmful substances.

Keratinocytes. Cells that produce keratin.

Ketone bodies. Substances produced in diabetic's blood when insulin levels are low.

Klinefelter's syndrome. When there is an extra sex chromosome resulting in a karyotype of 47,XXY.

Kupffer's cells. Specialized cells that line the blood spaces within the liver. They engulf and digest bacteria and other foreign substances, thus cleansing the blood.

Laparoscopy. A procedure in which an illuminated tube is inserted through a small incision or opening used to diagnose endometriosis.

Larynx. The voice box located at the entrance of the trachea.

Latent infection. A condition caused when viruses insert themselves in cells and do not reproduce.

Legionnaire's Disease. A lung infection caused by the bacterium, *Legionella pneumophila;* characterized by flu-like symptoms.

Leiomyomas. Benign tumors of the smooth muscle of the uterus, known as fibroid tumors.

Lesion. An abnormal tissue structure or function. May be the result of a wound, injury or pathologic condition.

Lethargy. A condition of drowsiness.

Leukemia. A cancer of white blood cells in which the bone marrow produces a large number of abnormal white blood cells.

Leukocytes. White blood cells, which are cellular components of blood.

Leukocytosis. The excessive production of white cells.

Leukopenia. An abnormal decrease in the number of circulating white blood cells; a side effect from chemotherapy.

Leukorrhea. A term for any vaginal discharge other than blood.

Ligaments. The substance that holds bones together.

Ligated. The tying off of various veins.

Lipase. A digestive enzyme which breaks down lipid or fat.

Lipoma. A soft, fatty, benign tumor that develops in adipose (fat) tissue.

Lipoproteins. A lipid fat that is water-soluble. It is packaged into particles that contain blood proteins, which do mix with water.

Lithotripsy. The crushing of kidney stones, replacing the need for surgery.

Low-density lipoproteins (LDL). The larger lipoprotein particles containing triglycerides.

Lower respiratory disease. Diseases affecting the lungs or bronchi.

Lumbar puncture. A procedure (spinal tap) used to diagnosis meningitis in which a hollow needle is inserted into the spinal canal between vertebrae near the L-4, or lumbar region.

Lumen. The inner space of a hollow organ such as a blood vessel or intestine.

Lumpectomy. Surgery to remove only the tumor from the breast.

Lymphadenopathy. Enlarged lymph nodes.

Lymphatic system. An important part of the body's immunity, it consists of a complex network of thin-walled capillaries carrying lymph fluid, nodes, and organs that help to maintain the internal fluid environment of the body.

Lymphocytes. A type of white blood cells consisting of T-lymphocytes and B-lymphocytes.

Lymphocytic. The type of leukemia which results from cancer of the lymphocytic stem cells, which are found both in the bone marrow and in the lymph nodes.

Lymphomas. Several types of malignancies of the lymphatic system.

Lyse. The infecting of cells by viruses.

Macular. Lesions on the skin that are flat.

Magnetic resonance imaging (MRI). A diagnostic-imaging technique used to make a diagnosis.

Malabsorption. The inability of a person to absorb substances from the small intestines.

Malignant melanoma. Skin cancer.

Malignant. Term used to describe a neoplasm or tumor that spreads and possibly causes death.

Mammography. Diagnostic x-ray for breast tissue that can detect small, early cancers.

Mast cells. Cells found in connective tissue and contain heparin, serotonin, bradykinin, and histamine.

Mastectomy. Surgery to remove the breast due to cancer.

Medullary cavity. A hollow cavity found in the long bones of the arms and legs that is filled with yellow bone marrow primarily consisting of fat.

Melanin. The dark pigment of the skin that protects the body from the harmful rays of the sun.

Melanocytes. Cells at the bottom of the epidermis that produce melanin.

Melena. Stool with a dark, tarry appearance, caused by blood from the upper part of the digestive tract.

Memory cells. B lymphocytes that do not become plasma cells but remain dormant until reactivated by the same antigen.

Menarche. The onset of menstruation, the beginning of a woman's reproductive life, occurring generally between ages 10 and 15.

Meninges. Three coverings that protect the delicate nerve tissue of the spinal cord.

Meningitis. An acute inflammation of the first two meninges that cover the brain and spinal cord.

Meningocele. A form of spina bifida noticeable at birth; the spinal cord is not involved in this defect.

Meningomyelocele. A form of spina bifida in which the nerve elements protrude into the sac and are trapped, thus preventing proper placement and development.

Menopause. The cessation of menstrual periods, the ending of a woman's reproductive life, which usually begins in the late 40s or early 50s.

Menorrhagia. Excessive or prolonged bleeding during menstruation.

Metaplasia. The conversion of normal tissue cells into an abnormal form after chronic stress or injury.

Metastasis. The spread of cancer to distant sites within the body.

Metastasize. To invade by metastasis.

Metrorrhagia. Bleeding between menstrual periods or extreme irregularity of the cycle.

Microliter. A volume equal to one-millionth of a liter.

Mineralocorticoids. A group of steroid hormones that regulate salt balance in the body.

Mitral stenosis. Occurs when the mitral valve opening is too small and the cusps that form the valve, become rigid and fuse together.

Mitral valve. The valve between the left atrium and left ventricle having two flaps, or cusps, that meet when the valve is closed.

Monocytes. A type of white blood cell that ingest dead cells and protect the body against many infective organisms.

Mons pubis. The pad of fat tissue located over the pubic symphysis that becomes covered with hair at puberty.

Mucosa. Secretes excessive mucus causing a runny nose and congestion.

Mucosal. Pertaining to the mucosa.

Mucus. A thick watery secretion.

Mutagens. Chemicals introduced to the lungs by cigarette smoking.

Mutated. The term for alteration to a gene.

Myasthenia gravis. A neuromuscular disorder in which neither nerves nor muscles are diseased at the myoneural junction.

Mycelia. Filaments in fungi specialized for absorption of nutrients.

Myelin. A lipid covering that insulates the fibers of sensory and motor neurons.

Myelocele. The most severe form of spina bifida.

Myelogenous. The type of leukemia in which the cancer originates in the bone marrow.

Myocardial infarction. A true heart attack.

Myocardium. The cardiac muscle found in the chamber walls of the heart.

Myoma. A tumor of the muscle that develops in smooth or involuntary muscle.

Myxedema. The condition of severe hypothyroidism, an inadequate level of thyroxine.

Necrotic. Dead tissue due to lack of blood.

Neoplasm. A mass of new cells that grows in a haphazard fashion with no useful function, a tumor.

Nephron. The functional unit of the kidney.

Nephrotripsy. A procedure using sonic vibrations to crush kidney stone in which the patient is not immersed in water for the procedure.

Neurogenic shock. Condition due to generalized vasodilation, resulting from decreased vasomotor tone.

Neutrophils. The most prevalent white blood cells and help protect the body against bacterial and fungal infections.

Nevus. A small, dark skin growth that develops from pigment-producing cells or melanocytes; a benign tumor.

Nitroglycerin. Medication used to dilate coronary arteries, permitting adequate blood flow.

Nocturia. The need to urinate during the night.

Noncommunicable. Infectious diseases that are not transmitted directly by humans.

Nondisjunction. The failure of two chromosomes to separate as the gametes, either the egg or the sperm, are being formed.

Normoblasts. Contain a nucleus but it begins to shrink as the cytoplasm fills with hemoglobin synthesized by the endoplasmic reticulum.

Nystagmus. Involuntary, rapid movement of the eyeball, characteristic of Wernicke's encephalopathy.

Obesity. A nutritional disorder in which an abnormal amount of fat accumulates in adipose tissue.

Occult blood. Blood detected in stool by means of a chemical test but not apparent to the naked eye.

Oliguria. A sudden drop in urine volume.

Oncogene. Any gene having the potential to induce a cancerous transformation.

Orchitis. Inflammation of the testes, can follow an injury or viral infection such as mumps.

Organic obstructions. The contents of the intestinal tract are unable to move forward due to material blockage.

Osteitis fibrosa cystica. In this disease, fibrous nodules and cysts form in the bones, which become very porous and decalcified.

Osteoarthritis. The most common form of arthritis, a chronic disease that accompanies aging and may affect only one joint.

Osteoblasts. A cell that works within the bone to form bone tissue.

Osteoclasts. A cell that works within the bone and which resorb bone.

Osteogenic sarcoma. A primary malignancy of the bone.

Osteoma. The most common benign tumor of the bone.

Osteomalacia. A bone disease in adults caused by the lack of vitamin D which results in a softening of the bones.

Osteomyelitis. An inflammation of the bone, particularly of the bone marrow in the medullary cavity and in the spaces of spongy bone.

Osteopenia. The loss or thinning of bone tissue.

Osteoporosis. The increased porosity of the bone.

Outbreak. Describes the sudden outbreak of a disease that occurs in unexpected numbers in a limited area and then subsides.

Ovaries. A part of the female reproductive system, they are small, oval-shaped glands that contain hundreds of thousands of ova which are present at birth.

Oxytocin. One of two hormones secreted by the posterior pituitary, causing smooth muscle, particularly that of the uterus, to contract and initiates milk secretions.

Paget's disease. A rare cancer involving inflammatory changes that affect the nipple and the areola.

Pallor. An abnormal paleness.

Palsy. Tremors caused by the degeneration of the brain that appears gradually and progresses slowly; Parkinson's disease.

Pancreatitis. A serious inflammation of the pancreas that occurs when the protein- and lipid-digesting enzymes become activated within the pancreas and begin to digest the organ itself. It can result in death.

Pandemic. Describes an epidemic that has spread to include several large areas worldwide.

Pap. A diagnostic technique for identifying cancer in the cervix by scraping cells from the cervix and examining them microscopically.

Papilloma. Also known as a polyp, it is an epithelial tumor that grows as a projecting mass on the skin, or from an inner mucous membrane; the common wart.

Papular. Lesions on the skin that are raised.

Paralytic obstructions. Caused when the contents of the intestinal tract are unable to move forward due to a decrease in peristalsis preventing propulsion of intestinal contents.

Parathormone. The hormone secreted by the parathyroids.

Paresis. A general paralysis associated with organic loss of brain function. It results in death if untreated.

Partial thromboplastin time. A method for measuring defects in coagulation.

Passive immunity. Doses of preformed antibodies from immune serum of an animal, usually a horse. This type of immunity is short-lived but acts immediately.

Patent ductus arteriosus (PDA). A common congenital disease in which the ductus arteriosus remains open and blood intended for the body flows from the aorta to the lungs overloading the pulmonary artery.

Pathogenesis. The source or cause of an illness or abnormal condition, and its development.

Pathogenic organisms. Bacteria, viruses, fungi or parasites that cause disease.

Pathogens. Microorganisms that cause disease.

Pathologic aspiration. The drawing of vomitus or mucus into the respiratory tract.

Pathology. The branch of medicine that studies the characteristics, causes, and effects of disease.

Pediculosis. Louse infestations that are classified into three categories: head lice, pubic lice, and body lice.

Peptic ulcers. Ulcers of the stomach and small intestine due, in part, to the action of pepsin, a proteolytic enzyme secreted by the stomach.

Perforation. An ulcer breaks through the intestinal or gastric wall causing sudden and intense abdominal pain.

Pericardium. The double membranous sac that encloses the heart.

Periosteum. A highly vascular layer of fibrous connective tissue that covers the surface of bones.

Peristalisis. Muscle contractions that propel food during the digestive process.

Peritonitis. Inflammation of the lining of the abdominal cavity, usually results when the digestive contents enter the cavity, because this material contains numerous bacteria.

Pernicious anemia. A vitamin B_{12} deficiency.

Petechiae. Tiny red or purple spots caused by minute blood vessels that rupture in the skin.

Petit mal. A mild form of epilepsy that usually disappears by the late teens or early 20s.

Phagocytes. Having the ability to engulf and digest bacteria and cellular debris.

Pharynx. The throat.

Phenylketonuria. Also called PKU, is caused by an autosomal recessive allele that lacks a specific enzyme that converts one amino acid, phenylalanine, to another, tyrosine.

Phlebitis. An inflammation of a vein, usually in the leg.

Phlebotomy. Drawing blood for diagnosis or treatment.

Photophobia. An abnormal sensitivity to light.

Phytochemicals. Substances contained naturally in fruits, vegetables, and grains that may be related to cancer protection.

Pipe-stem colon. Term used to describe the colon in patients suffering from chronic ulcerative colitis; colon appears straight and rigid.

Placenta. The interdigitation of embryonic and maternal tissue.

Plantar warts. Serious, painful warts, that form on the soles of the feet.

Plaque. Fatty deposits in the walls of arteries.

Plasma cells. Cells that develop from B cells and produce antibodies.

Platelets. Clotting elements of blood.

Pleura. A double membrane consisting of two layers that encases the lungs.

Pleural cavity. The space between the two layers of the pleura containing a small amount of fluid that lubricates the surfaces, preventing friction as the lungs expand and contract.

Pleurisy. The inflammation of the pleural membranes occurring as a complication of various lung diseases like pneumonia or tuberculosis.

Pneumonia. An acute inflammation of the lung in which air spaces in the lungs become filled with an inflammatory exudate.

Poliomyelitis. An infectious disease of the brain and spinal cord caused by a virus.

Polycystic kidney. A congenital anomaly, an error in development, usually involving both kidneys.

Polydactyly. An autosomal dominant disorder that causes extra fingers or toes.

Polydipsia. Extreme thirst.

Polymorphs. Certain white blood cells specialized to fight against invading agents or injuries.

Polyunsaturated. The term that refers to the component fatty acids in a triglyceride.

Polyuria. The excessive production of dilute urine.

Preeclampsia. Complication of pregnancy that involves hypertension, proteinuria, and edema.

Premenstrual syndrome (PMS). A group of severe symptoms, emotional, physical, and behavioral, that are associated with the menstrual cycle.

Prepuce. A flap of loosely attached skin covering the glans of the penis, also called the foreskin.

Prevalence. The number of existing cases of a disease.

Primary atypical pneumonia. Also known as "walking pneumonia." It is caused by a variety of microorganisms, including viruses and unusual bacterium called *Mycoplasma pneumoniae.*

Primary follicle. A single layer of cells that surround each ovum.

Proctoscope. An instrument consisting of a hollow tube with a lighted end used by physicians to observe the lining of the colon.

Proerythroblasts. An early stage of erythrocytes. It is a large, nucleated, primitive cell that possesses no hemoglobin.

Prognosis. The predicted course and outcome of a disease.

Progression. The third stage of cancer development.

Prolapse. Caused when a hemorrhoid comes through the anal opening; also when the terminal portion of the ureter slips into the bladder.

Promotion. The second stage of cancer development in which altered cells proliferate and resemble benign neoplasms, which can either regress to normal-appearing tissue or evolve into cancer.

Prostate. Male reproductive organ that produces semen.

Prostatitis. Inflammation of the prostate.

Prothrombin. An enzyme synthesized by the liver with the aid of vitamin K that initiates the chain reaction in the blood coagulation process.

Prothrombin time. A method for measuring defects of coagulation.

Pruritis. Itching which accompanies many skin diseases.

Psoriasis. A superficial recurring idiopathic skin disorder characterized by an abnormal rate of epidermal cell production and turnover.

Psychogenic factor. A psychological cause or component of a disease.

Puerperal sepsis. An infection of the endometrium after childbirth or an abortion.

Puerperium. The time period after childbirth when the endometrium is open and particularly susceptible to infection.

Pulmonary edema. A buildup of fluid in the lungs causing shortness of breath.

Pulmonary stenosis. The first cause of cyanosis in which the valve opening that leads into the pulmonary artery is too small and an inadequate amount of blood reaches the lungs to be oxygenated.

Purkinje fibers. The specialized heart tissue that conducts the impulse for contraction to the myocardium of the ventricles.

Purpura. Small hemorrhages into the tissue beneath the skin or mucous membranes.

Pustules. Lesions containing pus.

Pyelitis. An inflammation of the renal pelvis the juncture between the ureter and the kidney, caused by *E. coli* or other pus forming bacteria.

Pyelonephritis. A suppurative inflammation of the kidney and renal pelvis.

Pyloric sphincter. The sphincter muscle through which food passes from the stomach into the small intestine.

Pyloric stenosis. A congenital obstruction of the intestinal tract.

Pyogenic. The type of bacteria that causes pus.

Pyosalpinx. The outer ends of the fallopian tubes usually close and the tubes fill with pus as a result of an infection.

Pyuria. This condition is caused when abscesses in the kidney rupture and pus enters the renal pelvis and then appears in urine.

Quarantine. The separation of persons who may or may not be infected from healthy people until the period of infectious risk is passed.

Rabies. An infectious disease of the brain and spinal cord caused by a virus that is transmitted by the saliva of an infected animal.

Rales. Abnormal respiratory sounds detected with a stethoscope.

Raynaud's disease. The condition in which small arteries or arterioles in the fingers and toes constrict.

Recessive. Term used to describe an allele that manifests itself when the person is homozygous for the trait.

Reflux. The back-flow of the acid contents of the stomach causing inflammation of the esophagus.

Regional enteritis. An inflammatory disease of the intestine that most frequently affects young adults, particularly females.

Regurgitated. Passage of stomach contents into the esophagus.

Relapse. Occurs when a disease returns weeks or months after its apparent cessation.

Remission. The period of a chronic disease when signs and symptoms subside.

Renal pelvis. The juncture between the kidneys and the ureters; final urine from all collecting ducts empties here.

Renin. Secreted by cells that convert angiotensinogen to angiotensin, an active enzyme to help elevate blood pressure.

Reportable diseases. Certain diseases that are under constant surveillance and must be reported to the Centers for Disease Control and Prevention by physicians.

Reservoirs. The sources of a pathogen and a potential source of disease.

Respiratory epithelium. A mucous membrane that lines the entire respiratory tract.

Resuscitation. Assisting or reviving respiration to a person with a myocardial infarction.

Reticulocyte. The late stage of erythrocyte development.

Reye's syndrome. A potentially devastating neurologic illness that sometimes develops in young children after a viral infection.

Rhabomyosarcoma. A malignant tumor of the skeletal muscle.

Rh factor. Antigen on erythrocyte, used for blood typing.

Rhodopsin. The pigment that absorbs light in the rods of the retina.

Rickets. A disease of infancy and early childhood in which the bones do not properly ossify, or harden, generally caused by a vitamin D deficiency.

Ringworm. A skin condition that is caused by many fungi that reside in warm, moist areas of the body.

Roundworm. A worm-like animal that is relatively round in cross-section.

Salpingitis. An inflammation of the fallopian tubes.

Sarcoma. A less common type of cancer that spreads rapidly and is highly malignant.

Saturated. The term that refers to the component fatty acids in a triglyceride.

Scabies. A contagious skin disease called "the itch," and usually associated with poor living conditions.

Sclerosis. An abnormal hardening of a tissue.

Sclerotic. Have the condition of sclerosis.

Scrotum. A part of the male reproductive system, a saclike structure outside the body wall that contains the testes.

Sebaceous. Oil glands located within the dermis.

Seborrheic dermatitis. The excessive secretion of sebum from the sebaceous glands; chronic dandruff.

Sebum. Oily fluid released through the hair follicles.

Secondary Pneumonia. A pneumonia that develops as a secondary disorder from other diseases that weaken the lungs or the body's immune system.

Seizures. An uncontrolled nervous system activity manifested by uncoordinated motor action.

Seminal vesicle. An accessory gland found near the base of the urinary bladder in a male that forms the ejaculatory duct.

Seminiferous tubules. Highly coiled tubules contained within the testes in which sperm develop.

Seminoma. A cancer of the seminiferous tubules.

Senility. A disease that causes loss of mental, physical, or emotional control.

Septic embolism. An embolism that contains infected material from pyogenic bacteria.

Septicemia. A systemic infection of the blood.

Sequela. The aftermath of a particular disease such as permanent damage to the heart after rheumatic fever.

Serotonin. One of many neurotransmitters involved in regulating pain messages.

Sex-linked inheritance. Diseases that are usually confined to the male and are transmitted by the female.

Shingles. An acute inflammation of nerve cells caused by the chicken pox virus, herpes zoster.

Sickle cell anemia. A severe anemia, generally confined to blacks, in which the hemoglobin is abnormal, resulting in deformed sickle-shaped red blood cells.

Signs. The objective evidence of disease observed on physical examination, such as abnormal pulse or fever.

Sinoatrial node. The pacemaker of the heart, it is a small patch of tissue that initiates the heartbeat.

Spastic colon (irritable colon). A functional condition of the colon with diarrhea and cramping.

Spheroidal. An inherited disorder that results in spherical red blood cells rather than biconcave or disk-shaped.

Spider veins. Small, dense, red networks of veins.

Spina bifida. A condition in which one or more vertebrae fail to fuse, leaving an opening in the vertebral canal. The word *bifid* means a cleft or split into two parts, which is the condition of the vertebra in spina bifida.

Spirilla. Spiral-shaped bacterial cells.

Spirochetes. Corkscrew-shaped bacterial cells.

Spirometer. A simple instrument used to measure the movement of air in and out of the lungs.

Spirometry. A diagnostic procedure that measures and records changes in gas volume in the lungs, determining ventilation capacity and flow rate.

Splenomegaly. An enlarged spleen.

Spores. Microscopic fungal reproductive structures that can induce allergies.

Sporozoans. A form of protozoa; a single-celled not mobile eukaryotic microorganism.

Sprains. The result of the wrenching or twisting of a joint such as an ankle that injures the ligaments.

Spurs. Spicules of abnormal new bone development.

Squamous. A malignancy of the keratinocytes in the epidermis of people who have been excessively exposed to the sun; cell carcinoma.

Staghorn calculus. A kidney stone that becomes so large it fills the renal pelvis completely, blocking the flow of urine.

Standard precautions. Precautions such as gloves required of medical personnel when handling patients or bodily fluids.

Staphylococci. A type of bacterium associated with skin infections, toxic shock syndrome, and food poisoning.

Stasis. Slow blood flow that often causes infection.

Status asthmaticus. Life-threatening form of an asthma attack.

Strabismus. The condition of crossed eyes.

Strains. Pulled muscles that result from a tearing of a muscle and/or its tendon from excessive use or stretching.

Streptococci. A type of bacterium associated with infections of the ear, throat, skin, and heart valves.

Stroke. The term used broadly to include cerebral hemorrhages and blood-clot formation within cerebral blood vessels.

Subarachnoid. A tear in the surface membrane of the brain by a skull fracture.

Subdural. A hemorrhage under the dura mater, is from large venous sinuses of the brain rather than an artery.

Suppressor T cells. The type of T cell that controls the immune response.

Suppurative. A type of inflammation associated with pus formation.

Symptoms. An indication of disease perceived by the patient, such as pain, dizziness, and itching.

Syncope. Fainting caused by insufficient blood supply to the brain.

Syndrome. Combination of symptoms.

Synovial. The membrane that lines the joints.

Syphilis. A serious sexually transmitted disease caused by a spirochete.

Systemic lupus erythematosus (SLE). An autoimmune disease which affects not only the skin but also causes the deterioration of collagenous connective tissue.

Systole. The period of the heartbeat when the heart contracts and pumps the blood.

T lymphocytes. One of two types of lymphocytes that provide cell-mediated immunity and is processed by the thymus gland.

Tachycardia. When the heart rate increases significantly.

Tay-Sachs. An autosomal recessive condition that primarily affects families of Eastern Jewish origin.

Tendons. Substance that attaches skeletal or voluntary muscles firmly to bones.

Teratoma. A benign tumor of the ovary also known as a dermoid cyst.

Terminal. A disease ending in death.

Tetanus toxoid. A type of immunization that protects from the disease tetanus.

Tetany. A sustained muscular contraction.

Tetralogy of Fallot. One of the most serious congenital defects consisting of four *(tetra)* abnormalities.

Thrombi. Blood clots.

Thrombocyte. Platelets that initiate blood clotting.

Thrombocytopenia. A disease of platelets resulting in gastrointestinal and urogenital hemorrhages, as well as severe nosebleeds.

Thrombolytic. Agents that dissolve blood clots.

Thrombophlebitis. Thrombus formation in deep veins.

Thrombosis. The forming of blood clots on blood vessel walls.

Thrombus. A blood clot that forms in a blood vessel.

Thyroxine. One of the thyroid hormones.

Toxic shock syndrome (TSS). Caused by infection with *Staphylococcus aureus.*

Toxins. Substances that damage tissues and initiate an inflammatory response.

Toxoid. A chemically altered toxin, the poisonous material produced by a pathogenic organism.

Trachea. The windpipe.

Tracheotomy. A surgical procedure to open the trachea to facilitate passage of air or evacuation of secretions.

Tremors. A shakiness, particularly of the hands.

Trichomonas. A parasite that can be transmitted by sexual intercourse is one causative agent of vaginitis.

Tricuspid valve. The valve between the right atrium and right ventricle. It has three cusps.

Triglycerides. A lipid fat that is not water-soluble and, therefore, cannot mix with blood plasma.

Triiodothyronine. A thyroid hormone.

Trisomy 21. The condition of having chromosome 21 in triplicate, causing down's syndrome.

Tubercles. Lesions that are formed when tissue infected with tuberculosis heals with fibrosis and calcification, walling off the bacteria for months or many years.

Tuberculosis. A chronic infectious disease characterized by necrosis of vital lung tissue which can affect other body systems as well.

Tumor. A mass of new cells that grows in a haphazard fashion with no control or useful function.

Turner's syndrome. The condition caused when one of the sex chromosomes is missing resulting in a karyotype of 45,XO.

Ultrasound arteriography. Shows the anatomy of arteries, particularly the carotid bifurcation and the internal carotid artery.

Unsaturated. The term that refers to the component fatty acids in a triglyceride.

Upper respiratory diseases. Disorders of the nose and throat including common infections and allergies.

Urea. Nitrogen-containing waste products formed in the liver.

Uremia. A toxic condition of blood; the end result is kidney failure.

Ureterocele. An abnormally expanded ureter.

Ureters. The path urine takes between the kidney to the urinary bladder.

Urethra. The single tube through which urine empties to the outside from the urinary bladder.

Urethritis. Inflammation of the urethra.

Urinalysis. A simple diagnostic procedure which examines a urine specimen physically, chemically, and microscopically.

Urinary calculi. Stones formed primarily in the kidney when certain salts in the urine form a precipitate and grow in size.

Urticaria. Known as hives, results from a vascular reaction of the skin to an allergen.

Uterus. A part of the female reproductive system in which the embryo and fetus develops.

Vaccine. A substance given to a patient orally or by injection to prevent an infectious disease. Vaccines stimulate the immune system.

Vagina. A part of the female reproductive system, it is a tubular structure extending backward and upward to the cervix.

Vaginitis. An inflammation of the vagina; a common disease caused by several organisms.

Valvular insufficiency. Occurs when a valve opening is too large and does not prevent backflow.

Vas deferens. A duct that passes through the inguinal canal into the abdominal cavity of males.

Vasopressin. One of two hormones secreted by the posterior pituitary, also called antidiuretic hormone.

Vectors. Animals that transmit pathogenic microorganisms to humans.

Vegetations. Small nodular structures composed of bacteria and clots that form along the edge of cusps in a valve opening.

Venae cavae. The two largest veins of the body.

Ventricular fibrillation. Occurs when a series of uncoordinated impulses spread over the ventricles causing them to twitch or quiver rather than contract.

Verruca vulgaris. Warts caused by viruses affecting the keratinocytes of the skin, causing them to proliferate.

Vertical transmission. The route by which an infectious disease is transmitted from one generation to the next.

Very-low-density lipoproteins (VLDL). The lipoproteins that contain the most triglycerides. They are the largest and least dense.

Vesicles. Small, blisterlike eruptions on the skin.

Vibrios. Comma-shaped bacterial cells.

Vitiligo. A loss of melanin resulting in white patches of skin which are usually well demarcated and may cover large parts of the body.

Volvulus. A condition in which the intestine is twisted on itself.

Vulva. The external female genitalia that consists of the mons pubis, the labia majora and labia minora, the clitoris, and the vaginal opening.

Wellness. The condition of good physical and mental health, especially when maintained by proper diet, exercise, and habits that includes not just physical health but fitness and emotional well-being.

Wernicke's encephalopathy. A brain disease often associated with chronic alcoholism, in which the patient becomes mentally confused and disoriented and may suffer delirium tremens.

Wheals. Rounded elevations on the skin known as lesions, with red edges and pale centers, extremely pruritic, or itchy.

Wheezing. The sound of labored breathing as a result of narrowed tubes in the lungs.

Wilms' tumor. A malignant tumor of the kidney that develops in very young children.

Answers to Quick Self Study Questions

Chapter 1

Multiple Choice

1. D
2. C
3. D
4. A

True/False

1. F
2. F
3. F
4. T

Fill-ins

1. Prognosis
2. Idipathic
3. Exacerbation
4. Remission

Chapter 2

Multiple Choice

1. E
2. C
3. B
4. A

True/False

1. F
2. T
3. F
4. T

Fill-ins

1. T-4 helper
2. IgE
3. Memory cells
4. Cytotoxic or killer

Chapter 3

Multiple Choice

1. B
2. A
3. B
4. C

True/False

1. F
2. T
3. T
4. T

Fill-ins

1. Pathogenic microorganisms
2. Vaccination
3. Anthropods
4. Epidemiology

Chapter 4

Multiple Choice

1. D
2. C
3. B
4. C

True/False

1. T
2. T
4. F
5. F

Fill-ins

1. 15
2. Cyst
3. C—change in bowel or bladder habits
   A- a sore that does not heal
   U—unusual bleeding or discharge
   T—thickening or lump in breast or elsewhere
   I—indigestion or difficulty in swallowing
   O—obvious change in wart or mole
   N—ragging cough or harshness
4. Biopsy

Chapter 5

Multiple Choice

1. C
2. B
3. A
4. C

True/False

1. T
2. T
3. F
4. F

Fill-ins

1. Congenital
2. Hermaphrodites
3. Epilepsy, diabetes, allergy, cardiovascular problems
4. 50

Chapter 6

Multiple Choice

1. C
2. B
3. D
4. A

True/False

1. T
2. F
3. T
4. F
5. F

Fill-ins

1. Vitamin A
2. Osteomalacia
3. Vitamin C
4. Potassium

Chapter 7

Multiple Choice

1. B
2. C
3. A
4. A

True/False

1. T
2. T
3. F
4. F
5. T

Fill-ins

1. Aplastic
2. Pernicious
3. Hemolytic
4. Spheroidal

Chapter 8

Multiple Choice

1. B
2. D
3. C
4. B
5. B

True/False

1. T
2. F
3. F
4. T

Fill-ins

1. Echocardiography
2. Hypertrophy
3. Venae cavae
   Right ventricle
4. Aorta

Chapter 9

Multiple Choice

1. B
2. A
3. C
4. B
5. A

True/False

1. T
2. T
3. F
4. F

Fill-ins

1. Constriction
2. Systolic pressure
3. Recurrence, resolution, intravascular clotting
4. Unknown, known

Chapter 10

Multiple Choice

1. D
2. E
3. C
4. D

True/False

1. F
2. F
3. T
4. T
5. T
6. T
7. T

Fill-ins

1. Cystitis
2. Diabetic, nephropathy
3. Kidney stones
4. Lithotripsy
5. Polycystic kidney

Chapter 11

Multiple Choice

1. B
2. B
3. B
4. D

True/False

1. F
2. T
3. F
4. T

Fill-ins

1. Amoebic dysentery
2. Crohn's disease

3. Hernia
4. Endoscope

Chapter 12

Multiple Choice

1. D
2. C
3. B
4. A

True/False

1. T
2. F
3. F
4. F

Fill-ins

1. C
2. Gallstones
3. Bile duct
4. Ascites

Chapter 13

Multiple Choice

1. B
2. B
3. D
4. C

True/False

1. T
2. F
3. F
4. T

Fill-ins

1. Mantoux skin
2. Cyanosis
3. Tobacco
4. Pneumonia

Chapter 14

Multiple Choice

1. B
2. B
3. C
4. B

True/False

1. F
2. T
3. F
4. F
5. F
6. T
7. F
8. T

Fill-ins

1. Gigantism, acromegaly
2. Oxytocin; vasopressin (or ADH)
3. Addison's disease
4. Pheochromocytoma

Chapter 15

Multiple Choice

1. C
2. D
3. D
4. A

True/False

1. T
2. F
3. F
4. F

Fill-ins

1. Fibrocystic
2. Orchitis

3. Chlamydia

4. Cervical

Chapter 16

Multiple Choice

1. A

2. D

4. D

5. B

True/False

1. T

2. T

3. F

4. T

5. F

6. F

Fill-ins

1. Tetanus

2. EMG

3. MS

4. Parkinson's

Chapter 17

Multiple Choice

1. C

2. B

3. C

4. C

5. B

True/False

1. T

2. F

3. F

4. T

5. T

6. T

7. T

8. F

9. T

10. T

Fill-ins

1. Potts disease

2. Rickets

3. Osteoporosis

4. Gout, gouty, arthritis

Chapter 18

Multiple Choice

1. C

2. C

3. A

4. B

True/False

1. T

2. F

3. F

4. F

5. T

6. T

7. F

Fill-ins

1. Hives

2. The itch

3. Dandruff

4. Melanin

Chapter 19

Multiple Choice

1. C

2. B

3. A

4. A

True/False

1. T

2. F

3. F

4. T

Fill-ins

1. Anaerobic

2. C and E

3. Phytochemicals

4. Health

Chapter 20

Multiple Choice

1. C

2. B

3. A

4. A

True/False

1. T

2. F

3. F

4. T

Fill-ins

1. Anaerobic

2. C & E

3. Phytochemicals

4. Health

Index

Page numbers in *italics* denote figures; those followed by "t" denote tables.